Receptors and Recognition

Series A

Published

Volume 1 (1976)

M.F. Greaves (London), Cell Surface Receptors: A Biological Perspective
F. Macfarlane Burnet (Melbourne), The Evolution of Receptors and
    Recognition in the Immune System.
K. Resch (Heidelberg), Membrane Associated Events in Lymphocyte
    Activation
K.N. Brown (London), Specificity in Host-Parasite Interaction

Volume 2 (1976)

D. Givol (Jerusalem), A Structural Basis for Molecular Recognition: The
    Antibody Case
B.D. Gomperts (London), Calcium and Cell Activation
M.A.B. de Sousa (New York), Cell traffic
D. Lewis (London), Incompatibility in Flowering Plants
A. Levitski (Jerusalem), Catecholamine Receptors

Volume 3 (1977)

J. Lindstrom (Salk, California), Antibodies to Receptors for Acetylcholine
    and other Hormones
M. Crandall (Kentucky), Mating-type Interaction in Micro-organisms
H. Furthmayr (New Haven), Erythrocyte Membrane Proteins
M. Silverman (Toronto), Specificity of Membrane Transport

Volume 4 (1977)

M. Sonenberg and A.S. Schneider (New York), Hormone Action at the
    Plasma Membrane: Biophysical Approaches
H. Metzger (NIH, Bethesda), The Cellular Receptor for IgE
T.P. Stossel (Boston), Endocytosis
A. Meager (Warwick), and R.C. Hughes (London), Virus Receptors
M.E. Eldefrawi and A.T. Eldefrawi (Baltimore), Acetylcholine Receptors

In preparation

Volume 5 (1978)

P.A. Lehmann (Mexico), Stereoselectivity in Receptor Recognition
A.G. Lee (Southampton), Fluorescence and NMR Studies of Membranes
L. Kohn (NIH, Bethesda), Relationships in the Structure and Function of
    Receptors for Glycoprotein Hormones, Bacterial Toxins and Interferon

Series B

Published

The Specificity and Action of Animal, Bacterial and Plant Toxins (B1
edited by P. Cuatrecasas (Burroughs Wellcome, North Carolina)

Microbial Interactions (B3)
edited by J.L. Reissig (Long Island University, New York)

In preparation

Specificity of Embryological Interactions (B4)
edited by D. Garrod (University of Southampton)

Taxis and Behaviour (B5)
edited by G. Hazelbauer (Wallenberg Laboratory, Uppsala)

Virus Receptors (B6)
edited by L. Philipson and L. Randall (University of Uppsala), and
    K. Lonberg-Holm (Du Pont, Delaware)

Receptors and Recognition

General Editors: P. Cuatrecasas and M.F. Greaves

About the series

Cellular recognition — the process by which cells interact with, and respond to, molecular signals in their environment — plays a crucial role in virtually all important biological functions. These encompass fertilization, infectious interactions, embryonic development, the activity of the nervous system, the regulation of growth and metabolism by hormones and the immune response to foreign antigens. Although our knowledge of these systems has grown rapidly in recent years, it is clear that a full understanding of cellular recognition phenomena will require an integrated and multidisciplinary approach.

This series aims to expedite such an understanding by bringing together accounts by leading researchers of all biochemical, cellular and evolutionary aspects of recognition systems. The series will contain volumes of two types. First, there will be volumes containing about five reviews from different areas of the general subject written at a level suitable for all biologically oriented scientists (Receptors and Recognition, series A). Secondly, there will be more specialized volumes, (Receptors and Recognition, series B), each of which will be devoted to just one particularly important area.

Advisory Editorial Board

Receptors and Recognition

Series B Volume 2

Intercellular Junctions and Synapses

Edited by

J. Feldman
Department of Zoology, University College, London

N. B. Gilula
Biology Section, Rockefeller University, New York

J. D. Pitts
Department of Biochemistry, University of Glasgow, Glasgow

LONDON

CHAPMAN AND HALL

A Halsted Press Book

John Wiley & Sons, New York

First published 1978
by Chapman and Hall Ltd.,
11 New Fetter Lane, London EC4P 4EE

© *1978 Chapman and Hall Ltd*

Typeset by Josée Utteridge-Faivre of Red Lion Setters
and printed in Great Britain
at the University Printing House, Cambridge

ISBN 0 412 14820 X

Distributed in the U.S.A. by Halsted Press
A Division of John Wiley & Sons, Inc., New York

Library of Congress Cataloging in Publication Data

Main entry under title:
Intercellular junctions and synapses.
(Receptors and recognition, series B, V. 2).

    Includes index.
    1. Cell junctions. 2. Synapses.
    I. Feldman, J.   II. Gilula, N. B.   III. Pitts, J. D.
    IV. Series.
QH603.C4157   591.8'76   77-18542
ISBN 0-470-99372-3

Contents

Contributors

M.V.L. Bennett, Division of Cellular Neurobiology, Albert Einstein College of Yeshiva University, New York, U.S.A.

R. Dingledine, Department of Pharmacology, University of Cambridge Medical School, Cambridge, U.K.

J. Feldman, Department of Zoology, University College, London, U.K.

N.B. Gilula, Section of Cell Biology, Rockefeller University, New York, U.S.A.

J.S. Kelly, Department of Pharmacology, University of Cambridge Medical School, Cambridge, U.K.

A. Matus, Institute of Psychiatry, London, U.K.

J.D. Pitts, Department of Biochemistry, University of Glasgow, Glasgow, U.K.

J.D. Sheridan, Department of Zoology, University of Minnesota, Minneapolis, Minnesota, U.S.A.

C.R. Slater, The Muscular Dystrophy Group, Newcastle General Hospital, Newcastle-upon-Tyne, U.K.

L. Wolpert, Department of Biology as Applied to Medicine, Middlesex Hospital Medical School, London, U.K.

Preface

Intercellular communication is a fundamental requirement of complex multi-cellular organisms. This book describes two forms of such communication in animal tissues. One, the nervous system, provides a wide-ranging network of specialized cells connected by chemical synapses. The other allows direct communication between adjacent cells through permeable intercellular junctions (gap junctions).

The functional significance of the chemical synapse is clear — it provides a mechanism for the transfer of electrical signals from one cell to the next. However, the functional significance of the gap junction is less clear. Gap junctions contain channels which directly connect the cytoplasms of coupled cells and these channels are freely permeable to small cellular ions and molecules but are impermeable to cellular macromolecules. In some instances (e.g. in heart muscle), gap junctions behave as electrical synapses and, by ion transfer, permit the propagation of electrical impulses through coupled cell populations. Gap junctions though, are abundant in non-excitable tissues, where they are usually larger and more numerous than in nervous tissues. They may be necessary for the co-ordination of cellular activity and proliferation during embryonic development and in adult tissues.

Chemical synapses connect excitable cells in specific patterns but the mechanisms which determine specificity are not understood. The patterns of communication between cells through gap junctions are mostly undefined and it is not known if they are governed by rules of specificity.

This book has been planned to draw attention to the similarities and differences, in both structural and functional terms, between chemical synapses and gap junctions. The basis for the book originated at a meeting held in Cambridge, England in 1976 when research workers in the different fields were brought together to exchange ideas. A small number of authors were subsequently invited to review the important topics covered at the meeting in an attempt to provide a more cohesive and useful description of the current status of knowledge than would have been possible in a collection of shorter papers from all fifty or so participants.

The editors hope that these reviews, written in this form and at this time, will stimulate further research and point towards areas of joint interest to neuro-biologists, developmental biologists, cell biologists and biochemists.

September, 1977

J.D. Feldman
N.B. Gilula
J.D. Pitts

1 Structure of Intercellular Junctions

N. B. GILULA

Acknowledgements
The author has received support from the Irma T. Hirschl Trust, U.S.P.H.S. Grant HL 16507, and an R.C.D. Award (N.I.H.) HL 00110.

Intercellular Junctions and Synapses
(*Receptors and Recognition,* Series B, Volume 2)
Edited by J. Feldman, N.B. Gilula and J.D. Pitts
Published in 1978 by Chapman and Hall, 11 New Fetter Lane, London EC4P 4EE
© Chapman and Hall

1.1 INTRODUCTION

Specialized sites of cell-to-cell contact are generally referred to as intercellular junctions. Since the regions of intercellular contact are very small, they cannot be clearly resolved by light microscopy. Therefore, our appreciation of these specialized contacts has paralleled the development of appropriate techniques for electron microscopy. Virtually all of the major classes of cell junctions had been described on the basis of thin-section electron microscopic observations by 1970. At that time, the number of studies on cell junctions were limited because:

(1) the thin-section features of cell junctions were strikingly similar in different tissues and different organisms;
(2) 'classic' thin-section descriptions of the major junctions had already been provided; and
(3) it was difficult to expand the appreciation for structural details and function-related properties that had to be derived from studies on 'static' images in thin-sections. With the development of the freeze-fracture technique, it became possible to characterize the internal membrane modifications that correspond to the sites of intercellular contact. This technique was initially utilized to study various features of general membrane structure but, by 1970, it became an important approach for characterizing the structure of cell junctions. In addition, it became equally useful for identifying and quantitating junctional membranes in a variety of tissues. Since that time, there has been a significant increase in our appreciation of cell junctions, both in terms of their structure and function. In many respects, the freeze-fracture technique has provided a more 'dynamic' Gestalt about functional properties than was available previously through 'static' thin-section information alone.

The purpose of this chapter is to provide a representative overview of the state of affairs in the area of cell junction structure. Since our current knowledge of junctional structure has been intimately associated with the development and application of the freeze-fracture technique, much of the information has been generated since 1970. Several reviews that extensively deal with general and esoteric structural details of cell junctions are currently available (McNutt and Weinstein, 1973; Gilula, 1974b; Staehelin, 1974; Overton, 1974; Weinstein *et al.,* 1976; Griepp and Revel, 1977). These reviews should be utilized as resources to supplement the brief treatment of this area included in this chapter.

1.2 GAP JUNCTIONS

The gap junction has perhaps received the most attention in the past 10 years because it is present in most metazoan animals, and it has been strongly implicated as a structural pathway for cell-to-cell communication. There are two major types of gap junctions that have been characterized: one of these is present in most animal phyla, with the exception of Arthropoda, while the other has been extensively found in arthropod organisms. The two types of gap junctions have been treated separately in this chapter since their structural characteristics are distinctly different and, in turn, their physiological properties may be significantly different.

1.2.1 Ultrastructural features of non-arthropod gap junctions

The gap junction was resolved in its present form by Revel and Karnovsky in 1967 (for review of early history see McNutt and Weinstein, 1973). It is currently synonymous with the structure that was called the nexus by Dewey and Barr in 1962. In thin-section electron microscopy, the gap junction can be detected as a unique apposition between adjacent cells. At the site of contact, the junction can be resolved as a seven-layered (septilaminar) structure (Fig. 1.1). The entire width of the

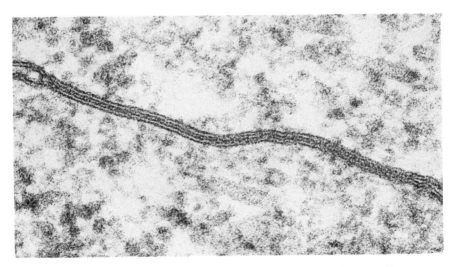

Fig. 1.1 Thin section appearance of a gap junction between insect cells (TN cell line) in culture. The junctional membranes are separated by a small 2–4 nm space or 'gap'. x 153 900.

septilaminar structure is 15–19 nm, or about 2–4 nm greater than the combined thickness of two 7.5 nm unit membranes. The septilaminar image represents the parallel apposition of two 7.5 nm unit membranes that are separated by a 2–4 nm 'gap' or electron-lucent space. This thin-section appearance led to the use of the term 'gap junction' to describe this structure. In many tissues the gap junction appears as a pentalaminar structure, and this created some confusion in the literature with another type of cell junction, the tight junction. Currently, practically all gap junctions can be resolved as septilaminar structures when they are treated with uranyl acetate staining *en bloc* (Revel and Karnovsky, 1967; Brightman and Reese, 1969; Goodenough and Revel, 1970; McNutt and Weinstein, 1970).

The precise clarification of the gap junctional structure in thin sections relied on the use of electron-opaque material, or tracer substances, that are able to fill the extracellular space. Currently, colloidal lanthanum hydroxide, pyroantimonate, and ruthenium red can all be utilized for this 'tracing' or 'staining' purpose (Revel and Karnovsky, 1967; Payton *et al.*, 1969; McNutt and Weinstein, 1970; Martinez-Palomo, 1970; Friend and Gilula, 1972a). The tracer substances are capable of penetrating a central region of the junction that corresponds to the location of the 'gap'. This fact clearly indicates that there is an extracellular continuity through the gap region of the junction, and it can be utilized as the basis for distinguishing between a tight junction (pentalaminar) and a gap junction (septilaminar). In oblique or *en face* views of tracer-impregnated gap junctions, it is possible to visualize a unique polygonal lattice of 7–8 nm subunits. The tracer outlines the subunits, which have a 9–10 nm center-to-center spacing, as a result of penetrating the regions of the lattice that are continuous with the extracellular space (Revel and Karnovsky, 1967). A 1.5–2 nm electron-dense dot is frequently present in the central region of these subunits, and it has been difficult to understand the manner in which the tracer material gains access to this internal region of the subunits. A similar lattice was described by Robertson (1963) at the site of an electrotonic synapse in a study that preceded the use of the tracer approaches. When gap junctions have been examined in detergent-treated isolated membrane fractions with negative stain procedures, a similar polygonal lattice of subunits has been observed (Benedetti and Emmelot, 1965, 1968; Goodenough and Revel, 1970; Goodenough and Stoeckenius, 1972; Goodenough, 1974, 1976) (Fig. 1.2).

The freeze-fracture technique has been utilized to obtain important complementary information about the gap junctional structure. Whereas the thin sections provide information about the relationship of the unit membranes and the intervening 'gap', the freeze-fracture procedure provides detailed information about the internal content of the junctional membranes. In general, specialized membranes, such as those present at the sites of cell junctions, have significant internal membrane structural modifications (for review, see McNutt and Weinstein, 1973; Staehelin, 1974). The freeze-fractured gap junctional membranes contain two complementary membrane halves or fracture faces (Fig. 1.3). The cytoplasmic or inner membrane half (fracture face P) contains a polygonal lattice of homogeneous 7–8 nm intramembrane particles. The extracellular or outer membrane half (fracture face E) contains a complementary arrangement of pits or depressions. In many instances, a 2–2.5 nm dot is detectable in the central region of these junctional particles. These

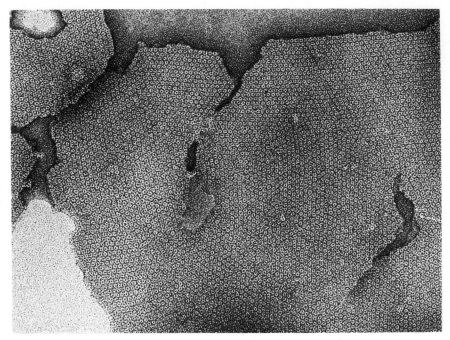

Fig. 1.2 Isolated gap junctions treated with negative stain. The isolated junctions are comprised of 8—9 nm particles that contain a central electron dense 1.5—2 nm dot. This central dot is a possible location of the low-resistance pathway or channel. x 179 550.

fracture face characteristics and membrane particle dispositions have now been documented as a constant feature of most non-arthropod gap junctions that have been examined (Goodenough and Revel, 1970; Chalcroft and Bullivant, 1970; McNutt and Weinstein, 1970; Friend and Gilula, 1972a; Staehelin, 1974). The junctional membrane lattices can exist in a variety of pleiomorphic forms, but the variations surround a single theme — a plaque-like or localized (focal) contact between interacting cells. Gap junctions are usually present as oval or circular plaques; however, a variety of forms, including linear strands (Raviola and Gilula, 1973) have been reported.

In general, the gap junction represents a unique paracrystalline lattice that is comprised of 7—8 nm particles or subunits that can be visualized with at least three independent techniques; tracer-impregnated thin section, freeze-fracturing and negative staining. Although the lattices are very attractive from a structural standpoint, it has been difficult to relate the size and arrangement of gap junctional units with a functional state. Thus far, gap junctions have been identified *in vivo* as aggregates of 2—3 particles as well as large plaques containing hundreds of particles.

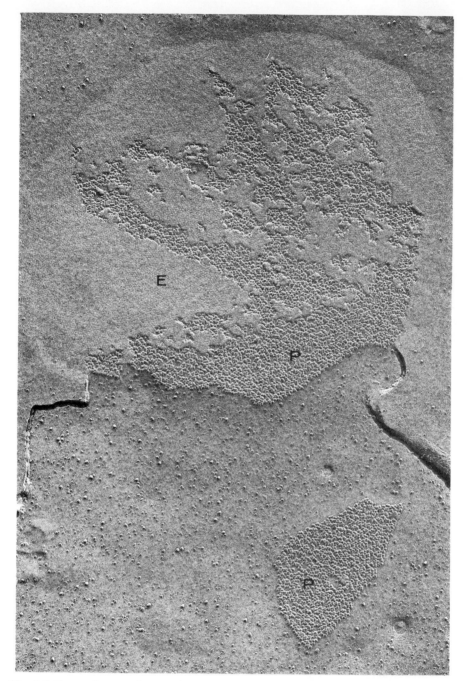

Fig. 1.3 Freeze-fracture image of gap junctions between granulosa cells in a rat ovarian follicle. The junctional membranes contain a polygonal lattice of intramembrane particles on the P fracture face and a complementary arrangement of pits on the E fracture face. x 64 260.

The gap junctions are structurally resistant to treatments with proteases and other agents that are used to dissociate intact tissues. When tissues are dissociated by such treatments, the gap junctions are retained as intact complexes on the single dissociated cells (Muir, 1967; Berry and Friend, 1969; Amsterdam and Jamieson, 1974). This response indicates that the gap junctional membranes are tightly bound into a cohesive unit or complex, and the binding is not simply explained by divalent cation salt linkages. With time, the gap junctional remnants are either ingested by the cells or re-utilized for establishing contact between single cells.

At the present time, there has been only one satisfactory procedure for 'splitting' or separating the gap junctional membranes in intact tissues. This procedure involves the perfusion of tissues with hypertonic sucrose solutions (Barr *et al.*,1965, 1968; Dreifuss *et al.*, 1966; Goodenough and Gilula, 1974). In intact mouse liver, the junctional membranes are separated by this treatment somewhere in the central region of the extracellular 'gap' (Goodenough and Gilula, 1974). The separated junctional membranes still contain the characteristic particle lattices in freeze–fracture replicas, and the particles appear to be more tightly packed when the membranes are separated. Furthermore, the junctional membrane particle lattices respond to this treatment as intact domains rather than as a membrane sector comprised of independent particles or units. In essence, the interactions between junctional membrane particles are strengthened, if anything, by this treatment, while the interactions between the two junctional membranes are definitely weakened to result in separation. Although this treatment results in a radical disruption of the gap junction, it must be considered relatively mild or physiologically significant since the entire process can be easily reversed by simply replacing the hypertonic sucrose with a normal salt solution.

1.2.2 Ultrastructural features of arthropod gap junctions

Gap junctions have been described in a variety of arthropod tissues with both thin-section and freeze-fracture techniques (Flower, 1972; Peracchia, 1973b; Johnson *et al.*, 1973; Satir and Gilula, 1973; Gilula, 1974b; Dallai, 1975). The structural features of the arthropod gap junctions are sufficiently different from non-arthropod gap junctions to be considered as a unique structural variation.

In thin sections, the arthropod gap junctions are quite similar to non-arthropod gap junctions (Fig. 1.1), although the intercellular 'gap' is slightly larger (about 3–4 nm) (Payton *et al.*, 1969; Hudspeth and Revel, 1971; Rose, 1971; Peracchia, 1973a). Also, in lanthanum-impregnated specimens, the subunit lattice has slightly larger dimensions (Hudspeth and Revel, 1971; Johnson *et al.*, 1973; Peracchia, 1973a). In freeze-fracture replicas, the structural differences in the arthropod gap junctions are very striking (Fig. 1.4). The gap junctional membranes contain two complementary fracture faces: the inner membrane half (fracture face P) contains pits or depressions; and the outer membrane half (fracture face E) contains a plaque-like arrangement of intramembrane particles. The junctional membrane

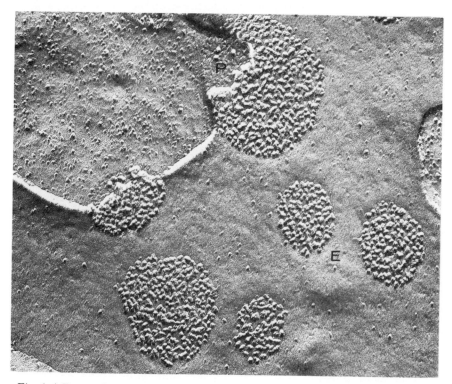

Fig. 1.4 Freeze-fracture image of gap junctions between arthropod epithelial cells (crayfish hepatopancreas). Note that the intramembrane particles are associated with the E fracture face, and the complementary pits with the P fracture face. x 100 000.

particles are large (11 nm or larger in diameter) and often heterogeneous in size; and they are frequently present as fused aggregates of two or more particles. In addition, the particles are not usually in a highly ordered polygonal array (Flower, 1972; Johnson *et al.*, 1973; Dallai, 1975).

1.2.3 Distribution

Gap junctions are widely distributed in the animal kingdom. These structures have been observed in many vertebrate as well as invertebrate organisms. In vertebrate organisms, the junctions have been described between all types of cells (epithelial, connective, neuronal and muscle) and the junction can connect both homologous and heterologous cells in these tissues. For example, gap junctions can be observed between mucous-secreting and absorptive cells in the small intestine. In the nervous system, the gap junction has been identified as the site of the electrotonic or electrical synapse (see Bennett, 1973) and in the myocardium it is a conspicuous element of the elaborate cell surface specialization, the intercalated disc (McNutt and Weinstein, 1973). At the present time, gap junctions have not been ultrastructurally identified and characterized between slime mold cells and sponge cells (Porifera).

In early stages of embryonic development, gap junctions are widely distributed throughout the embryo. However, as organogenesis proceeds, there is a pattern of uncoupling that reflects the generation of the individual organ systems. This uncoupling pattern was initially described in the squid embryo (Potter *et al.*,1966). From recent reports, it is clear that the mammalian embryos are capable of expressing gap junctions even prior to fertilization; for gap junctions have been described between mammalian oocytes and follicular cells (Epstein *et al.*, 1976; Anderson and Albertini, 1976).

Gap junctions are present between most cells in vertebrate organisms; however, there are certain cell types that do not appear to express gap junctional structures, or at least the junctions are expressed at a very low frequency. Such cells include mature skeletal muscle fibers (innervated), erythroid cells, lymphoid cell and many differentiated neurons.

It is important to note that ionic coupling has been reported in some instances between stimulated lymphoid cells (Hülser and Peters, 1971; Oliveira-Castro *et al.*, 1973); however, no typical gap junctional structures have yet been reported in these systems. Coupling (dye transfer) has also been reported between target and killer cells in cytotoxicity interactions (Sellin *et al.*, 1971), and no gap junctions have been detected yet between these cells. In these lymphoid cell systems, it is reasonable to consider the possibility that ionic coupling can occur between cells (perhaps on a short time-scale) without the generation of a gap junctional structure. In fact, there is no reason to expect a gap junctional structure to be detectable in every instance where a low-resistance pathway is generated. Certainly, transient low-resistance mechanisms must exist that do not require an elaborate gap junctional structure.

1.2.4 Formation and turnover

There have been several recent studies both *in vivo* and in culture that have described a sequence of structural events that are associated with the formation of gap junctions (Revel *et al.*, 1973; Johnson *et al.*, 1974; Decker and Friend, 1974; Benedetti *et al.*, 1974; Albertini and Anderson, 1974; Decker, 1976). The formation process in freeze-fracture replicas generally consists of the following stages:

(1) the appearance of formation plaques;
(2) the appearance of large 'precursor' particles with a reduction of the intercellular space;
(3) the appearance of smaller 'junctional' particles in polygonal arrangements; and
(4) the enlargement of junctions. The formation plaques are difficult to identify in

thin sections since there is no apparent modification of the cytoplasmic or extra-cellular surfaces in these regions. There is no information available yet about the biochemical or structural relationship of the large precursor particles to the smaller gap junctional particles. One can assume, at present, that mature junctional particles with low-resistance properties are not present in the plasma membrane prior to initiating junctional formation, since the normal resistance properties of the surface membranes are maintained in single intact cells. However, junctional precursors, probably in a different conformational state, do exist in intact cells since it has been difficult, if not impossible, in most systems to inhibit the generation of communica-tion between cells by inhibiting protein synthesis (Epstein *et al.,* 1977). There has been only one reported exception (Decker, 1976) and, in this system, the formation of gap junctions that is apparently hormonally induced is inhibited by inhibiting protein and RNA synthesis.

In several studies, it has been reported that the gap junctional size and frequency may be influenced by treatments with hormones (Merk *et al.,* 1972; Decker, 1976), vitamins (Elias and Friend, 1976) and hepatectomy (Yee, 1972). In epithelial systems, there is also an apparent structural relationship between gap junctional particles and tight junctional elements during the formation process; in some cases the two junctional elements arise in close association with each other (Yee, 1972; Revel *et al.,* 1973; Decker and Friend, 1974; Albertini *et al.,* 1975; Montesano *et al.,* 1975). This raises the interesting possibility that there may be a biochemical and/or functional relationship between gap and tight junctions.

Gap junctions must be regarded as unusually stable (or static) elements of cell surface plasma membranes. This statement can be made primarily on the basis of a study on the relative degradation rates of mouse liver surface membrane proteins (Gurd and Evans, 1973). This study indicated that the degradation of proteins in a subcellular fraction containing gap junctions occurred very slowly. Gap junctions have been frequently observed as internalized elements or 'annular gap junctions' in a number of different tissues (Merk *et al.,* 1973; Albertini *et al.,* 1975; Amsterdam *et al.,* 1976), and in some instances the internalized structures are incorporated into phagolysosomal vacuoles. However, there has been no report of lysosomal enzyme activity in these vacuoles.

1.2.5 Isolation and biochemical characterization

Gap junctions have been isolated as enriched subcellular fractions primarily from rat and mouse liver (Benedetti and Emmelot, 1968; Goodenough and Stoeckenius, 1972; Evans and Gurd, 1972; Gilula, 1974a; Duguid and Revel, 1975; Goodenough, 1974; 1976). The gap junctional fractions have been obtained by starting with a plasma membrane fraction and reducing the non-junctional membrane elements by treatment with detergents, such as deoxycholate or sarkosyl. Unfortunately, the detergent-resistant fraction that contains the gap junctions, is heavily contaminated with several elements [such as collagen, amorphous protein, uricase crystals] that interfere with the final enrichment on sucrose density gradients. Therefore, enzymatic treatments have been used to reduce the contaminating material; collagenase and hyaluronidase (both containing some non-specific protease activity) have frequently been employed for this purpose. At present, all of the gap junctional fractions that have been isolated from liver have been exposed to enzymatic treatments, so the reported polypeptide contents may be significantly altered by this treatment (see Duguid and Revel, 1975, for a discussion of the proteolysis). Since no endogenous activity has been detected in the junctional fraction, ultrastructural analysis (with thin sections and negative staining) is the major criterion for purity.

In the isolated gap junction fractions both protein and lipid are present, but no carbohydrate has been reported. In spite of the possible proteolysis, it appears that a 25 000 daltons polypeptide can be detected, together with other polypeptides, as a prominent component in both mouse and rat liver preparations. Dunia *et al.* (1974) have isolated a fraction of junctions from bovine lens fibers, and they report the presence of a prominent 34 000 dalton polypepide in this fraction. From a study on the lipids extracted from isolated gap junctions, Goodenough and Stoeckenius (1972) reported the presence of phosphatidylcholine, some phosphatidylethanolamine, and some neutral lipid (probably cholesterol).

The isolated mouse liver gap junctions have been analyzed by X-ray diffraction (Goodenough *et al.,* 1974) and both meridional and equatorial reflections have been phased. From the meridional reflections, the authors interpret the electron density profile to indicate the presence of two lipid bilayers (42 Å peak-to-peak) that are spanned by protein, with protein also present in the 'gap'. In addition, gap junctional subunits with a six-fold substructure have been deduced from the equatorial reflections.

1.2.6 Physiological significance

The role of gap junctions in excitable tissues has been recognized for several years; however, the role of these structures in development, differentiation, and maintenance of non-excitable tissues has not been easy to determine. In excitable tissues, the gap junction can be regarded as the low-resistance pathway for electrotonic coupling; in fact, it serves as the structural definition for the electrical synapse (for reviews, Bennett, 1973; McNutt and Weinstein, 1973; Gilula, 1974b). The most direct evidence for this fact in excitable tissues has been obtained from studies on vertebrate myocardium where the gap junctions (nexus) were reversibly and selectively dissociated concomitant with a reversible perturbation of electrotonic coupling (Barr *et al.,* 1965; Dreifuss *et al.,* 1966). In non-excitable tissues, the gap junction has also been implicated as the structural pathway for ionic and metabolic coupling from studies in a co-culture system where a gap junctionally defective cell type was demonstrated to be communication-defective (Gilula *et al.,* 1972). Since gap junctions are widely distributed in non-excitable tissues, it has been tempting to speculate that they are responsible for permitting the flow of regulatory information (in the form of low-molecular weight molecules) between cells. However, attempts to speculate about function solely on the basis of structural identification should be cautioned, because, at the present time, we have no basis for determining whether or not a gap junctional structure is predictably coupled or uncoupled.

There have been several attempts to relate the structure of gap junctions directly to low-resistance physiological properties (see Bennett, 1973). In general, it has been virtually impossible to relate specific resistances or permeability measurements to the number of presumptive channels that can be detected ultrastructurally. The difficulties have been related primarily to the problem of finding a well-defined system (preferably a two-cell system) where the coupling and other membrane properties are relatively stable, and where the number of gap junctional particles can be reliably quantitated. Even with such a system, there are certain assumptions that must be made, and these must include some consideration of the low-resistance properties of each junctional particle that is observed. When one assumes that every junctional particle contains a functional low-resistance pathway (about 2 nm in diameter), then there have always been too many junctional particles present to account for the low-resistance measurements. Therefore, all of the junctional particles must not be equivalent with respect to low-resistance properties. It is quite possible that some of the particles provide a low-resistance pathway for current transmission, some provide a polar pathway for metabolite transmission, and some may actually not participate in cell—cell coupling under certain conditions. At the present time, it is not possible to conclude that the channels involved in current flow are the same as those involved in metabolite and dye transfer.

The precise location of the low-resistance channel in the gap junctional lattice has never been demonstrated with either ultrastructural or molecular probes. However, on the basis of the ultrastructural appearance of the gap junctional lattice, it has been suggested that the channel is located in the central region of the junctional particles (Payton *et al.,* 1969; McNutt and Weinstein, 1970). More recently, continuous electron-dense 'channels' at this site have been observed in negative stain preparations of isolated gap junctions (Gilula, 1974a; Goodenough, 1976). The penetration of aqueous stain into this region of the junctional particles is certainly consistent with the localization of a polar 'channel' within the junctional lattice. The actual demonstration of the polar channel in the future will rely on a molecular and X-ray crystallographic analysis of the junctional lattice.

The most striking gap junctional variation has been found in arthropod tissues as indicated previously. This variation does not appear to detectably influence the general ionic coupling properties that are observed, since coupling is easily detected in arthropod tissues. In fact, most of the information on the regulation of junctional permeability has been obtained from studies on arthropods (Payton *et al.,* 1969; Rose and Loewenstein, 1975; Gilula and Epstein, 1976). This is important to note since the dramatic structural differences may indicate some important regulatory differences in communication in arthropod and non-arthropod systems (Gilula and Epstein, 1976).

1.3 TIGHT JUNCTIONS

The tight junction is a cell contact that is normally present between most vertebrate epithelial and endothelial cells. This structure was referred to as the zonula occludens by Farquhar and Palade (1963) to indicate the form and distribution of the structure, as well as its potential physiological role. This junction is characterized in thin sections by a series of focal fusions between the membranes of adjacent cells (Fig. 1.5). The junctional membranes have a combined width of 14—15 nm at the

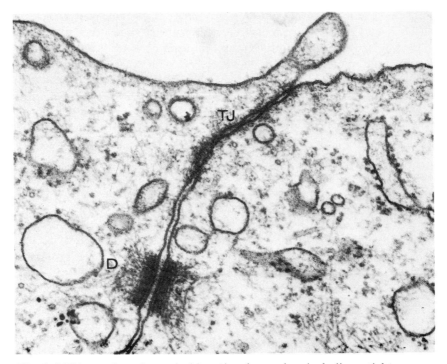

Fig. 1.5 Thin section of an apical junctional complex, including a tight junction (TJ) and desmosome (D) in 7 day chicken embryonic otocyst epithelium. (Micrograph courtesy of Rosemary D. Ginzberg.) x 57 900.

points of fusion. The tight junction may exist as a belt-like structure (zonula) or as an isolated band of membrane fusion (fascia). The zonular element can be an effective occluding barrier to the diffusion of large molecules between cells, as indicated by the use of electron-dense 'tracer' materials (Miller, 1960; Farquhar and Palade, 1963; Brightman and Reese, 1969; Goodenough and Revel, 1970; Friend and Gilula, 1972a).

In freeze-fracture replicas, the tight junction can be characterized by two internal membrane fracture face components that are complementary (Fig. 1.6). The inner membrane half (fracture face P) contains a mesh-like or anastomosing arrangement of ridges or strands (8–9 nm in diameter), while the outer membrane half (fracture face E) contains a complementary arrangement of grooves. These fracture

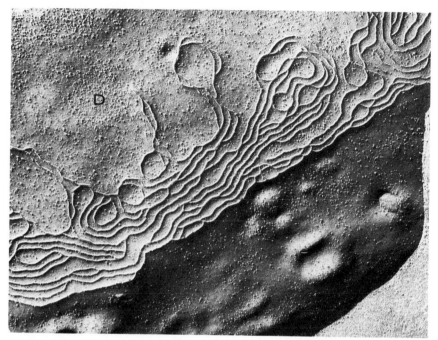

Fig. 1.6 Freeze-fracture appearance of the anastomosing tight junctional membrane ridges and desmosomal membrane plaque (D) in the adult chicken semicircular canal epithelium. (Micrograph courtesy of Rosemary D. Ginzberg.) x 45 900.

face components correspond to the form and distribution of the membrane fusions that are observed in thin sections (Chalcroft and Bullivant, 1970; Friend and Gilula, 1972a; Claude and Goodenough, 1973; Staehelin, 1973; Wade and Karnovsky, 1974). Tight junctional membrane elements often co-exist with gap junctional elements; in fact, gap junctional particles may be completely sequestered within tight junctional ridges (Friend and Gilula, 1972a; Goodenough and Stoeckenius, 1972).

As indicated above, the term zonula occludens was used to describe the potential role of this structure, in addition to its form and distribution (Farquhar and Palade, 1963). On the basis of analyzing the complexity (strand number) of the tight junctions in epithelia with varying transepithelial permeability properties, Claude and Goodenough (1973) suggested that there was a direct relationship between strand number and the electrical resistance of an epithelial layer. For example, a 'tight' epithelium would have tight junctions comprised of several strands, while a 'leaky' epithelial tight junction would have few complete strands. Recently, a couple of studies have suggested that the permeability of tight junctions is not regulated by the number of strands, but by other, yet to be determined, properties of the tight junctional membranes (Martinez-Palomo and Erlij, 1975; Mollgard *et al.*, 1976).

Tight junctions are almost exclusively found in vertebrate organisms (Gilula, 1974b; Staehelin, 1974); however there has been a report that a similar structure may exist as part of the blood-brain barrier in the insect nervous system (Lane and Swales, 1976). A tight junctional variant called the Sertoli cell junction has been described in the region of the blood-testis barrier between Sertoli cells in the mammalian testis (Gilula *et al.*, 1976; Nagano and Suzuki, 1976a, 1976b). Also, some fascia or single ridge-like elements resembling tight junctions have been described in the vertebrate nervous system in association with myelin (Dermietzil, 1974; Mugnaini and Schnapp, 1974).

The formation of tight junctions has recently been examined in a variety of epithelia with freeze-fracturing. From these studies, it appears that individual intramembrane particles are arranged into linear segments that fuse to become short linear ridges (Hull and Staehelin, 1974; Montesano *et al.*, 1975; Elias and Friend, 1976; Porvaznik *et al.*, 1976). These short ridges, in turn, fuse with other ridge segments to form anastomosing networks that eventually become complete belts or zonulae. When the zonule is completed, 'tracers' are excluded and the permeability barrier is formed (Ducibella *et al.*, 1975; Larsson, 1975).

At the present time, the possibility still exists that the tight junction may play a role in electrotonic coupling between cells. Unfortunately, no analysis of coupling has been made on a cellular system that contains only tight junctions; as indicated previously, they usually co-exist with gap junctions. In addition, it is quite possible that there is a close biochemical relationship between intramembrane particles that comprise tight and gap junctions since the two junctional elements may be so intimately associated with each other under normal conditions (Friend and Gilula, 1972a) and during the formation process in epithelial tissues (Montesano *et al.*, 1975).

1.4 SEPTATE JUNCTIONS

The septate junction has primarily been identified in invertebrate tissues (Wood, 1959; Gilula *et al.*, 1970; Danilova *et al.*, 1969, and Noirot-Timothee and Noirot, 1973). Septate-like junctions that have been described in vertebrate tissues (Lasansky, 1969; Gobel, 1971) appear to be a distinctly different cell surface specialization (Friend and Gilula, 1972b).

In thin sections, the septate junction has a distinct 'railroad track' appearance as a result of a periodic arrangement of electron-dense bars or septa that join the two adjacent plasma membranes (Fig. 1.7a). The spacing between septa may vary, but the

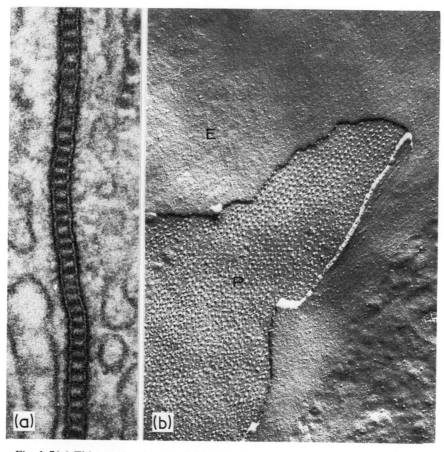

Fig. 1.7(a) Thin section image of the septate junction in molluscan gill epithelium. x 160 000.

(b) Freeze-fractures of the septate junctional membranes in the molluscan gill epithelium. Parallel rows of intramembrane particles are associated with the P fracture face, while complementary rows are present on the E fracture face. x 60 000.

septal widths are quite constant. The septal sheets form a complete belt around the cells and the sheets may be flat or pleated. The interaction of adjacent pleated sheets may produce a series of hexagonal units. The morphology of the septal sheets may vary considerably in different invertebrate systems (Staehelin, 1974).

In freeze-fracture replicas, the septate junctional membranes are characterized by two complementary internal membrane fracture faces (Fig. 1.7b). The inner membrane half (fracture face P) contains rows of individual 85 Å particles, while the outer membrane half (fracture face E) contains interrupted rows of depressions. The particles within a row are 21 nm apart, and the particles between rows are not in register. The particle rows are usually parallel; however the arrangement and distribution of the particle rows are predictably similar to that of the intercellular septa. An assembly process for the formation of septate junctions in sea urchin embryos has also been described with freeze-fracturing (Gilula, 1973).

The physiological role of the septate junction is rather unclear at the present time. It has been proposed as a candidate for electrotonic coupling (Gilula *et al.,* 1970; Loewenstein and Kanno, 1964; Bullivant and Loewenstein, 1968), a transepithelial permeability barrier (Dan, 1960) and a device for cell—cell adhesion (Wood, 1959). It has been difficult to determine the potential role of the septate junction in electrotonic coupling because gap junctions have also been present in the tissues that have been analyzed (Hudspeth and Revel, 1971; Gilula and Satir, 1971; Hand and Gobel, 1972). Therefore, a system must be analyzed that only contains septate junctions between the cells in order to determine the possible cell-to-cell low resistance properties of this structure.

1.5 DESMOSOMES

Desmosomes are probably the largest class of cell—cell contacts. There are several types of desmosomes that are present in a variety of both invertebrate and vertebrate tissues. The three most prominent mammalian desmosomes have been referred to as:

(1) the macula adhaerens (desmosome);
(2) the zonula adhaerens; and
(3) the fascia adhaerens (Farquhar and Palade, 1963). The structural and developmental aspects of these cell contacts have been thoroughly reviewed recently (McNutt and Weinstein, 1973; Staehelin, 1974; Overton, 1974).

The macula adhaerens structure is characterized in thin sections by a bipartite arrangement of material on the cytoplasmic surfaces of the desmosomal membranes (Fig. 1.5). The cytoplasmic surface of the desmosomal membranes contains a dense plaque, and the intervening intercellular space (about 20—30 nm wide) contains a condensation of dense crystalline material. The dense plaque frequently serves as the insertion site for filaments. The macula adhaerens is a plaque-like structure, while the zonula adhaerens is a belt-like structure and the fascia adhaerens is a band-like element. The zonula adhaerens is an important insertion site for the microfilaments of the epithelial cell terminal web. In some instances, desmosomal membranes have a detectable freeze-fracture specialization that is present as a non-polygonal arrangement of closely packed particles or granules (Fig. 1.6). These fracture-face components can be detected on both the inner and outer membrane fracture faces (McNutt *et al.,* 1971; Breathnach *et al.,* 1972; Staehelin, 1974).

There has been one extensive study by Skerrow and Matoltsy (1974a,b) on the isolation and biochemical characterization of desmosomes from the bovine snout. In this study they report that the desmosomal plaque contains two high molecular weight polypeptides (230 000 and 210 000 daltons). The crystalline material of the intercellular space probably contains several carbohydrate-containing polypeptides (140 000 and 120 000 daltons), and three major polypeptides (90 000, 75 000 and 60 000 daltons) that appear to be integral components of the desmosomal membrane.

Desmosomes are most prominent in tissues that undergo significant stress, such as stratified squamous epithelium and myocardium. In these tissues, the desmosomes are primarily responsible for maintaining cell-to-cell adhesion. Their role in cell adhesion has been clearly indicated by studies that have utilized selective disruption of desmosomes to facilitate the dissociation of intact tissue (Muir, 1967; Berry and Friend, 1969). These structures definitely do not participate in low-resistance cell-to-cell communication, since they can be disrupted without affecting low-resistance permeability (Dreifuss *et al.,* 1966).

1.6 CONCLUSIONS

During the past 5—10 years, there has been significant progress in characterizing various junctional structures with electron microscopic techniques, in particular with freeze-fracturing. In most instances, a structure-function relationship has been established for cell junctions with little direct and much indirect evidence. In the future, more direct evidence for the structure-function relationships will rely on an integration of physiological, genetic, and molecular information with the structural characterization of various cell junctions.

REFERENCES

Albertini, D.F. and Anderson, E. (1974), *J. Cell Biol.,* **63**, 234—250.
Albertini, D.F., Fawcett, D.W. and Olds, P.J. (1975), *Tissue and Cell,* **7**, 389—405.
Amsterdam, A. and Jamieson, J.D. (1974), *J. Cell Biol.,* **63**, 1037—1056.
Amsterdam, A., Josephs, R., Lieberman, M.E. and Lindner, H.R. (1976), *J. Cell Sci.,* **21**, 93—105.
Anderson, E. and Albertini, D.F. (1976), *J. Cell Biol.,* **71**, 680—686.
Barr, L., Berger, W. and Dewey, M.M. (1968), *J. gen. Physiol.,* **51**, 347—368.
Barr, L., Dewey, M.M. and Berger, W. (1965), *J. gen. Physiol.,* **48**, 797—823.
Benedetti, E.L., Dunia, I. and Bloemendal, H. (1974), *Proc. natn. Acad. Sci., U.S.A.,* **71**, 5073—5077.
Benedetti, E.L. and Emmelot, P. (1965), *J. Cell Biol.,* **26**, 299—305.
Benedetti, E.L. and Emmelot, P. (1968), *J. Cell Biol.,* **38**, 15—24.
Bennett, M.V.L. (1973), *Fedn Proc. fedn Am. Socs exp. Biol.,* **32**, 65—75.
Berry, M.N. and Friend, D.S. (1969), *J. Cell Biol.,* **43**, 506—520.
Breathnach, A.S., Stolinski, C. and Gross, M. (1972), *Micron,* **3**, 287—304.

Brightman, M.W. and Reese, T.S. (1969), *J. Cell Biol.*, **40**, 648−677.

Bullivant, S. and Loewenstein, W.R. (1968), *J. Cell Biol.*, **37**, 621−632.

Chalcroft, J.P. and Bullivant, S. (1970), *J. Cell Biol.*, **47**, 49−60.

Claude, P. and Goodenough, D.A. (1973), *J. Cell Biol.*, **58**, 390−400.

Dallai, R. (1975), *J. Submicros. Cytol.*, **7**, 249−257.

Dan, K. (1960), *Int. Rev. Cytol.*, **9**, 321.

Danilova, L.V., Rokhlenko, K. and Bodryagina, A.V. (1969), *Z. Zellforsch.*, **100**, 101−117.

Decker, R.S. (1976), *J. Cell Biol.*, **69**, 669−685.

Decker, R.S. and Friend, D.S. (1974), *J. Cell Biol.*, **62**, 32−47.

Dermietzel, R. (1974), *Cell Tiss. Res.*, **148**, 565−576.

Dewey, M.M. and Barr, L. (1962), *Science*, **137**, 670−672.

Dreifuss, J.J., Girardier, L. and Forssman, W.G. (1966), *Pflugers Arch.*, **292**, 13−33.

Ducibella, T., Albertini, D.F., Anderson, E. and Biggers, J.D. (1975), *Dev. Biol.*, **45**, 231−250.

Duguid, J.R. and Revel, J.P. (1975), *Symp. Quant. Biol.*, **40**, 45−47.

Dunia, I., Sen, K., Benedetti, E.L., Zweers, A. and Bloemendal, H. (1974), *FEBS Letters*, **45**, 139−144.

Elias, P.M. and Friend, D.S. (1976), *J. Cell Biol.*, **68**, 173−188.

Epstein, M.L., Beers, W.H. and Gilula, N.B. (1976), *J. Cell Biol.*, **70**, 302a.

Epstein, M.L., Sheridan, J.D. and Johnson, R.G. (1977), *Exp. Cell. Res.*, **104**, 25−30.

Evans, W.H. and Gurd, J.W. (1972), *Biochem, J.*, **128**, 691−700.

Farquhar, M.G. and Palade, G.E. (1963), *J. Cell Biol.*, **17**, 375−412.

Flower, N.E. (1972), *J. Cell Sci.*, **10**, 683−691.

Friend, D.S. and Gilula, N.B. (1972a), *J. Cell Biol.*, **53**, 758−776.

Friend, D.S. and Gilula, N.B. (1972b), *J. Cell Biol.*, **53**, 148−163.

Gilula, N.B. (1973), *Am. Zool.*, **13**, 1109−1117.

Gilula, N.B. (1974a), *J. Cell Biol.*, **63**, 111a.

Gilula, N.B. (1974b), *Cell Communication* (Cox, R.P., ed), John Wiley, New York.

Gilula, N.B., Branton, D. and Satir, P. (1970), *Proc. natn. Acad. Sci., U.S.A.*, **67**, 213−220.

Gilula, N.B. and Epstein, M.L. (1976), *Soc. exp. Biol. Symp.*, **30**, 257−272.

Gilula, N.B., Fawcett, D.W. and Aoki, A. (1976), *Dev. Biol.*, **50**, 142−168.

Gilula, N.B., Reeves, O.R. and Steinbach, A. (1972), *Nature*, **235**, 262−265.

Gilula, N.B. and Satir, P. (1971), *J. Cell Biol.*, **51**, 869−872.

Gobel, S. (1971), *J. Cell Biol.*, **51**, 328−333.

Goodenough, D.A. (1974), *J. Cell Biol.*, **61**, 557−563.

Goodenough, D.A. (1976), *J. Cell Biol.*, **68**, 220−231.

Goodenough, D.A., Caspar, D.L.D., Makowski, L. and Phillips, W.C. (1974), *J. Cell Biol.*, **63**, 115a.

Goodenough, D.A. and Gilula, N.B. (1974), *J. Cell Biol.*, **61**, 575−590.

Goodenough, D.A. and Revel, J.P. (1970), *J. Cell Biol.*, **45**, 272−290.

Goodenough, D.A. and Stoeckenius, W. (1972), *J. Cell Biol.*, **61**, 575−590.

Griepp, E.B. and Revel, J.P. (1977), *Intercellular Communication*, (De Mello, ed), Plenum Press, New York.

Gurd, J.W. and Evans, W.H. (1973), *Eur. J. Biochem.*, **36**, 273−279.

Hand, A.R. and Gobel, S. (1972), *J. Cell Biol.*, **52**, 397−408.

Hudspeth, A.J. and Revel, J.P. (1971), *J. Cell Biol.*, **50**, 92–101.

Hull, B.E. and Staehelin, L.A. (1976), *J. Cell Biol.*, **68**, 688–704.

Hülser, D.F. and Peters, J.H. (1971), *Eur. J. Immunol.*, **1**, 494–495.

Johnson, R.G., Hammer, M., Sheridan, J. and Revel, J.P. (1974), *Proc. natn. Acad. Sci. U.S.A.*, **71**, 4536–4540.

Johnson, R.G., Herman, W.S. and Preus, D.M. (1973), *J. Ultrastruct. Res.*, **43**, 298–312.

Lane, N.J. and Swales, L.S. (1976), *J. Cell Biol.*, **70**, 590a.

Larsson, L. (1975), *J. Ultrastruct. Res.*, **52**, 100–113.

Lasansky, A. (1969), *J. Cell Biol.*, **40**, 577–581.

Loewenstein, W.R. and Kanno, Y. (1964), *J. Cell Biol.*, **22**, 565–586.

Martinez-Palomo, A. (1970), *Lab. Invest.*, **22**, 605–614.

Martinez-Palomo, A. and Erlij, D. (1975), *Proc. natn. Acad. Sci. U.S.A.*, **72**, 4487–4491.

McNutt, N.S., Hershberg, R.A. and Weinstein, R.S. (1971), *J. Cell Biol.*, **51**, 805–825.

McNutt, N.S. and Weinstein, R.S. (1970), *J. Cell Biol.*, **47**, 666–687.

McNutt, N.S. and Weinstein, R.S. (1973), *Prog. Biophys. Mol. Biol.*, **26**, 45–101.

Merk, F.B., Albright, J.T. and Botticelli, C.R. (1973), *Anat. Rec.*, **175**, 107–125.

Merk, F.B., Botticelli, C.R. and Albright, J.T. (1972), *Endocrinol.*, **90**, 992–1007.

Miller, F. (1960), *J. Biophys. Biochem. Cytol.*, **8**, 689–718.

Mollgard, K., Malinowska, D.H. and Saunders, N. (1976), *Nature*, **264**, 293–294.

Montesano, R., Friend, D.S., Perrelet, A. and Orci, L. (1975), *J. Cell Biol.*, **67**, 310–319.

Mugnaini, E. and Schnapp, B. (1974), *Nature*, **251**, 725–727.

Muir, A.R. (1967), *J. Anat.*, **101**, 239–262.

Nagano, T. and Suzuki, F. (1976a), *Anat. Rec.*, **185**, 403–415.

Nagano, T. and Suzuki, F. (1976b), *Cell Tiss. Res.*, **166**, 37–48.

Noirot-Timothee, C. and Noirot, C. (1973), *J. Microscopie*, **17**, 169–184.

Oliveira-Castro, G.M., Barcinski, M.A. and Cukierman, S. (1973), *J. Immunol.*, **111**, 1616–1619.

Overton, J. (1974), *Prog. Surface Memb. Sci.*, **8**, 161–208.

Payton, B.W., Bennett, M.V.L. and Pappas, G.D. (1969), *Science*, **166**, 1641–1643.

Peracchia, C. (1973a), *J. Cell Biol.*, **57**, 54–65.

Peracchia, C. (1973b), *J. Cell Biol.*, **57**, 66–76.

Porvaznik, M., Johnson, R.G. and Sheridan, J.D. (1976), *J. Ultrastruct. Res.*, **55**, 343–359.

Potter, D.D., Furshpan, E.J. and Lennox, E.S. (1966), *Proc. natn. Acad. Sci., U.S.A.*, **55**, 328–336.

Raviola, E. and Gilula, N.B. (1973), *Proc. natn. Acad. Sci. U.S.A.*, **70**, 1677–1681.

Revel, J.P. and Karnovsky, M.J. (1967), *J. Cell Biol.*, **33**, C7–C12.

Revel, J.P., Yip, P. and Chang, L.L. (1973), *Dev. Biol.*, **35**, 302–317.

Robertson, J.D. (1963), *J. Cell Biol.*, **19**, 201–221.

Rose, B. (1971), *J. Memb. Biol.*, **5**, 1–19.

Rose, B. and Loewenstein, W.R. (1975), *Nature*, **254**, 250–252.

Satir, P. and Gilula, N.B. (1973), *Ann. Rev. Entomol.*, **18**, 143–166.

Sellin, D., Wallach, D.F.H. and Fischer, H. (1971), *Eur. J. Immunol.*, **1**, 453–458.
Skerrow, C.J. and Matoltsy, A.G. (1974a), *J. Cell Biol.*, **63**, 515–523.
Skerrow, C.J. and Matoltsy, A.G. (1974b), *J. Cell Biol.*, **63**, 524–530.
Staehelin, L.A. (1973), *J. Cell Sci.*, **13**, 763–786.
Staehelin, L.A. (1974), *Int. Rev. Cytol.*, **39**, 191–283.
Wade, J.B. and Karnovsky, M.J. (1974), *J. Cell Biol.*, **60**, 168–180.
Weinstein, R.S., Merk, F.B. and Alroy, J. (1976), *Adv. Cancer Res.*, **23**, 23–89.
Wood, R.L. (1959), *J. Biophys. Biochem. Cytol.*, **6**, 343–352.
Yee, A.G. (1972), *J. Cell Biol.*, **55**, 294a.

2 Junctional Permeability

M. V. L. BENNETT

Intercellular Junctions and Synapses
(*Receptors and Recognition,* Series B, Volume 2)
Edided by J. Feldman, N.B. Gilula and J.D. Pitts
Published in 1978 by Chapman and Hall, 11 New Fetter Lane, London EC4P 4EE
© Chapman and Hall

2.1 INTRODUCTION

The observation that cells are electrically coupled raises two immediate questions

(1) Do the ions pass between cells by a private pathway not involving extracellular space? and
(2) What substances pass between cells, in particular how big and with what charge?

Both questions are relevant to junctional structure, and are important in delimiting the roles that the junctions might play in non-electric communication. There is now little doubt that the gap junction is the principal morphological substrate of electrical coupling, although instances of coupling by way of extracellular space and by cytoplasmic continuity are also known (see below).

To speak to the historical point intercellular movement of fluorescein was the first observation of non-electrical transfer between cytoplasms that was presumed to be mediated by the same pathway as that which mediated electrical coupling (Loewnstein and Kanno, 1964). Shortly afterwards, movement of this dye was observed between coupled neurons, and cells in tissue culture (Pappas and Bennett, 1966; Furshpan and Potter, 1968).

It was suggested to me by E.J. Furshpan (in the discussion of a meeting presentation) that the fluorescein might actually be crossing extracellular space between cells. Failure to see leakage out of the apposition between the cells was not a critical test, because of the possibility of rapid dilution. Indeed, we had calculated that close apposition of low resistance membrane could produce significant coupling that would not be electrically distinguishable from coupling by way of a private pathway (cf. Bennett, 1973). Further testing showed that the dyes we had used up until that time did penetrate the cells from the outside, and so movement across extracellular space could not really be excluded.

An initial resolution of what may be termed the private pathway question was provided by the dye Procion yellow (Payton et al., 1969a). This dye did cross the junctions we had been studying under normal conditions, but it did not penetrate the cells from the outside, even after prolonged soaking. We could be confident on the failure of the dye to penetrate, because it is a reactive dye that binds to amino groups of proteins, and following fixation by ordinary histological techniques, no dye was present inside intact cells, although it was readily observed in the cytoplasm of cells that had been cut open prior to soaking. (Although Procion yellow does enter cardiac muscle cells from the outside, it apparently leaks out more slowly and intercellular movement can be observed; Imanaga, 1974). One gets into some nasty questions of sensitivity of measurement here, but for gap junctions in general the existence of a private pathway seems in little doubt. In experiments to be described below the basic criterion of intercellular spread without entry from the exterior is well established in several additional systems.

The structure of the gap junction, the probable location of the physiologically characterized channel, and even the possible visualization of the transmembrane channel in the electron microscope are discussed in the preceding chapter (Gilula, 1978).

2.2 EVIDENCE THAT GAP JUNCTIONS MEDIATE ELECTRICAL COUPLING AND INTERCELLULAR TRANSFER OF MOLECULES

The basis on which gap junctions are identifiable as a coupling pathway may be briefly summarized, since both electric current and identifiable molecules can pass between cells by other means. Furthermore, cells with gap junctions often have large areas of non-specialized apposition as well as other junctions, specifically desmosomes, maculae or zonulae adherentes (intermediate junctions), zonulae occludentes (tight or occluding junctions), or, in invertebrates, septate desmosomes.

Where cells are coupled, gap junctions are commonly found, or at least there are close appositions which are putative gap junctions, i.e. the appositions have been shown to have the more or less periodic substructure which distinguishes them tight junctions and the artifactual close appositions that sometimes appear to result from fixation (cf. Bennett *et al.*, 1967; Brightman and Reese, 1969). Where coupling is demonstrably or presumably absent, gap junctions are absent or rare. At sites where coupling is close, gap junctions can sometimes be seen to be more common than at sites where coupling is weak, but the quantitative correlation is not very good and there remains considerable uncertainty as to the actual value of the electrical resistivity of gap junction membrane. Measured values are if anything rather larger than would be calculated from channel diameter estimated from permeability and channel density per unit area. (A channel 100 Å long, 10 Å in diameter and filled with 100 mho resistivity solution would have a resistance of $10^{10}\,\Omega$. Spaced 100 Å apart the membrane resistivity would be about 0.01 $\Omega\,cm^2$).

Several cultured cell lines that form gap junctions are coupled whereas related cell lines that don't form gap junctions, but otherwise exhibit similar appositional regions, are not coupled (Gilula *et al.*, 1972). (In these systems, coupling is also correlated with metabolic co-operation, see below).

In the septate axon of the crayfish the appositional region between adjacent segments is largely occupied by glial cells and a fibrillar layer (Pappas *et al.*, 1969a). Axonal processes extend through small windows in this layer to form gap junctions, and there is little true apposition between the cells other than gap junction. Thus the case for mediation of both coupling and intercellular transfer of material via the junctions is strengthened.

There are a number of studies in which experimental treatments uncouple cells

and there is a corresponding loss of gap junctions. In septate axon several treatments
that cause uncoupling also cause separation of junctional membranes; recovery of
coupling is associated with reappearance of gap junctions (Asada and Bennett, 1971;
Pappas *et al.*, 1971). Similar results have been obtained in cardiac and smooth
muscle in which, however, it is not possible to be confident in actual junctional
resistances (Barr *et al.*, 1965, 1968; Dreifuss *et al.*, 1966).

There are a number of negative cases. DNP treatment and cooling increase
junctional resistance in the septate axon, but do not cause the junctions to separate
(Payton *et al.*, 1969b; Politoff and Pappas, 1972). Uncoupling is reported to produce
no effect on junctions in *Chironymus* salivary gland (Rose, 1971). Several treatments
increase the regularity of the gap junctional lattice in different tissues; it is suggested
that these are associated with uncoupling (Peracchia, 1977, Peracchia and Dulhunty,
1976). Aldehyde fixation is a very effective method of increasing junctional resistance
and except for fast frozen gap junctions (Landis and Reese, 1974), probably all gap
junctions examined in fixed tissue are of high resistance (Bennett, 1973). (There is
some doubt about the resistance of isolated gap junctions).

In addition to the private pathway question, one may ask whether intercellular
transfer of tracer molecules is by the same pathway as electrical coupling. In septate
axon (Pappas and Bennett, 1966) and *Chironymus* salivary gland (Simpson *et al.*,
1977) experimental treatments that disrupt coupling also block movement of larger
molecules, which suggests that a single pathway is involved. Furthermore, the non-
specific permeability to relatively large hydrophilic molecules suggests mediation by
aqueous channels (Bennett, 1973).

Although one concludes that gap junctions are a structure mediating chemical
communication, other mechanisms exist. Some cells such as neurons and endocrine
cells do communicate chemically by way of extracellular space, sometimes quite
non-specifically (Specht and Grafstein, 1973). Glial or other cells will accummulate
some transmitters released by neurons, although no direct communicative function
can be assigned to this uptake. Also glia can provide proteins to the squid giant axon
(Lasek *et al.*, 1974) although the cells are presumably not electrically coupled and
movements across gap junctions would not be expected in any case (see below). A
possible morphological basis is provided by micrographs of endocytosis by axons
localized to cytoplasmic regions of sheath cells (Waxman, 1968). Also certain specific
proteins can be taken up by particular cells (e.g. Neufeld, 1974).

A further possibility is that electronic coupling can be mimicked in one direction
at least by chemical synapses that are tonically releasing transmitter (cf. Bennett,
1977). This chemically mediated coupling could in principle be reciprocal although
only unidirectional coupling has been studied physiologically. The existence of both
electrical and chemical transmission at a single synapse presents possibilities for
more complex interactions (cf. Bennett, 1977) and inhibitory synapses even allow
coupling which is in effect negative in sign (Spira *et al.*, 1976).

Another important qualification in evaluating coupling is the possibility of
syncytia, either normal or artifactual. Dividing cells can retain mid-pieces for

some time after cleavage is complete to superficial examination, and these structures could mediate considerable coupling or intercellular transfer (a one micron hole connecting two cells would have a resistance of the order of 1 MΩ). A further complication is that small regions of cytoplasmic continuity can develop during fixation. Thus, cells may uncouple and then recouple in the course of fixation (Bennett, 1973). In *Fundulus* blastomeres, at least, formation of new channels in fixation is not accompanied by an increase in leakage to the outside; the electrical evidence strongly suggests that fusion occurs on a microscopic scale (Bennett and Spira, 1973). While in terms of electrical measurements, coupling via gap junctions is indistinguishable from coupling via relatively macroscopic cytoplasmic bridges, larger molecules can pass in the latter case. Also morphological criteria can be applied. However, the generation of continuity by fixation complicates the interpretation of intercellular movement assayed after fixation, as it is in fact in the case of the horse-radish peroxidase method (Graham and Karnovsky, 1965, Bennett, 1973).

In certain specific instances electrical coupling occurs across extracellular space. This occurs most dramatically if shorting out through the clefts between cells is prevented by zonulae occludentes (Bennett and Trinkaus, (1970), but significant pick-up of extracellular fields probably also occurs without any specialized junctional arrangements (Ishii *et al.,* 1971; Nelson, 1966; cf. Bennett, 1977). At the Mauthner cell axon hillock region, altered resistivity in the surrounding tissue leads to coupling of the electrical inhibitory neurons across extracellular space (Korn and Faber, 1975).

One may ask if other junctional types mediate coupling. Certainly many cell types joined by adhering junctions (Gilula *et al.,* 1972) or the 'active zones' of chemical synapses are not coupled. It is difficult to exclude that tight junctions and septate desmosomes mediate coupling. No tissue joined by tight junctions is known that is not coupled, but since these are all epithelia, gap junctions are also very likely to be present, and without freeze fracture, gap junctions are very difficult to identify if they are intercalated within a tight junction web. Brightman and Reese (1969) argued that olfactory epithelial neurons which are joined by tight junctions should not be coupled to each other or to supporting cells as this would decrease specificity. The argument becomes less convincing in view of coupling between photoreceptor cells (Fain *et al.,* 1975) and the apparent coupling of hair cells to supporting cells (Weiss *et al.,* 1974) where one would expect that the same adaptive value of independence would apply. Similarly, no tissues with septate desmosomes have been shown not to be coupled. Again, the problem is the parallel occurrence of gap junctions. In respect to both tight junctions and septate desmosomes, one may presume that coupling is absent on grounds of simplicity and the absence of morphological data for a cytoplasmic channel corresponding to those from gap junctions.

Pinocytosis involves uptake of a variety of materials from extracellular space which could involve proteins secreted by neighboring or even distant cells. Whether such activity involves any communicative function is obscure; pinocytosed material is after all still membrane-bounded. Nevertheless a cell body knows quite quickly when its axon has been cut and when the normal retrograde transport of pinocytosed material is interrupted. That colchicine can mimic axotomy suggests a microtubule-dependent transport system and also membrane-bounded messages.

2.3 CHARACTERIZATION OF CHANNEL PERMEABILITY

The simplest and most direct test of junctional permeability is the observation of movement of directly visualizable molecules, either through fluorescent or ordinary transmission microscopy. Somewhat more involved technically is observation of radio-isotope movement by direct isolation of post-junctional structures or by radio-autography. Getting substances into the cells may involve simple injection, preloading by soaking, or more subtle methods. The measurements of junctional permeability can be viewed from two perspectives; a few dyes have been used extensively; a few junctions have been studied in depth (Table 2.1).

The salivary gland of the midge, *Chironymus*, is the most completely characterized. Its cells are joined by gap junctions (Rose, 1971), presumably of the arthropod type, which show several differences from vertebrate junctions. The former have a larger gap and in freeze fracture show a reduced density of particle packing. Also the particles adhere to the E face rather than the P face (Chapter 1, this volume). The gland cells are joined by extensive septate desmosomes as well as gap junctions. A number of oligopeptides have been labeled with fluorescein, lissamine rhodamine B or dansyl chloride (Simpson *et al.*, 1977). $(Leu)_3(Glu)_2$ with lissamine rhodamine label on the amino end (mol. wt. 1158) generally crosses and many smaller molecules cross. $(Leu)_3(Glu)_2$ with fluorescein label on the amino end (mol. wt. 1004) rarely crosses. Fluorescein-labeled fibrinopeptide A (mol. wt. 1926) and fluorescein-labeled insulin A chain (mol. wt. 2921) fail to cross. By use of smaller lissamine rhodamine B-labeled compounds which have distinctively different fluorescent emission or by electrophysiological criteria, junctional permeability was shown to be high even in the experiments where negative results were obtained with larger molecules. Of permeant molecules larger ones tended to have lower rates of trans-junctional movement. The control of lack of penetration from the external medium of compounds crossing the junctions verifies that the intercellular transfer is via a private pathway. Permeant molecules treated with cytoplasm failed to reveal any changes in paper electrophoresis patterns indicating that there is no breakdown intracellularly.

The labeled peptides were all acidic, i.e. negatively charged. Fluorescent-labeled oligosaccharides up to a mol. wt. of 1058 were also preliminarily reported to cross (Loewenstein, 1975). While junctions may or may not be permeable to positively charged molecules of similar sizes, the proposition is difficult to test because of binding to cytoplasmic constituents.

The conclusion was reached that the channel is about 14 Å in diameter (assuming spherical configuration of the tracers) or somewhat less if an extended configuration

Table 2.1 Electrotonically coupled cells and representative permeant molecules. Gap junctions have been described for all except leech and *Asterias*

Probe (mol. wt.)	*Chironymus* salivary gland (31, 46, 48)	Vertebrate cultured cells (18, 33, 43)	Crayfish septate axon (5, 37, 38)	Novikoff hepatoma (25)	Vertebrate heart (23, 52, 55)	Dogfish retina horizontal cells (26)	Leech Retzius cells (45)	*Xenopus* neurula (47)	Blastomeres *Fundulus* (5, 7, 11)	Blastomeres *Xenopus* (47)	Blastomeres *Asterias* (53)
Na^+, Cl^-, SO_4^{2-} (96)			+								
K^+ (39)			+		+						
Co^{2+}			+								
Amino acids (75–131)		+					+				
Uridine (244)		+					+				
Fluorescein (332)	+	+	+	+				+	+	?	?
cAMP (347)					+						
Dansyl glutamate (380)	+				+						
Procion yellow (630)	+		+	+	+						?
Fluo. maltose (725)	+										
Fluo. (Glu)$_3$ (794)	+										
Dansyl (Leu)$_3$(Glu)$_2$ (849)	+										
Fluo. maltotriose (899)	+										
Fluo. maltotetriose (1058)	+										
IrB (Leu)$_3$(Glu)$_2$ (1158)	+			permeant							
Sugar phosphates nucleotides, folic acid (tetraglu.?) (1020)		+									
Fluo. (Leu)$_3$(Glu)$_2$ (1004)	−										
Fluo. firbinopeptide A (1926)	−			impermeant							
Fluo. insulin A chain (2921)	−										
Proteins	−	−	−				−				
RNAs, DNA	−						−				

Fluo. − labeled with fluorescein; IrB − labeled with lissamine rhodamine B; Glu − glutamate; Leu − leucine is assumed. The smallest impermeant molecules would, if spherical, have diameters of 16 to 18 Å.

Other junctions or rather a class of junctions well-characterized in terms of permeability are those formed in tissue culture between vertebrate epithelial cells and fibroblasts. The initial method of detection of transjunctional movement was in principle a bioassay. A cell line that was unable to make a compound essential for growth could grow when co-cultured with a cell that could make that compound. The phenomenon was termed metabolic co-operation when first described (cf. Chapter 4, this volume). Further, the defective cell line might not be able to use the compound when it was applied in the medium, which indicates again that communication is by way of a private pathway not involving extracellular space. Movements of fluorescein were also noted between cultured cells (Furshpan and Potter, 1968; Michalke and Loewenstein, 1971).

These results have been greatly extended by using a variety of methods of prelabeling a population of cells and allowing them to contact target cells (Pitts and Finbow, 1977). One cell group can be cultured with appropriate materials taken up by those cells, washed and then plated with other cells to see if that substrate or any of its metabolic products are transmitted. Amino acids are readily loaded into cells and are transferred rapidly and in large amounts to co-cultured cells. (An extracellular pathway is a little difficult to exclude in this particular kind of experiment for some degree of transfer by extracellular space is likely to occur in any case, cf. Specht and Grafstein, 1973). Similar experiments can be done with vitamins and co-factors, and nucleic acid precursors. To date, the largest molecule observed to cross is folic acid which if it occurs in the usual tetraglutamate form has a molecular weight of about 1020.

Of equal importance are the molecules that do not move between cells. Labeled proteins (with a cold amino acid chase to avoid spread of breakdown products) do not move between cells. DNA and RNA including transfer RNA similarly do not cross the junctions. It is difficult to give a precise lower limit for permeation, because of sensitivity questions and lack of knowledge of the amount of low molecular weight polypeptides in the labeled cell cytoplasm. As for the salivary gland cells one would anticipate a channel size of around 10–14 Å. The correspondance between permeabilities of these vertebrate and invertebrate junctions is somewhat surprising given the difference in structure.

Junctions in the septate axon of the crayfish are permeable to small anions and cations and to fluorescein, neutral red, sucrose and Procion yellow (Bennett, 1973; Pappas and Bennett, 1966; Payton *et al.*, 1969). They are not permeable to horseradish peroxidase (Bennett *et al.*, 1973) or to fluorescein-labeled bovine serum albumin (unpublished). In this case channel diameter is less well-characterized, but it can be concluded to lie between 10 and 20Å.

Cultured Novikoff hepatoma cells become coupled and movement of fluorescein, dansyl-*l*-glutamate and dansyl-*dl*-aspartate occurs between them (Johns and Sheridan, 1971). No uptake was observed with brief external application.

Vertebrate cardiac muscle junctions pass K^+ (Weidman, 1966) and Procion yellow (Imagana, 1974). Cyclic AMP also appears to move across the junctions (Tsien and Weingart, 1976). Procion yellow passes between coupled horizontal cells in the dogfish retina (Kaneko, 1971).

Transfer between the coupled Retzius cells of the leech was observed for fucose, glucosamine, glycine, leucine, orotic acid and uridine (Rieske *et al.,* 1975). Puromycin injected into the transjunctional cell blocked labeling in that cell but not in the donor cell indicating that the injected substrates and not their macromolecular products were transferred. This study is the only one showing intercellular movement of substances in annelids in which interneuronal gap junctions have yet to be demonstrated (cf. Coggeshall, 1974).

The inferred channel sizes are consistent with electron microscopic observations in lanthanum or otherwise stained thin-sectioned material, in negatively stained isolated junctions, and in freeze-fracture images (cf. Chapter 1, this volume). That is the lattice comprising the junction contains a central specialization that is roughly 10–20 Å across. Also the interchannel spacing is roughly 100 Å (in vertebrate material, somewhat greater in arthropods). Two walls of the coupling channel and an extracellular space of some 20 Å must be fitted into this periodicity. The walls are very non-leaky and whatever they are made of, there is obviously not much room for a larger channel. Of course molecular weight goes up roughly as the cube of the diameter, so a small change in channel size could produce a very significant change in molecular weight of permeable molecules.

Although junctional permeability in the different systems so far described appears reasonably uniform, there are other reports of differences. Impermeability to fluorescein or Procion yellow has been asserted for several coupled embryonic systems: *Xenopus* blastulae (Slack and Palmer, 1969), isolated and reaggregated *Fundulus* blastomeres (Bennett *et al.,* 1972; Bennett, 1973) and blastomeres of the starfish *Asterias* (Tupper and Sanders, 1972). We have recently found that the *Fundulus* junctions are permeable to fluorescein and to another fluorescent dye Lucifer yellow (Bennett *et al.,* 1977). The latter (synthesized by W.W. Stuart) is a substituted 4-amino naphthalimide with two sulfonate groups and a molecular weight of 476. The non-junctional membranes of the cells are quite impermeable to this dye and passage between coupled cells is easily measured. In contrast, fluorescein leaks out of the cells, and demonstration of intercellular movement requires use of very well-coupled cells and long waiting times. The difficulty in measuring fluorescein permeation is in marked contrast to its ready demonstration in other tissues. However, our earlier failures seem more likely to result from loss from the cells and relatively small junctional area rather that impermeability of the junctions to larger molecules.

In *Xenopus,* fluorescein permeability was clearly demonstrated in the neurula stage, but results with blastomeres were somewhat equivocal (Sheridan, 1971). Re-examination is desirable, but similar results to those with *Fundulus* blastomeres would not now be surprising. The failure of the dyes to pass between coupled

Asterias blastomeres (Tupper and Saunders, 1972) must also be suspect. The coupling coefficients were comparable to those cases in *Fundulus* which failed to show fluorescein transfer and apparently there was a relatively large autofluorescence which would have tended to obscure any dye movement. Injection of EGTA into one blastomere of the 2-celled *Xenopus* egg blocks cleavage in that blastomere only (Baker and Warner, 1972). Aside from a requirement for Ca in cleavage, one might infer that the junctions between cells were impermeable to Ca (as well as EGTA) for the EGTA should either be saturated by Ca flowing from the uninjected cell, or the uninjected cell should have its Ca reduced below the level required for cleavage. At this point quantitative factors rather than qualitative impermeability of the junctions seem likely to account for the results.

The rectifying synapses between lateral and motor giant fibers of the crayfish nerve cord appear to be impermeable to fluorescein (Keeter *et al.*, 1974). This point needs to be checked during tetanic stimulation, since the junctions have a relatively high resistance in the resting condition. Because of the presence of a voltage–sensitive gating mechanism a difference in permeability would not be surprising.

Ultrastructural studies by both thin section and freeze fracture fail to reveal any difference between gap junctions in embryonic, rectifying, and ordinary adult junctions (Bennett and Gilula, 1974; Keeter *et al.*, 1974; Hanna *et al.*, 1976). This failure is not surprising, if the commonly accepted model of gap junction structure is correct because a small change in channel diameter would probably not be recognizable, particularly if it occurred at only a short region of the intercyto-plasmic channel.

To recapitulate, gap junctions are very common, and occur where intercellular movement of molecules rather than charges appears to be the relevant property. The junctions generally admit molecules up to a molecular weight of about 1000 of both neutral and negatively charged molecules. The junctions are permeable to small positive ions, but upper size limits are difficult to evaluate for positively charged molecules because of binding to cytoplasmic constituents.

The permeability limits are consistent with models of junctional structure involving a 10–20 Å hydrophilic channel, and are not inconsistent with measurements of electrical resistivity (which is very poorly known).

The restrictive permeability provides a framework in which the significance of communication by way of the junctions must be evaluated. Other modes of communication are also known that can mediate different functions.

REFERENCES

1. Asada, Y. and Bennett, M.V.L. (1971), Experimental alteration of coupling resistance at an electrotonic synapse. *J. Cell Biol.*, **49**, 159–172.
2. Baker, P.F. and Warner, A.E. (1972), Intracellular calcium and cell cleavage in early embryos of *Xenopus laevis*. *J. Cell Biol.*, **53**, 579–581.

3. Barr, L., Berger, W. and Dewey, M.M. (1968), Electrical transmission at the nexus between smooth muscle cells. *J. gen Physiol.,* **51**, 347–369.
4. Barr, L., Dewey, M.M. and Berger, W. (1965), Propagation of action potentials and the structure of the nexus in cardiac muscle. *J. gen. Physiol.,* **48**, 797–823.
5. Bennett, M.V.L. (1973), Permeability and structure of electrotonic junctions and intercellular movement of tracers. In: *Intracellular Staining Techniques in Neurobiology* (Kater, S.D. and Nicholson, C., eds.), pp. 115–133. Elsevier, New York.
6. Bennett, M.V.L. (1977), Electrical Transmission: a functional analysis and comparison with chemical transmission. In: *Cellular Biology of Neurons* (Vol. I, Sec. I. *Handbook of Physiology: The Nervous System.*) (Kandel, E.R., ed.), Williams and Wilkins, Baltimore, (In press).
7. Bennett, M.V.L., Feder, N., Reese, T.S. and Stewart, W. (1973), Movement during fixation of peroxidases injected into the crayfish septate axon. *J. gen Physiol.,* **61**, 254–255.
8. Bennett, M.V.L. and Gilula, N.B. (1974), Membrane and junctions in developing *Fundulus* embryos, freeze fracture and electrophysiology. *J. Cell Biol.,* **63**, 21a.
9. Bennett, M.V.L., Pappas, G.D., Giménez, M. and Nakajima, Y. (1967), Physiology and ultrastructure of electrotonic junctions. IV. Medullary electromotor nuclei in gymnotid fish. *J. Neurophysiol.,* **30**, 236–300.
10. Bennett, M.V.L. and Spira, M.E. (1973), Effects of fixatives for electron microscopy on electrical coupling and tracer movement between embryonic cells. *J. Cell Biol.,* **59**, 23a.
11. Bennett, M.V.L., Spira, M.E. and Pappas, G.D. (1972), Properties of electrotonic junctions between embryonic cells of *Fundulus. Dev. Biol.,* **29**, 419–435.
12. Bennett, M.V.L., Spira, M. and Spray, D.C. (1977), Permeability of electrotonic junctions between embryonic cells, a reevaluation . *J. Cell Biol.,* **75**, in press (abstract).
13. Bennett, M.V.L. and Trinkaus, J.P. (1970), Electrical coupling between embryonic cells by way of extracellular space and specialized junctions. *J. Cell Biol.,* **44**, 592–610.
14. Brightman, M.W. and Reese, T.S. (1969), Junctions between intimately apposed cell membranes in the vertebrate brain. *J. Cell Biol.,* **40**, 648–677.
15. Coggeshall, R.E. (1974), Gap junctions between identified glial cells in the leech. *J. Neurobiol,* **5**, 463–468.
16. Dreifuss, J.J., Girardier, L. and Forssmann, W.G. (1966), Etude de la propagation de l'excitation dans le ventricule de rat au moyen de solutions hypertoniques. *Pfügers Arch.,* **292**, 13–33.
17. Fain, G.L., Gold, G.H. and Dowling, J.E. (1975), Receptor coupling in the toad retina. *Cold Spring Harbor Symp. Quant. Biol.,* **40**, 547–561.
18. Furshpan, E.J. and Potter, D.D. (1968), Low-resistance junctions between cells in embryos and tissue culture. In: *Current Topics in Developmental Biology, Vol. 3,* (Moscona, A.A. and Montroy, A. eds.), Academic Press, New York.
19. Gilula, N.B. (1978), Structure of intercellular junctions. In. *Intercellular Junctions and Synapses,* (Feldman, J.D., Gilula, N.B. and Pitts, J.D. eds.), Chapman and Hall, London.
20. Gilula, N.B., Reeves, O.R. and Steibnach, A. (1972), Metabolic coupling, ionic coupling and cell contacts. *Nature,* **235**, 262–265.

21. Graham, R.C. and Karnovsky, M.J. (1965), The early stages of absorbtion of injected horse-radish peroxidase in the proximal tubules of mouse kidney: ultrastructural cytochemistry by a new technique. *J. Histochem. Cytochem.,* **14**, 221–302.
22. Hanna, R.B., Keeter, J.S. and Pappas, G.D. (1976) Comparison of the fine structure of a rectifying and a non-rectifying synapse. *J. Cell Biol.,* **70**, 151a.
23. Imanaga, I, (1974), Cell to cell diffusion of Procion yellow in sheep and calf Purkinje fibres. *J. Memb. Biol.,* **16**, 381–388.
24. Ishii, Y., Matsuura, S. and Furukawa, T. (1971), An input-output relation at the synapse between hair cells and eighth nerve fibers in goldfish. *Jap. J. Physiol.,* **21**, 91–98.
25. Johnson, R.G. and Sheridan, J.D. (1971), Junctions between cancer cells in culture: ultrastructure and permeability. *Science,* **174**, 717–719.
26. Kaneko, A. (1971), Electrical connections between horizontal cells in the dogfish retina. *J. Physiol.,* **213**, 95–105.
27. Keeter, J.S., Deschenes, M., Pappas, G.D. and Bennett, M.V.L. (1974), Fine structure and permeability studies of a rectifying electrotonic synapse. *Biol. Bull.,* **147**, 485–486.
28. Korn, H., and Faber, D.S. (1975), An electrically mediated inhibition in goldfish medulla. *J. Neurophysiol.,* **38**, 452–471.
29. Landis, D.M.D. and Reese, T.S. (1974), Membrane structure in rapidly frozen, freeze-fracture cerebellar cortex. *J. Cell Biol.,* **63**, 184a.
30. Lasek, R.J., Gainer, H. and Przybylski, R.J. (1974), Transfer of newly synthesized proteins from Schwann cells to the squid giant axon. *Proc. natn. Acad. Sci., U.S.A.,* **71**, 1188–1192.
31. Loewenstein, W.R. (1975), Permeable junctions. *Cold Spring Harbor Symp. Quant. Biol.,* **40**, 49–63.
32. Loewenstein, W.R. and Kanno, Y. (1964), Studies on an epithelial (gland) cell junction. I. Modification of surface membrane permeability. *J. Cell Biol.,* **22**, 565–586.
33. Michalke, W. and Loewenstein, W.R. (1971), Communication between cells of different types. *Nature,* **232**, 121–122.
34. Nelson, P.G. (1966), Interaction between spinal motoneurons of the cat. *J. Neurophysiol.,* **29**, 275–287.
35. Neufeld, E.F. (1974), Uptake of lyzosomal enzymes by fibroblasts: studies of mucopolysaccharidoses and I-cell disease. In: *Cell Communication* (Cox, R., ed.), pp. 217–231, Wiley, New York.
36. Pappas, G.D., Asada, Y and Bennett, M.V.L. (1971), Morphological correlates of increased coupling resistance at an electrotonic synapse. *J. Cell Biol.,* **49**, 173–188.
37. Pappas, G.D. and Bennett, M.V.L. (1966), Specialized junctions involved in electrical transmission between neurons. *Ann. N.Y. Acad. Sci.,* **137**, 495–508.
38. Payton, B.W., Bennett, M.V.L. and Pappas, G.D. (1969a), Permeability and structure of junctional membranes at an electrotonic synapse. *Science,* **166**, 1641–1643.
39. Payton, B.W., Bennett, M.V.L. and Pappas, G.D. (1969b), Temperature-dependence of resistance at an electotonic synapse, **165**, 594–597.

40. Peracchia, C. (1977), Gap junctions. Structural changes after uncoupling procedures. *J. Cell Biol.,* **72**, 628−641.
41. Peracchia, C. and Dulhunty, A.F. (1976), Low resistance junctions in crayfish. Structural changes with functional uncoupling. *J. Cell Biol.,* **70**, 419−439.
42. Pitts, J.D. (1978), Gap junctions and cellular growth control. In: *Intercellular Junctions and Synapses* (Feldman, J.D., Gilula, N.B. and Pitts, J.D. eds.), Chapman and Hall, London.
43. Pitts, J.D. and Finbow, M. (1977), Junctional permeability and its consequences. In: *Intercellular Communication,* (De Mello, W.C. ed.), pp. 61−68, Plenum, New York.
44. Politoff, A. and Pappas, G.D. (1972), Mechanisms of increase in coupling resistance at electrotonic synapses of the crayfish septate axon. *Anat. Rec.,* **172**, 384−385.
45. Rieske, E., Schubert, P. and Kreutzberg, G.W. (1975), Transfer of radioactive material between electrically coupled neurons of the leech central nervous system. *Brain Res.,* **84**, 365−382.
46. Rose, B. (1971), Intercellular communication and some structural aspects of membrane junctions in a simple cell system. *J. Memb. Biol.,* **5**, 1−19.
47. Sheridan, J.D. (1971), Dye movement and low resistance junctions between reaggregated embryonic cells. *Dev. Biol.,* **26**, 627−636.
48. Simpson, I., Rose, B. and Loewenstein, W.R. (1977), Size limit of molecules permeating the junctional membrane channels. *Science,* **195**, 294−296.
49. Slack, C., and Palmer, J.F. (1969), The permeability of intercellular junctions in the early embryo of *Xenopus laevis* studied with a fluorescent tracer. *Exp. Cell Res.,* **55**, 416−419.
50. Specht, S.C. and Crafstein, B. (1973), Accumulation of radioactive protein in mouse cerebral cortex after injection of ^{3}H-fucose into the eye. *Exp. Neurol.,* **41**, 705−722.
51. Spira, M.E., Spray, D.C. and Bennett, M.V.L. (1976), Electrotonic coupling: effective sign reversal by inhibitory neurons. *Science,* **194**, 1065−1067.
52. Tsien, R.W. and Weingart, R. (1976), Inotropic effect of cyclic AMP in calf ventricular muscle studied by a cut end method. *J. Physiol.,* **260**, 117−141.
53. Tupper, J.T. and Saunders, J.W. Jr. (1972), Intercellular permeability in the early *Asterias* embryo. *Dev. Biol.,* **27**, 546−554.
54. Waxman, S.G. (1968), Micropinocytotic invaginations in the axolemma of peripheral nerves. *Z. Zellforsch.,* **86**, 571−573.
55. Weidmann, S. (1966), The diffusion of radiopotassium across intercalated disks of mammalian cardiac muscle. *J. Physiol.,* **187**, 323−342.
56. Weiss, T.F., Mulroy, M.J. and Altmann, D.W. (1974), Intracellular responses to acoustic clicks in the inner ear of the alligator lizard. *J. Acoust. Soc. Am.* **55**, 606−619.

3 Junction Formation and Experimental Modification

J . D . SHERIDAN

Acknowledgements

The author wishes to thank Ms. Sarah Lindahl for typing the manuscript. The unpublished work reported in this review was supported in part by N.I.H. grants CA 16335 and HL 06314. The author is a Career Development awardee of the N.C.I.

Intercellular Junctions and Synapses
(*Receptors and Recognition,* Series B, Volume 2)
Edited by J. Feldman, N.B. Gilula and J.D. Pitts
Published in 1978 by Chapman and Hall, 11 New Fetter Lane, London EC4P 4EE
© Chapman and Hall

3.1 INTRODUCTION

Much of the evidence concerning the structure and permeability of 'low resistance' junctions depicts them as relatively static structures. The purpose of this chapter is to show that this view may be misleading. In fact these junctions can be quite dynamic in their turnover (i.e. formation and breakdown) and possibly in their regulation by intracellular molecules. Investigation of these more dynamic aspects of 'low resistance' junctions has been spurred on by two hopes: on the one hand, that the relation between structure and permeability might be further clarified and, on the other, that clues to biological function and perhaps tools for approaching function more directly might be discovered. The first hope is gradually being realized, whereas the second remains elusive.

3.2 JUNCTION FORMATION

3.2.1 Electrical coupling

'Low resistance' junctions were first detected by their ability to couple cells electrically (Furshpan and Potter, 1958; Loewenstein and Kanno, 1964; Kuffler and Potter, 1964). It is appropriate, therefore, to begin our discussion with electrical coupling which remains the earliest detectable sign of junction formation.

The rapid development of electrical coupling between reaggregating cells was first demonstrated by Loewenstein (1967a) using dissociated sponge cells. In the prescence of calcium (and the appropriate aggregation factor), coupling appeared within minutes after cells had been manipulated into contact. Similarly, rapid development of coupling between amphibian blastomeres (Ito and Loewenstein, 1969) and cultured cells (Johnson *et al.*, 1974) has been shown directly with microelectrodes. Using an indirect approach, that infers coupling by the onset of synchronous contractions, Hirakow and DeHaan (1970) showed that cardiac myoblasts in culture become electrically coupled within a few minutes after coming into contact. Thus, from all these studies it appears that only a few minutes are required for 'low resistance' junctions to form.*

* Two recent reports (Ito *et al.*, 1974a; Bennett and Spira, 1975) that embryonic cells, uncoupled by physical separation, can recouple in seconds is apparently an artefact. The cells remain connected by fine cytoplasmic bridges whose high internal resistance isolates the cells electrically. When the cells are reapproximated, the bridges retract and coupling returns.

The conversion of the normally high resistance, non-junctional membrane into a low resistance junctional membrane in such a brief time is quite remarkable. It is even more remarkable considering the number of events which must take place within and between the membranes as the junctions are assembled (see Section 3.2.3 below).

Although coupling is detectable within a few minutes, the degree of coupling increases progressively with time, suggesting that formation involves a rather rapid initiation phase followed by a maturation or growth phase. Ito *et al.* (1974a,b) conclude from their studies on amphibian blastomeres, that the initiation phase involves the opening of a small number of low resistance junctional channels into the extracellular space and the maturation phase involves the continued accretion of junctional channels and the development of a 'perijunctional insulation,' isolating each channel from the extracellular space. Although their data can be interpreted in other ways (Sheridan, 1976), the structural implications of this idea are important. As we will see below, the early steps in formation of gap junctions provide an interesting parallel with the electrical events.

In suitable systems, the measurements of electrical coupling and input resistance provide enough data for estimating the conductance of the junctional elements as they are formed. Bennett *et al.* (1972) used four intercellular electrodes to determine junctional and non-junctional resistances for reaggregated cells from *Fundulus* blastulae. Although this method provides the optimal electrical information, only a few junctional resistance values were given, ranging from 1.3 to 8.5×10^6 Ω (or 7.7 to 1.2×10^{-7} mhos for conductance). The precise time coupling first appeared after contact was not given, but the authors comment that at least one-half hour was routinely allowed for coupling to occur.

Ito *et al.* (1974b) report that the conductance of each junctional membrane at the time when coupling is first detected is about 3.5×10^{-8} mhos. This is equivalent to about 0.35 μm^2 for each junctional membrane if the figure of 2×10^2 mhos cm^{-2} is used for specific junctional conductance (value for 'half' junction). In our Novikoff system, we can detect coupling when the junctional conductance is about 0.5×10^{-8} mhos which is equivalent to 0.005 μm^2 (unpublished data). Again, as we discuss below, these values are consistent with junctional sizes determined ultrastructurally.*

* The apparent difference in detection limit is due in part to differences in the equivalent electrical circuit used for the two estimates. Ito *et al.* (1974b) include a shunt resistance term whereas we do not. As a result, their estimated junctional conductance is higher than ours for a comparable coupling coefficient and input resistance. Thus, in their Fig. 4, at about 28 min post-contact, our model would give a junctional conductance of 1.5×10^{-8} mhos whereas they give a figure of 8.3×10^{-8} mhos. Even with this correction, however, our limit of detection appears lower.

3.2.2 Transfer of small molecules

In many systems, electrically coupled cells can also exchange a variety of small molecules besides inorganic ions. It is natural, then, to ask when this exchange first becomes possible during junctional formation. Surprisingly little attention has been given to this question. Azarnia and Loewenstein (1971) showed that some cultured cells can transfer fluorescein after being in contact for 2 hours, but no studies at earlier times were reported. Cells from *Xenopus* gastrulae and neurulae can exchange fluorescein after as little as 20 min of reaggregation (Sheridan, 1971). Reaggregated *Fundulus* blastomeres, however, fail to pass fluorescein or Procion yellow, although they become effectively electrically coupled as early as one-half hour after being placed in contact (Bennett *et al.,* 1972). Although the *Fundulus* experiments have been interpreted as evidence for a physiological restriction of junctional permeability to molecules larger than inorganic ions in early embryos, it is possible that the lack of dye transfer represents a stage in junction development or reflects a quantitative problem due to the large size of the cells (Sheridan, 1976).

We have studied the transfer of fluorescein between reaggregating Novikoff cells and have found the following: (a) coupled cells often pass fluorescein, but many do not, (b) the cells that pass fluorescein are generally better coupled than those that do not, (c) some well-coupled cells fail to pass fluorescein at early times, (d) consequently, the increase in percentage of coupled cells and in mean coupling coefficient precedes the increase in percentage of cells passing fluorescein. These results suggest that the ability to pass fluorescein in most cases is correlated with the degree of electrical coupling, and presumably with the ionic permeability (conductance) of the junctions. The well-coupled cells failing to pass fluorescein resemble those in the *Fundulus* experiment, and have two possible explanations: the cells may have qualitative differences in their junctions or may have junctions at an earlier stage in formation. Parallel ultrastructural observations (see below) suggest that in a sense both explanations are correct in part. Briefly the idea is that the immature gap junction ('formation plaque), which differs qualitatively from the 'mature form,' can electrically couple cells without permitting transfer of other small molecules. Support for this idea will be discussed later.

Another, rather elegant approach to testing junctional permeability during formation involves the use of radioactive precursors. Most of these methods test the ability of junctions to pass nucleotides, although methods for study of other metabolites have been recently devised. (Pitts discusses these methods in greater detail in his chapter). Although most cultured cells can transfer nucleotides, again little study has been made of the development of this capability. Recently, Pederson (Pederson *et al.,* 1976) in my lab has shown that the transfer of uridine nucleotides between reaggregated Novikoff hepatoma cells can be detected as early as 1 hour after the cells are plated out. He finds a progressive increase in percentage of cells receiving labeled nucleotides from donors as the reaggregation time is extended to two and four hours.

3.2.3 Structural features of gap junction formation

The earlier chapters describe the basis for our current belief that gap junctions serve as the primary if not exclusive sites for junction communication. It is then appropriate to begin this section with a brief summary of gap junction structure to establish the structural 'end-point' of the formation process.

The gap junction, or 'nexus,' has the following distinctive features: (a) there is a regular and greatly reduced extracellular space of 2.0—4.0 nm (as viewed in thin section), (b) the space separates two junctional membranes which contain complementary aggregates of 6—10 nm intramembranous particles (IMP's) (as viewed in freeze-fracture), (c) each particle in one membrane is believed to extend into the extracellular space and attach to the extension of a comparable particle from the opposing membrane (the extracellular components are viewed with negative staining).

The structure of the gap junction clearly defines the prerequisites for formation, i.e. reduction of the extracellular space, assembly of two sets of intramembranous subunits and interaction of these subunits across the extracellular space. Many mechanisms are conceivable for each of these steps and we have only recently begun to sort them out.

The first clues came from studies on embryos in which morphogenetic movements and cell rearrangements accentuate breakdown and reformation of gap junctions. These initial studies on chick (Revel *et al.*, 1973) and amphibian (Decker and Friend, 1974) embryos suggested that the newest gap junctions are quite small, consisting of loose or tight aggregates of as few as 6—10 particles. These small junctions, it was suggested, enlarge by accretion of nearby particles or insertion of new particles directly into the junctional membranes. The continued aggregation of particles moving in the plane of the membrane is a particularly attractive consequence of the fluid-mosaic organization of the membrane.

A primary difficulty with these systems, however, is the intrinsic ambiguity between junctional formation and breakdown as well as the presence of another junctional type, the tight junction, which undergoes complex changes at the same time. The developing lens appears to be a less complicated model for studying gap junction formation. Benedetti *et al.* (1974) have shown that epithelial cells in the calf lens, which are joined by typical gap junctions, begin to form extensive gap-like junctions as they elongate and differentiate into cortical fibers. Formation begins with interlacing rows of IMP's that encircle relatively particle-deficient membrane patches. Subsequently, the patches become filled with particles until large regions of membrane are covered with junctional aggregates. The authors are reluctant to use the term 'gap' junction because the particles (and corresponding E-face pits) are packed in groups, but similar arrangements have been seen in other systems (see below).

In order to avoid the problem of junctional breakdown and possible confusion with tight junction changes, yet hopefully to provide a clearer description of the stages of gap junction formation, we began a study of reaggregating Novikoff hepatoma cells. In earlier studies, we showed that these cells grow as clumps in suspension culture and are connected by gap junctions with typical structure and permeability (Johnson and Sheridan, 1971). Though epithelial in origin, these cells lack tight junctions, thus providing a simpler system than most epithelia *in vivo*.

We have obtained evidence for a sequence of inter- and intramembranous events leading to gap junctions (Johnson *et al.*, 1974). Formation begins in small regions of cell apposition, which we have termed 'formation plaques.' The plaques are a few tenths of a micron in diameter, and are characterized by a general decrease in density of IMP's less than about 9 nm in diameter and a clustering (with perhaps an increased density) of 'large' IMP's, 9–11 nm in diameter. The plaques are often 'flatter' than surrounding membrane which aids in delimiting their boundaries.

The formation plaques are apparently initiated in pairs, one in each apposed membrane. It is significant that they appear before the extracellular space (ECS) is narrowed, which suggests that they are probably connected in some way across a rather wide space. The most economical possibility is that the 'large' particles in the apposed plaques have extracellular extensions which interact in the gap. The inter- actions might have a number of consequences, perhaps even leading to development of the plaques in the first place. For example, the interaction might trigger changes in the lipids, promoting loss or exclusion of smaller intramembranous particles and/or accumulation of 'large' particles. Alternatively, by maintaining the membranes at a fixed, and perhaps slightly reduced distance, negatively charged glycoproteins might be displaced laterally due to charge repulsion, thereby producing the particle- deficient region.

Once the plaques have been formed, the extracellular space must be reduced. Again the 'large' particles might be involved: i.e. reduction of the space might result from conformational changes in the 'large' particles leading to shortening of their extracellular extensions. Occasionally, the space between formation plaques is narrowed, but we have never observed a wide space between apposed particle aggregates, suggesting that the reduction of the space can precede particle aggrega- tion. If so, the reduction of the space must be followed almost immediately by particle aggregation. This is strongly suggested by certain larger plaques that contain small aggregates, and have a breakthrough crossing both the aggregate and the rest of the plaque. Generally, the space narrows only between the apposed aggregates and widens between the adjacent plaque areas.

Such a sequence implies that the particles are unable to aggregate until the space is reduced. This would be harder to imagine if the particles were free to move independently in each formation plaque than if they had to move in pairs, one particle from each plaque, as our model contends.

Although the large particles may begin to aggregate rapidly following reduction of the ECS, the initial aggregates are generally small, incorporating only a small percentage of the large particles of the plaques. (The first aggregates we see have total areas/interface of the order of 0.001 to 0.005 μm^2 and thus are fully compatible with our estimates of junctional conductance — see Section 3.2.1 above). Frequently, two or more aggregates occur in single plaques, but it is only later that larger aggregates are seen. In some cases, these larger aggregates are composed of 'domains' of small aggregates separated by narrow, particle-free aisles. It seems possible that the domains represent smaller aggregates that became closely associated but failed to fuse. Similar arrangements are seen in many of the very large, 'mature' junctions of the undissociated cells, suggesting that the 'domains' of mature junctions also arise during formation from arrangements of many small, individual aggregates.

We have not followed the formation process beyond three hours. At that time some junctions appear completed, that is they have a very regular perimeter and only a very narrow particle-free 'halo.' Some junction formation may continue, however, since changes in permeability to tracers (see above) still occur after two hours and larger junctions are often seen between undissociated cells.

The most striking feature of our model for gap junction formation is the formation plaque. It is clear in retrospect that similar structures were seen in the earlier embryonic studies. However, it is equally clear that there were differences. In the chick (Revel *et al.,* 1973), the formation plaques nearly always contain aggregates which might reflect an acceleration of the initial steps of formation. In the amphibian (Decker and Friend, 1974), the 'formation plaques' begin with a greater deficiency of particles and there is a clearer enrichment of large particles as formation proceeds. Formation plaques are also seen when granulosa cells in the ovary are induced to form junctions (Albertini and Anderson, 1974, 1975).

3.2.4 Formation of 'tight' junctions and potential role in coupling

Because of the strong evidence for the gap junction as the site of intercellular transfer, it might seem that consideration of 'tight' junctions is out of place. However, the formation of tight junctions not only occurs in close association with gap junctions in many cases but also has some interesting similarities. In fact, the similarities are sufficiently striking to raise the possibility that developing tight junctions might provide intercytoplasmic channels and so, initially, provide electrical coupling.

The mature tight junction usually occurs as a belt-like structure connecting the apical membranes of epithelial cells (Staehelin, 1973). These junctions vary considerably in complexity, but have the following characteristic features: (a) the external laminae of the apposed membranes are fused, generally intermittently (as seen in thin section), (b) the fusions obliterate the ECS and prevent the movement of extracellular tracers, such as colloidal lanthanum, from the luminal to serosal compartments, (c) in freeze-fracture, the junction consists of a network of interlacing fibrils or ridges (on the P-face) and complementary grooves (on the E-face).

Thus, the mature tight junction differs markedly from the gap junction and, aside from involving a very close linkage between the two cell membranes, provides very little structural reason for suggesting a role in cell-to-cell transfer.

However, quite a different picture is seen when the tight junction is forming.

Montesano *et al.* (1975) have described the formation of tight junctions in fetal liver. They find that the early stages in formation occur in relatively particle-deficient regions and involve strands of regularly spaced particles that gradually assemble into interlocking networks. Coincident with the arrangement into a network, the particles appear to fuse leading to the production of the typical tight junction fibrils. Because the E-face counterpart of the early stage appears to be a network of grooves rather than rows of distinct pits, the authors make no reference to an ambiguity in distinguishing the developing tight junctions from gap junctions. However, Porvaznik (unpublished) has found similar P-face views of developing tight junctions between H4IIE hepatoma cells in culture as well as rows of corresponding pits in E-faces. In the hepatoma system, there is no means for clearly distinguishing immature tight and 'linear' gap junctions and in fact, often at intersections of the particulate strands, there are larger accumulations of P-face particles (and E-face pits) resembling gap junctions. The particles in the strands ultimately fuse to form fibrils, and only at this point do the tight junctions and 'intercalated' gap junctions become clearly distinguishable.

These studies add further support to the suggestion (Elias and Friend, 1976) that the particles going into tight and gap junctions come from a common pool. If so, the regulation of formation of the two junctions must be even more complex than previously imagined. Perhaps the intrinsic polarity of the cells and separation of compartments with different ionic composition somehow trigger the formation of tight junctions in preference to gap junctions. Since tight junctions have a prominent association with cytoplasmic microfilaments (which are apparently absent from gap junctions), it is conceivable that the arrangement of the particles in rows rather than larger aggregates depends on the action of these filaments. The subsequent fusion of the tight junction particles, however, must depend on more than just a linear arrangement. An early stage in the formation of gap-like junctions in the lens involves networks of particle strands (see above), yet these particles never fuse to form fibrils.

The unclear distinction between developing tight junctions and 'linear' gap junctions naturally raises the possibility that particles in both junctions have hydrophilic channels and can permit cell-to-cell transfer of small molecules. There have been no direct tests of this possibility, but some results are highly suggestive. For example, H4IIE cells are weakly, but rather frequently coupled electrically (unpublished observation). The high frequency of coupling is hard to explain by the low frequency of gap junctions, but might be explained if tight junctions also served as low resistance pathways.

The distinction between gap and developing tight junctions is similarly blurred by the apparent ability of linear particle strands to couple vertebrate visual receptors (Raviola and Gilula, 1973; Baylor *et al.*, 1971). Furthermore, cells in the neural plate of chick embryos are coupled (Sheridan, 1966, 1968), but apparently are joined only by short strands of particles or tight junction-like fibrils (Revel *et al.*, 1973).

3.2.5 Minimal structure required for 'coupling'

The possibility raised by the previous section is that certain intramembranous particles can form intercytoplasmic channels whether they are arranged in linear strands or in groups typical of gap junctions. An even more basic question concerns the time the particles first develop their high permeability, i.e. what is the minimal structure required for the increased membrane permeability in the junction ?

As discussed in Section 3.2.1, above, Ito *et al.* (1974b) suggest that the junctional conductance increases before the extracellular space is sealed off. In terms of the structural stages we suggest for gap junction formation, their electrical model implies that the large particles in the formation plaques have hydrophilic channels prior to their aggregation and to the reduction of the extracellular space (see Section 3.2.3). In our initial study of reaggregating Novikoff cells, we argued that single formation plaques were unlikely to couple cells since most cells had plaques by 30 min whereas only about 50–60% of the interfaces were electrically coupled (Johnson *et al.*, 1974). We concluded provisionally that particle aggregates probably mediated coupling, although we left open the possibility that two or more plaques might couple an interface. Recently, with more quantitative data, we have found that with only 5 min of aggregation in loose pellets, more than 80% of the cells tested were coupled (Hammer and Sheridan, unpublished). When coupling by way of alternate cellular pathways is taken into account (Johnson *et al.*, 1974), this figure implies that about 50% of the interfaces have low resistance 'junctions.' The percentage of coupling in these recent experiments is higher than in the earlier ones because we tested coupling using only one electrode in each cell, thereby avoiding uncoupling of weakly coupled cells. (When a third electrode was subsequently inserted into each of the current-injected cells, the percentage of coupling fell to the value seen earlier).

From freeze-fracture studies of cells reaggregated for 15 min we know that only 27% of the interfaces have particle aggregates whereas 44% have aggregates and/or aggregate-free formation plaques. Thus, coupling by way of formation plaques appears necessary to reconcile the electrophysiological and ultrastructural data.

As described in Section 3.2.3, formation plaques at early times are separated by a relatively wide space. It is thus reasonable to ask whether plaque particles with a conductance similar to that of aggregated particles could couple cells when electrically shunted by the extracellular space. Preliminary calculations based on an electrical model of this system indicate that detectable coupling could be produced by at least some of the plaques of the sizes we see (Kam and Sheridan, unpublished).

If the plaque particles have hydrophilic channels opening into the extracellular space, it occurred to us that a tracer such as Procion yellow, which can cross the junction but not the non-junctional membrane, might be able to enter the cell via the plaque particles. In a number of experiments to test this idea, however, no increased uptake of Procion yellow was seen during reaggregation. These results suggest that, if our model is correct, the plaque particles must have narrower channels than aggregated particles or the channels must be continuous across and isolated from the space. A restriction in the size of the channels seems more likely and would explain our findings that some well-coupled Novikoff cells fail to transfer fluorescein; i.e. these cells are coupled by large and multiple formation plaques impermeable to fluorescein. A similar explanation might be given for the lack of fluorescein transfer between reaggregated, well-coupled *Fundulus* cells (see Section 3.2.2 above).

Formation plaques are relatively transient structures even in our Novikoff system and are unlikely to account for a significant part of the junctional conductance of undissociated cells. There are two other systems, however, in which structures similar to formation plaques occur and might provide a physiologically important means of electrical coupling. The first system involves the association between the plasma membrane and sarcoplasmic reticulum in muscle. A number of studies with freeze-fracture have shown that the contact regions lack gap junction-like particle aggregates, but do have loosely clustered large particles in an otherwise particle-deficient membrane (e.g. Franzini-Armstrong, 1974; Henkart *et al.*, 1976). It is reasonable to suggest that a limited amount of electrical coupling might occur in these regions, acting as the elusive link in excitation-contraction coupling.

The second system involves the interaction between T-lymphocytes activated by plant lectins. These cells reputedly become electrically coupled (Hülser and Peters, 1972; Oliveira-Castro *et al.*, 1973), but the structural basis for the coupling is unclear. Recently, Lenne and Kapsenberg (1976) have described both an 'inverted' gap junction, occurring at low frequency, and a general clustering of large particles, occurring at higher frequency. The uniformity of coupling is best explained if both of the 'structures' act as low resistance junctions. These are clearly speculative ideas, but perhaps they will stimulate further work.

3.2.6 Regulation of junction formation

The sizes of individual gap junctions as well as the total junctional areas per interface vary considerably in different tissues and organisms, and at different stages in embryogenesis. The control of these variations has attracted increasing attention over the past few years.

We have approached this problem at the most basic level by attempting to define the conditions essential for formation to occur. Our results, based on studies of electrical coupling, indicate that formation of junctions between Novikoff cells is minimally affected by inhibiting protein synthesis for up to 12 hours preceding and including the reaggregation period (Epstein *et al.*, 1977). Similarly, reduction of ATP levels (with iodoacetate) to 5% of normal has little effect on formation. These results are consistent with a self-assembly of preformed junctional precursors, perhaps already present in the membrane.

We have found that formation has an unusual serum dependency: 5% calf serum gives optimal formation; 10% gives decreased formation and 2, 1, and 0.5% give progressively lower formation. Interestingly, 5% bovine serum albumin will completely replace calf serum in supporting formation as tested electrophysiologically

(Hammer, unpublished) and electron microscopically (R. Meyer, unpublished). High pH and/or lower CO_2 reduce formation markedly. Temperature is quite important: E. Kam (unpublished) has demonstrated a progressive decrease in formation as the temperature is lowered below $30°C$.

In an attempt to find more physiological agents affecting formation, we have carried out an extensive study of the effects of cyclic nucleotide derivatives. With electrophysiological techniques (Sheridan *et al.,* 1975), we have found that the time course of the development of coupling is altered transiently in opposite directions by dibutyryl cAMP (dbcAMP; 10^{-3} M) and 8Bromo-cGMP (8BrcGMP; 10^{-8} to 10^{-7}M): dbcAMP generally increases formation whereas cGMP inhibits it. The effects are maximal at 30 min of reaggregation at which time the dbcAMP-treated samples have 89% coupling, the controls have 61%, and the 8BrcGMP-treated samples only 45%. Minimal effects are seen when both agents are added together and breakdown products of the derivatives do not reproduce the effects. The effects at 15 min and 60 min are smaller, but qualitatively in the same direction. By 120 min the effects have subsided.

The effects on the percentage of coupled cells are accompanied by more complex effects on the degree of coupling. Both dbcAMP and 8BrcGMP produce increases in the mean coupling coefficient, but the increase produced by dbcAMP is generally greater. The effects of the 8BrcGMP are superficially discordant with its inhibitory effects on the percentage of coupling. However, a clue to the explanation lies in the time course of the mean coupling coefficients seen in control samples. The mean coupling coefficient is lower at 30 min than 15 min, a result attributable to an accelerated formation of new, and thus smaller, junctions during the 15–30 min reaggregation period. The relative increase in smaller junctions (and perhaps formation plaques, see Section 3.2.5, above) reduces the mean. In the 8BrcGMP sample, however, the new formation is greatly restricted during the 15–30 min period and thus, the mean coupling coefficient is less affected by new and smaller junctions. Following the same line of reasoning the increase in coupling coefficient with dbcAMP must reflect a substantial increase in the sizes of all junctions since there is also an increased rate of formation of new junctions.

These conclusions are supported by parallel ultrastructural observations (Preus, Meyer, Johnson and Sheridan, unpublished). At 30 min, the mean area of particle aggregates per interface is nearly doubled in the dbcAMP-treated material. The areas for the 8BrcGMP and control preparation are similar, but the number of control interfaces with formation plaques alone greatly exceeds that for the cGMP material (see below). If these formation plaques act as small, low resistance junctions, then the lower mean coupling coefficient in the control can be explained.

Our recent observations that up to 50% of interfaces initiate junction formation by 5 min may explain another feature of the 8BrcGMP effects. In both 15 min and 30 min material treated with 8BrcGMP, most formation plaques have aggregates. Furthermore, the percentage of all interfaces with aggregates changes very little between 15 min and 30 min. It is reasonable to suggest that many, if not most, of these formation plaques were initiated during the first 5 min or so of reaggregation, before the 8BrcGMP could exert its effect. This implies that the 8BrcGMP completely prevents new formation during the period of 5–30 min. The gradual increase in the percentage of coupling can be explained simply by assuming that the aggregates increase in size during this time, raising junctional conductance in some interfaces to detectable limits.

The Novikoff system has advantages for studying basic properties of gap junction formation. The use of reaggregating tumor cells, however, is doubly removed from normal cells *in vivo*. The use of more normal systems is clearly desirable even though these are more complex and often beset with an ambiguity between junction formation and breakdown.

A few systems show promise for studying the regulation of junction formation in a more normal context. The early amphibian larva has been used to advantage by Decker (1976) to demonstrate the effect of a hormone, thyroxine, on gap junction formation *in vivo*. The ependymoglial cells in hypophysectomized *Rana* larvae are stimulated to differentiate in response to thyroid hormone. Decker finds that a prominent feature of the differentiation is a proliferation of gap junctions. Qualitatively, 16–20 hours after treatment, extensive formation plaques develop, followed 4–8 hours later by gap junctions. There also appears to be a quantitative increase in formation plaque and gap junction areas even above the values from normal, non-hypophysectomized animals. The extent of the increase is unclear, however, since the quantitative figures do not measure areas of plaque or junction/interface, but only areas/100 μm^2 of A-face membrane containing some plaque or junction. The response to thyroxine is blocked by actinomycin-D or cycloheximide, in contrast to formation in the Novikoff system (see above). Although this could indicate a need for the synthesis of new junctional precursors, it is equally possible that synthesis of non-junctional protein, e.g. protein necessary for cell adhesion, is required for the formation to proceed.

A similar effect of inhibiting protein synthesis has been shown by Griepp and Bernfield (unpublished; see abstract, this volume). They have studied the synchronization of the beating of cardiac myoblasts in culture. Aggregates of cardiac cells are allowed to attach to monolayers of similar cells. Usually the aggregates and layers initially beat asynchronously, but become synchronized within 2–24 hours. The acquisition of synchrony, taken as a reflection of junction formation, is blocked reversibly by cycloheximide (or puromycin). This result differs from Goshima's (1971), which demonstrated that minimally trypsinized cardiac myoblasts became synchronized in the presence of puromycin. Thus, Griepp and Bernfield's observation may indicate a need for increased numbers of junctional precursors, or perhaps just for some critical non-junctional protein.

Chick embryonic epidermis provides another interesting system for studying the formation of both gap and tight junctions. Elias and Friend (1976) have recently shown that Vit A induces a marked metaplasia of this epidermis in organ culture. There is a rapid development of gap junctions, beginning as early as one day following introduction of Vit A. The gap junctions begin as small aggregates that merge into larger junctions while retaining particle-free aisles (similar to those observed in the Novikoff junctions; Section 3.2.3 above). As the cells move distally, the gap junctions regress and tight junctions expand, prompting the suggestion that common precursors are used for both junctions.

The stimulation of gap junction formation in the epidermis resembles in some ways the effects of gonadotrophin and estrogens on gap junctions between granulosa cells in the mammalian ovary (Merk *et al.*, 1972). In hypophysectomized rats, there are only small gap junctions between granulosa cells. Administration of gonadotrophin or estrogen (diethylstilbestrol) leads to proliferation of granulosa cells accompanied by formation of gap junctions. The junctions become very extensive, resembling the highly developed junctions of the normal, mature ovaries. The tremendous increase in gap junction area seen in the embryonic epidermis and the ovary would seem likely to require synthesis of new junctional precursors. However, in neither system have the effects of inhibitors of protein synthesis been tested.

It is clear that our understanding of the factors regulating the formation of gap (and tight) junctions is still fragmentary. This is likely to be a particularly fruitful area of future investigations.

3.3 EXPERIMENTAL MODULATION OF JUNCTIONAL PERMEABILITY AND STRUCTURE

3.3.1 Junctional permeability

Most workers have been impressed with the fact that damaged cells readily uncouple from undamaged neighbors. It is likely that this uncoupling serves to isolate damaged cells and to prevent the effects of damage from spreading to undamaged neighbors. Whereas this uncoupling occurs in vertebrates as well as invertebrates, the clues as to the basis of the effects have come almost exclusively from arthropods.

Insect salivary gland

Based primarily on studies of insects, Loewenstein (1967b) has proposed that uncoupling under a variety of conditions depends upon a decreased junctional permeability (i.e., increased junctional resistance) produced by an increase in Ca^{2+} concentration at the cytoplasmic side of the junction. He proposes further that intracellular Ca^{2+} normally regulates junctional permeability in a dynamic fashion. This is a provocative and far-reaching hypothesis if true, and its experimental basis deserves a detailed analysis.

Support for the 'Ca^{2+} hypothesis' has come predominantly from experiments on *Chironomus* salivary glands carried out in Loewenstein's laboratory. In the earliest experiments (Loewenstein *et al.*, 1967; Politoff *et al.*, 1969), a variety of chemical and physical treatments were used to 'uncouple' cells (the term 'uncouple' is a bit misleading for often the cells remained significantly coupled, though at a reduced level). Uncoupling was produced by treating the cells with EGTA, high pH, trypsin, hypertonic solutions, membrane perforation in the presence of extracellular Ca^{2+} (or Mg^{2+}), decreased temperature, and various metabolic inhibitors. It was suggested that these diverse treatments operated through a common mechanism: An increase in the intracellular Ca^{2+} concentration. However, uncoupling was nearly always accompanied or preceded by depolarization. As we will see, distinguishing which (if either) of these two alternatives, i.e. increased intracellular Ca^{2+} or depolarization, is primarily responsible for uncoupling has remained a major experimental question.

The next series of experiments offered in support of the Ca^{2+} hypothesis came from the work of Rose and Loewenstein (1971). They studied in some detail the effects of extracellular Li^+ on electrical coupling and fluorescein exchange in salivary glands. The rationale for these experiments was that extracellular Li^+ leads to an accumulation of intracellular Ca^{2+} in some systems (e.g. Baker *et al.*, 1971). Replacement of Na^+ by Li^+ in a Ca^{2+}, Mg^{2+}-free medium consistently produced uncoupling. The decrease in coupling ratio occurred much faster (within about 18 min) than in Ca^{2+}, Mg^{2+}-free medium with Na^+ (83—120 min) or in Ca^{2+}, Mg^{2+}-containing medium with Li^+ (70—105 min). Uncoupling was signalled first by an increase in input resistance in the cell receiving current pulses while the voltage in the second cell remained relatively constant. Then the voltage in the second cell decreased. This result implies an increase in junctional resistance provided the non-junctional resistances of the two cells remain constant or change the same way.

In Rose and Loewenstein's experiments, as in the earlier studies, uncoupling was routinely accompanied (and often preceded) by depolarization. The relation between membrane potential and coupling was further illustrated by the observation that repolarization of the non-junctional membrane could reverse uncoupling. The restoration by repolarization was immediate and uncoupling returned as soon as the repolarizing current ceased. Repolarization was effective no matter what condition produced the uncoupling, e.g. DNP poisoning, Li^+ medium, Ca^{2+}, Mg^{2+}-free Li^+- and Ca^{2+}, Mg^{2+}-free Na^+-medium. This result is even more intriguing in light of the observation by Socolar and Politoff (1971) that depolarization by passage of outward current with a microelectrode could produce uncoupling between salivary gland cells. The effects of membrane potential are far from simple, however, since depolarization with high extracellular K^+ did not produce uncoupling though it could accelerate uncoupling by other treatments. (It should be added that the effects of K^+ were only followed for 18 min, a rather brief time [uncoupling might have occurred later]).

In an accompanying paper, Oliveira-Castro and Loewenstein (1971) approached the Ca^{2+} hypothesis more directly. They perforated the membrane of one of the salivary gland cells, making a hole large enough and stable enough to allow entry of extracellular material. They then tested the coupling of the 'perforated' cell with its neighbors while exposing the gland to media of different ionic compositions. When the external medium had 5×10^{-5} M Ca^{2+} or greater (or somewhat higher concentration of Mg^{2+}, Sr^{2+}, Ba^{2+} and Mn^{2+}) the perforated cell became uncoupled from its neighbors (although the threshold of the effect was given as 5×10^{-5} Ca^{2+}, most experiments shown were done with 12×10^{-3} M Ca). The interpretation of these experiments assumed that the extracellular ions equilibrated with the inside of the perforated cell, although the degree of equilbration was not directly measured. The uncoupling could not be reversed by replacing the uncoupling medium with Ca^{2+}, Mg^{2+}-free medium, but could be reversed partially by repolarizing the membrane of the undamaged cell. This reversal occurred only in the presence of Ca^{2+}, Mg^{2+}-free medium. The effect of repolarization in these experiments, however, is puzzling (see their Fig. 13B). Although the brief test pulses in the undamaged cell produced a small potential change in the perforated cell, there was no potential change in the perforated cell when the longer, repolarizing pulse was applied to the undamaged cell. This result seems inconsistent with the fact that the repolarizing pulse produced about the same potential change (15 mV) in the undamaged cell as did the test pulse (16 mV).

The uncoupling produced by damage in medium with high concentrations of divalent cations was usually restricted to the immediate neighbors of the damaged cells. However, when the divalent cation medium was replaced by Ca^{2+}, Mg^{2+}-free medium, often other cells became uncoupled. The authors contend that this uncoupling was a general effect of the Ca^{2+}, Mg^{2+}-free medium rather than movement of the Ca from the damaged cell to its neighbors. Yet the alternative suggestion was given in explanation of earlier observation of nonlocal uncoupling by Ca^{2+} injection (Loewenstein *et al.*, 1967). Whereas more recent studies with Ca^{2+} injection into cells containing aequorin (see below) suggest that large amounts of Ca^{2+} do not move from cell to cell, there is no direct data ruling out small amounts of transfer and subsequent uncoupling non-locally.

An unexplained complication in the damage experiments is the 'transient' uncoupling that occurred immediately after the cell was perforated. Again this term is misleading since the damage, by lowering the membrane resistance of the cell, automatically lowers the coupling coefficient for pulses applied in an adjacent cell (Sheridan, 1973). The authors in fact used the term to refer to the time when the input resistance of the cell next to the damaged cell increased transiently. This 'transient' uncoupling occurred in Ca^{2+}, Mg^{2+}-free medium and thus, if it involved Ca^{2+}, the Ca^{2+} must have come from internal stores. It is not possible to be certain that the increase in input resistance in the undamaged cell was totally due to the decrease in junctional conductance. It may have had a component of increased non-junctional resistance perhaps due to transient sealing around the electrodes.

Both Rose and Loewenstein (1971) and Oliveira-Castro and Loewenstein (1971) showed that uncoupling is accompanied by loss of junctional permeability to fluorescein. Their observations were extende by Deleze and Loewenstein (1976) who demonstrated that fluorescein transfer could be blocked or slowed by Ca^{2+} injections causing a minimal decrease in electrical coupling. They contend that this simply reflects the very non-linear relationship between electrical coupling and junctional permeability when the coupling is high (coupling coefficient greater than 0.9). In this range a large decrease in junctional conductance is required to produce a small decrease in coupling coefficient. As the authors point out, however, it would be wrong to conclude from these studies that junctional permeability to different molecules is being changed selectively. Even though the coupling was not detectably affected, the movement of ions was conceivably restricted in exact proportion to the decrease in junctional permeability to fluorescein.

Again the Deleze and Loewenstein (1976) study re-emphasizes the tight correlation between membrane depolarization and electrical uncoupling: uncoupling was always accompanied by extensive depolarization and never occurred when depolarization was limited. In fact, even the slowing or blockage of fluorescein transfer was accompanied by depolarization, though less than seen with electrical uncoupling.

The most recent test of the Ca^{2+} hypothesis has been reported in an important paper by Rose and Loewenstein (1976). Using aequorin to detect changes in intra-cellular Ca^{2+} concentration, they showed that in most (but not all; see below) experimental treatments leading to electrical uncoupling, there was an associated rise in aequorin luminescence detectable visually and photometrically. Uncoupling only occurred when the size and extent of the luminescent region seemed to touch a lateral cell boundary.

Qualitatively, the results are in agreement with earlier work and support the basic Ca^{2+} hypothesis. However, there are reasons to question quantitative aspects of the studies. As clearly stated by Blinks *et al.* (1976) in a recent review, and earlier by Baker *et al.* (1971), there is no satisfactory method for quantitating the aequorin response intracellularly. Rose and Loewenstein do not show their calibration curves for luminescence vs. $[Ca^{2+}]$, but the approach they describe has a number of draw-backs: (a) No account is taken of the rather substantial inhibitory effect of physio-logical (mM) concentrations of Mg^{2+} on the Ca^{2+} aequorin reaction. (b) Injection of large volumes of Ca^{2+}/EGTA solutions (for calibration) lead to different aequorin concentrations, different Mg^{2+} concentrations, and different ionic strength in the area of the injection than with smaller injection or in regions to which the Ca^{2+} diffuses. (c) Variations in aequorin concentrations in different experiments necessitate calibration in each case, but it is not clear that this was done. (d) The preparative technique used for the aequorin does not adequately remove EDTA, thus exaggerating the discrepancy between Ca^{2+} levels produced with small and with large injected volumes and potentially altering the true cytoplasmic Ca^{2+} levels produced with given treatments, e.g. Ca^{2+} iontophore. Thus, it is essentially im-possible for the authors to determine from the luminescence what the local Ca^{2+} concentration was in the cell.

The authors also make debatable statements about the spatial resolution of their detection system. They contend that their system has a spatial resolution of 1 μm, but this is misleading. Although the luminescence shows an abrupt spatial cutoff, which can be resolved by their microscope, the Ca^{2+} concentration almost certainly falls off more gradually, producing an abrupt change in luminescence only due to the non-linear relation between Ca^{2+} concentration and light output. The quantitative problems discussed above would make the spatial relationship even more difficult to define. These problems are especially critical for determining whether or not Ca^{2+} crosses the junction.

The problem of quantitating the concentration of Ca^{2+} is important in another regard. In the Deleze and Loewenstein (1976) paper the amounts of Ca^{2+} injected by pressure were enormous, producing a calculated free Ca^{2+} concentration, assuming free diffusion, *at the junction* of $10^{-3} - 10^{-2}$ M. The authors contend that the sequestering ability of the cell, however, probably restricted the Ca^{2+} increase to the immediate region of the micropipette tip. They support this contention by citing the Rose and Loewenstein (1975) statements that a Ca^{2+} concentration of 10^{-4} M could be maintained within a 5 μm radius of the center of the cell while the concentration was less than 10^{-5} M, 50 μm away at the junctions. As we've seen, however, these statements depend on a questionable quantitation of the aequorin response. Furthermore, the situations in the experiments are not strictly comparable. In the Rose and Loewenstein data cited, the reported concentration near the micropipette was one to two orders of magnitude lower than that quoted for the calculated value *near* the junction in the Deleze and Loewenstein paper. Presumably the value near the micropipette in the Deleze and Loewenstein experiments was considerably higher, perhaps another order of magnitude. Thus there may be a real discrepancy between the Deleze and Loewenstein experiments and the Rose and Loewenstein experiments, which remains to be satisfactorily resolved.

Depolarization was again found by Rose and Loewenstein (1976) to accompany uncoupling in most cases. An attempt was made (though the number of experiments was not given) to dissociate depolarization and uncoupling by 'voltage clamping' the cell into which Ca^{2+} had been injected. The 'clamp' was 'loose' so that superimposed current pulses produced some voltage change in both cells. In the experiment shown there was a small uncoupling (a change in coupling coefficients from 0.95 to 0.64) accompanied by a small depolarization. This experiment was submitted as evidence against a primary role of depolarization in uncoupling. However, in a similar experiment carried out by Oliveira-Castro and Loewenstein (1971; cf. their Fig. 4), the membrane potential was maintained by inward current and the transient uncoupling was blocked. This discrepancy is important, but received no comment.

Depolarization by extracellular K^+ was repeated in these experiments (as in Rose and Loewenstein, 1971) and again no uncoupling was seen in the absence of increased intracellular Ca^{2+}. In these experiments, however, there was not as great a depolarization as seen in many of the uncoupling situations and in the earlier K^+ experiments.

Significantly, Rose and Loewenstein (1976) reported that Ca^{2+} transients were not detectable with all conditions leading to uncoupling. Li^+ treatment in Ca^{2+}, Mg^{2+}-free solutions gave no aequorin response in 8/9 experiments (or even in experiments in which mitochondrial reuptake of Ca^{2+} and Mg^{2+} was presumably blocked by drugs). Similarly, in 3/4 experiments in Ca^{2+}-free, Na^+ medium, and 2/2 experiments in medium with propionate replacing Cl, uncoupling was unaccompanied by an aequorin response. Though not stated explicitly in all cases, depolarization presumably occurred. These are important experiments that cannot be lightly dismissed. Either the aequorin technique is insufficiently sensitive or Ca^{2+} increases are not necessary for uncoupling. No matter which interpretation is correct, without further study these results are important challenges to the Ca^{2+} hypothesis.

Thus, taken as a whole, the experiments on insect salivary gland provide support for the Ca^{2+} hypothesis, but a secondary or even primary role of membrane depolarization has not been ruled out.

Other systems

Evidence for a role of intracellular Ca^{2+} in regulating junctional permeability in other systems is quite sparse. The crayfish septal synapse is quite labile and is readily uncoupled by lowered temperature, EDTA treatment, and replacement of Cl by propionate (Payton *et al.*, 1969; Asada and Bennett, 1971). Aside from the similarity between the effects of these treatments in the synapse and salivary gland, there is no evidence for an involvement of intracellular Ca^{2+} in uncoupling at the synapse.

The evidence for Ca^{2+}-induced uncoupling of vertebrate cells is even less clear. Gilula and Epstein (1976) have shown that the Ca^{2+} ionophore readily uncouples cultured insect cells, but has little effect on cultured mammalian fibroblasts or heart muscle cells. The lack of effect on the mammalian cells, especially heart cells, contrasts with De Mello's (1975) report that Ca^{2+} injection into cardiac cells uncouples them. It is interesting that decreased temperature, which lowers the coupling between insect salivary gland cells and crayfish axon segments, has no effect on the longitudinal resistance (which includes junctional resistance) of cardiac Purkinje fibers (see Payton *et al.*, 1969) other than that attributable to a decrease in diffusion constant. Many of the other techniques shown to uncouple arthropod junctions, e.g. Ca^{2+} ionophore, metabolic poisons, hypertonicity, depolarization, do not noticeably alter coupling between cultured Novikoff hepatoma cells (Epstein and Sheridan, unpublished).

Uncoupling of mammalian cells *in situ* can be produced by hypertonicity in some cases (Barr *et al.*, 1965, 1968). It appears likely that this uncoupling results from separation of the cells at the junctions, possibly an 'unzippering' of the apposed sets of particles (see below).

Thus, there is insufficient data to justify extrapolating from the insect studies to vertebrate (or even other non-arthropod) junctions. It is even possible that arthropod junctions are unusually labile, reflecting perhaps their unusual structure and fracturing characterisitics (Satir and Gilula, 1973).

3.3.2 Junctional structure

The gap junction is quite stable and more resistant to many agents, e.g. trypsin, detergents, and EDTA, than tight junctions, desmosomes, or non-junctional membrane (Bennedetti and Emmelot, 1967; Goodenough and Revel, 1970). The resistance to enzymes and detergents in fact forms the basis for the purification of gap junctions (Goodenough and Stoekenius, 1972; Goodenough, 1974). There are, however, some treatments that in some systems have been shown to alter the gap junction directly. In two important papers in the 60's, Barr and colleagues showed that hypertonic solutions ruptured 'nexuses' between cardiac (Barr *et al.,* 1965) and smooth muscle (Barr *et al.,* 1968) cells, leading to loss of electrical coupling.

Hypertonic solutions also rupture gap junctions between liver cells *in situ* (Goodenough and Gilula, 1974) although associated electrophysiological changes have not been tested. The junctions apparently separate down the middle of the extracellular 'gap,' with a set of aggregated junctional particles remaining with each half junctional membrane. It is possible that a similar 'unzippering' of gap junctions occurs when the crayfish synapse is experimentally uncoupled and the cells separate (Pappas *et al.,* 1971). When the junctions unzipper, they must rapidly increase their resistance or there would be a massive loss of ions and other small molecules to the exterior.

Cells can separate and lose their coupling in other ways. For example, as shown first by Muir (1967) for EDTA-treated cardiac muscle, the gap junction can remain with one cell after being torn out of the membrane of the other; in the presence of normal Ca^{2+} the hole seals, restoring the disrupted membrane.

Unzippering or tearing away of junctions are drastic processes. Recently Perrachia and Dulhunty (1976) have reported more subtle alterations in gap junctions correlating with decreased coupling and increased junctional resistance. After EDTA-treatment followed by return to normal and Ca^{2+}-containing salt solution, crayfish septal synapses have greatly reduced coupling (Asada and Bennett, 1971). In some cases the loss of coupling is irreversible, and the cells have been shown to be totally separated (Pappas *et al.,* 1971). In other cases the effects are reversible. Studying such reversible uncoupling, Peracchia and Dulhunty show that the gap junctions have the following changes: (a) decreased extracellular space; (b) decreased particle diameter; (c) decreased center-to-center spacing and increased regularity of packing of particles. Similar changes are seen with DNP-induced decrease in coupling. (The authors suggest that the junctional particles shrink in size at the expense of the intercytoplasmic channels, thus leading to increased junctional resistance.) Although data for only the septal synapses are given, similar findings were seen in rat gastric mucosa treated with DNP or made anoxic (Peracchia and Dulhunty, 1974). The vertebrate data may bear no relationship to uncoupling *per se,* however, there are no physiological data on the effects of DNP or anoxia on coupling in mammalian tissues *in situ.* Furthermore, Goodenough and Gilula (1974) reported no changes in lattice spacing or particle sizes in 'unzipped' gap junctions in liver (see above).

The elegant studies fail to provide one key link in the correlation between the structural changes and the loss of coupling. There is no information given on the total area of gap junction/system remaining after uncoupling. A loss of 95% of the junctional area (necessary to explain a x 20 increase in junctional resistance) should have been very obvious, but a smaller decrease in area might have been missed without careful quantitation. It is surprising in fact that the authors saw no cases where irreversible uncoupling occurred with an obvious separation of pre- and post-synaptic cells as seen by Pappas *et al.* (1971).

These reservations prompt a general comment that ties together studies of formation and junctional modification. Theoretically, junctional permeability can be decreased by decreasing the channel size or decreasing the number of channels (i.e. junctional area). If two attached cells are rapidly turning over their junctions, then any effect on coupling could simply be due to an effect on formation without an effect on breakdown. Nearly all the effects on coupling described in Sections 3.1.4 and 3.2 could be explained by a decreased rate of formation. In the absence of quantitative data on junctional area, this alternative explanation must be kept in mind.

3.4 CONCLUSIONS

Our understanding of the processes of gap junction formation and modification by experimental manipulations is still quite rudimentary. We can make general statements about the structural and permeability changes accompanying formation but we have little concrete information about the molecular mechanisms or about regulation. We can reduce junctional permeability in some systems, but the effects are not specific and even if the Ca^{2+} hypothesis proves true, the mechanisms are unclear. Lack of a specific method for altering junction formation or permeability is the most serious obstacle to an understanding of the physiological function of these interesting and ubiquitous structures. Finding such a method is an important goal for future research, and may, we hope, be achieved as we learn more about junction formation and dynamics.

REFERENCES

Albertini, D.F. and Anderson, E. (1974), *J. Cell Biol.*, **63**, 234–250.
Albertini, D.F. and Anderson, E. (1975), *Anat. Rec.*, **181**, 171–194.
Asada, Y. and Bennett, M.V.L. (1971), *J. Cell Biol.*, **49**, 159–172.
Azarnia, R. and Loewenstein, W.R. (1971), *J. Memb. Biol.*, **6**, 368–385.
Baker, P.F., Hodgkin, A.L. and Ridgeway, E.B. (1971), *J. Physiol.*, **218**, 709–755.
Barr, L., Berger, W. and Dewey, M. (1965), *J. gen. Physiol.*, **48**, 797–823.
Barr, L., Berger, W. and Dewey, M. (1968), *J. gen. Physiol.*, **51**, 347–368.

Baylor, D.A., Fuortes, M.G.F. and O'Bryan, P.M. (1971), *J. Physiol.*, **214**, 265–294.
Benedetti, E.L., Dunia, I. and Bloemendal, H. (1974), *Proc. natn. Acad. Sci. U.S.A.*, **71**, 5073–5077.
Benedetti, E.L. and Emmelot, P. (1967), *J. Cell Sci.*, **2**, 499–512.
Bennett, M.V.L. and Spira, M.E. (1975), *J. Cell Biol.*, **67**, 27a.
Bennett, M.V.L., Spira, M.E. and Pappas, G.D. (1972), *Dev. Biol.*, **29**, 419–435.
Blinks, J.R., Prendergast, F.G. and Allen, D.G. (1976), *Pharm. Rev.*, **28**, 1–93.
Decker, R.S. (1976), *J. Cell Biol.*, **69**, 669–685.
Decker, R. and Friend, D. (1974), *J. Cell Biol.*, **62**, 32–47.
Deleze, J. and Loewenstein, W.R. (1976), *J. Memb. Biol.*, **28**, 71–86.
DeMello, W.C. (1975), *J. Physiol.*, **250**, 231–245.
Elias, P.M. and Friend, D.S. (1976), *J. Cell Biol.*, **68**, 173–188.
Epstein, M.L., Sheridan, J.D. and Johnson, R.G. (1977), *Exp. Cell Res.*, **104**, 25–30.
Franzini-Armstrong, C. (1974), *J. Cell Biol.*, **61**, 501–513.
Furshpan, E.J. and Potter, D.D. (1958), *J. Physiol.*, **145**, 289–325.
Gilula, N.B. and Epstein, M.L. (1976), *Symp. Expt. Biol.*, **30**, 257–272.
Goodenough, D.A. (1974), *J. Cell Biol.*, **61**, 557–563.
Goodenough, D.A. and Gilula, N.B. (1974), *J. Cell Biol.*, **61**, 575–590.
Goodenough, D.A. and Revel, J.P. (1970), *J. Cell Biol.*, **45**, 272–290.
Goodenough, D.A. and Stoeckenius, W. (1972), *J. Cell Biol.*, **54**, 646–656.
Goshima, K. (1971), *Exp. Cell Res.*, **65**, 161–169.
Henkart, M., Landis, D.M.D. and Reese, T.S. (1976), *J. Cell Biol.*, **70**, 338–347.
Hirakow, R. and DeHaan, R.L. (1970), *J. Cell Biol.*, **47**, 88a.
Hülser, D.F. and Peters, J.H. (1972), *Exp. Cell Res.*, **74**, 319–326.
Ito, S., Sato, E. and Loewenstein, W.R. (1974a), *J. Memb. Biol.*, **19**, 305–338.
Ito, S., Sato, E. and Loewenstein, W.R. (1974b), *J. Memb. Biol.*, **19**, 339–355.
Ito, S. and Loewenstein, W.R. (1969), *Dev. Biol.*, **19**, 228–243.
Johnson, R.G. and Sheridan, J.D. (1971), *Science*, **174**, 717–719.
Johnson, R., Hammer, M., Sheridan, J. and Revel, J.P. (1974), *Proc. natn. Acad. Sci. U.S.A.*, **71**, 4536–4540.
Kuffler, S.W. and Potter, D.D. (1964), *J. Neurophysiol.*, **27**, 290–320.
Lenne, W. and Kapsenberg, M.L. (1976), *J. Cell Biol.*, **70**, 345a.
Loewenstein, W.R. (1967a), *Dev. Biol.*, **15**, 503–520.
Loewenstein, W.R. (1967b), *J. Colloid. Sci.*, **25**, 34–46.
Loewenstein, W.R. and Kanno, Y. (1964), *J. Cell Biol.*, **22**, 565–586.
Loewenstein, W.R., Nakas, M. and Socolar, S.J. (1967), *J. gen. Physiol.*, **50**, 1865–1891.
Merk, F.B., Botticelli, C.R. and Albright, J.T. (1972), *Endocrinol.*, **90**, 992–1007.
Montesano, R., Friend, D.S., Perrelet, A. and Orci, L. (1975), *J. Cell Biol.*, **67**, 310–319.
Muir, A.R. (1967), *J. Anat.*, **101**, 239–261.
Oliveira-Castro, G.M.D., Barcinski, M.A. and Cukierman, S. (1973), *J. Immunol.*, **111**, 1616–1619.
Oliveira-Castro, G.M.D. and Loewenstein, W.R. (1971), *J. Memb. Biol.*, **5**, 51–77.
Pappas, G.D., Asada, Y. and Bennett, M.V.L. (1971), *J. Cell Biol.*, **49**, 173–188.

Payton, B.W., Bennett, M.V.L. and Pappas, G.D. (1969), *Science*, **165**, 594−597.
Pederson, D.C., Sheridan, J.D. and Johnson, R.G. (1976), *J. Cell Biol.*, **70**, 338a.
Peracchia, C. and Dulhunty, A.F. (1974), *J. Cell Biol.*, **63**, 263a.
Peracchia, C. and Dulhunty, A.F. (1976), *J. Cell Biol.*, **70**, 419−439.
Politoff, A.L., Socolar, S.J. and Loewenstein, W.R. (1969), *J. gen. Physiol.*,
    53, 498−515.
Raviola, E. and Gilula, N.B. (1973), *Proc. natn. Acad. Sci. U.S.A.*, **70**, 1677−1681.
Revel, J.P., Yip, P. and Chang, L.L. (1973), *Dev. Biol.*, **35**, 302−317.
Rose, B. and Loewenstein, W.R. (1971), *J. Memb. Biol.*, **5**, 20−50.
Rose, B. and Loewenstein, W.R. (1975), *Science*, **190**, 1204−1206.
Rose, B. and Loewenstein, W.R. (1976), *J. Memb. Biol.*, **28**, 87−119.
Satir, P. and Gilula, N.B. (1973), *Ann. Rev. Entomol.*, **18**, 143−166.
Sheridan, J.D. (1966), *J. Cell Biol.*, **31**, c1−c5.
Sheridan, J.D. (1968), *J. Cell Biol.*, **37**, 650−659.
Sheridan, J.D. (1971), *Dev. Biol.*, **26**, 627−636.
Sheridan, J.D. (1973), *Am. Zool.*, **13**, 1119−1128.
Sheridan, J.D. (1976), *The Cell Surface in Animal Embryogenesis and Development*,
    (Poste, G. and Nicholson, G.L., eds.), Elsevier North-Holland, New York.
Sheridan, J.D., Hammer, M.G. and Johnson, R.G. (1975), *J. Cell Biol.*, **67**, 395a.
Socolar, S.J. and Politoff, A.L. (1971), *Science*, **172**, 492−494.
Staehlin, A. (1973), *J. Cell Sci.*, **13**, 763−786.

4 Junctional Communication and Cellular Growth Control

J. D. PITTS

Acknowledgement
This work was supported by research grants from the Cancer Research Campaign.

Intercellular Junctions and Synapses
(*Receptors and Recognition,* Series B, Volume 2)
Edited by J. Feldman, N.B. Gilula and J.D. Pitts
Published in 1978 by Chapman and Hall, 11 New Fetter Lane, London EC4P 4EE
© Chapman and Hall

INTRODUCTION

Many types of animal cells, both *in vivo* and in culture, form intercellular junctions which are freely permeable to small ions and molecules but which are impermeable to macromolecules. The permeability of these junctions has been characterized by both biochemical and electrophysiological methods and the results from the two approaches are in good agreement.

As a consequence of junctional communication, all the cells in a coupled population (i.e. a tissue or a culture of communicating cells) share their small ions and metabolites and thus mixtures of cells with different metabolic capacities (i.e. different enzyme activities due to different genotypes or differences in gene expression) become phenotypically indistinguishable. However, the identities of the individual cells in such coupled populations are maintained by their macromolecules which remain in the cells where they were synthesised (or their daughters). The genotypes of coupled cells are therefore unchanged and the characteristic phenotypes of the cells reappear immediately the cells are separated (Pitts, 1971).

It is generally believed that the physical basis of the permeable junction is the gap junction seen by electron microscopy (see Chapter 1). The structure of the gap junction, determined by electron microscopy and by chemical and physical analysis of isolated junction preparations, is consistent with the observations on its permeability. The junctions are composed of subunits and each subunit appears to contain an aqueous channel which directly connects the cytoplasms of coupled cells. The diameter of the channel has been estimated to be between 10 and 20 Å Goodenough, 1975; Simpson *et al.* 1977; Gilula, Chapter 1) but because the chemical nature and conformation of the groups which presumably line the channel are unknown, it is impossible to predict which water-soluble molecules will pass through the channels and which will be excluded. However, such a transfer mechanism, depending on passive diffusion through narrow channels, offers a simple explanation for the observation that the only specificity of junctional transfer lies in the physical size of the transferred ions and molecules.

Despite the recent advances is understanding the structure and permeability of intercellular junctions, very little is known about their functions.

Partly because they were discovered by electrophysiologists, the terms electronic junction and electrical synapse have frequently been used and they have often been referred to simply as sites of electrotonic coupling. In some excitable tissues, such as heart, there seems little doubt that these permeable junctions do indeed provide intercellular pathways for the propagation of electrical impulses (DeHaan and Sachs, 1972). However, these junctions occur widely in non-excitable tissues (where they are often larger and more numerous than those found in the nervous tissues) and now that they have been shown to be permeable to intermediate metabolites and small control molecules as well as to current-carrying ions, it seems likely that their functions may be more varied than was first expected.

Several authors have speculated on the possible functions of junctional communication (Pitts, 1972; 1977; Sheridan, 1974; 1976; Loewenstein, 1973; 1975; Pitts and Finbow, 1977). Junctions could, for example, provide a communication system for the co-ordination of cell proliferation and cell activity during embryogenesis and in adult tissues (Pitts, 1971; 1976; Loewenstein, 1973). They could allow co-ordination and amplification in target tissues of hormonal responses mediated by second messengers (Pitts, 1972; Sheridan, 1974). They could be required for embryonic induction (Saxen *et al.*, 1976; Pitts, 1977). During embryogenesis they could provide the pathways by which gradients of positional information are established (see Chapter 5).

This chapter will review the work that implicates junctional communication in cellular growth control. The first and largest part of the chapter will examine the different approaches which have been used in attempts to elucidate the role of junctions in the control of cell proliferation and cell activity. As most of this work has been done in tissue culture, the last part of the chapter will discuss the relation of the findings in cultured cells to growth control *in vivo*.

The approaches which have been used to examine the functions of junctional communication can be conveniently divided into direct and indirect approaches. The direct approaches include attempts to find drugs which specifically inhibit junctional communication and attempts to select mutant cells which are defective in junctions formation. The indirect approaches include defining junctional permeability, establishing the patterns of communication specificity and analysing model systems.

4.1 INHIBITORS OF JUNCTIONAL COMMUNICATION

Several authors have reported attempts to find specific inhibitors of junctional communication but so far no one has achieved undisputed success.

There is no doubt that there are a number of treatments (e.g. treatment with EDTA) which will break junctional communication between cells, but cell detachment and separation also occur and it is difficult to distinguish breakdown consequent on these processes from specific inhibition. It is perhaps worth noting at this point that cell death (loss of ability to proliferate) does not in itself inhibit junction formation or cause junction breakdown. X-irradiated and mitomycin C-treated cells (often used as feeder layers for the culture of primary cells) form junctions as well as do untreated cells (Simms and Pitts, unpublished observations).

Cytochalasin B has been shown by Cox *et al.* (1974) to inhibit junction-mediated nucleotide transfer between human and hamster fibroblasts in culture. However, the concentration of the drug which was used ($10 \mu g\ ml^{-1}$) disturbed cell morphology and caused some retraction of cell processes so it is difficult to decide how specific the inhibition is.

Stoker (1975) discovered this effect independently and showed that the drug inhibits junction formation between hamster and mouse fibroblasts in culture at much lower concentrations (1.0 μg ml^{-1}). However, this concentration only partially affects preformed junctions (Cox *et al.* added the drug to cells which were already coupled by junctions) and otherwise is reported to affect only glucose uptake and cell locomotion (Brownstein *et al.*, 1975). It is thought (Stoker, 1975) to have no effect (determined by light microscopy) on the extent of contact between cells; it acts rapidly and the inhibition of formation is reversible so he suggests it should be a useful tool for the investigation of intercellular communication but, as yet, there are no reports of functional studies using this drug.

Ito *et al.* (1974) found that cytochalasin B (1 μM) had no significant effect on electrical coupling between newt embryo cells. At this concentration, the drug blocked the movement of cellular processes and cytokinesis (but not nuclear division) and made it difficult to achieve successful electrode penetrations, but in experiments with imposed intercellular contact (by micromanipulation) coupling was established, though coupling onset took longer than in the absence of the drug.

Unpublished work in this laboratory (part of a screening programme to find specific junction inhibitors which has so far proved unsuccessful) has shown that cytochalasin B (1.0 μg ml^{-1}) has no detectable effect on nucleotide transfer between hamster fibroblasts in culture, when the drug is added after junctions have been allowed to form. Addition of the drug before the cells are mixed (i.e. before junctions are formed) prevents junction formation and also prevents normal cell spreading. The inhibition of junction formation may therefore be a secondary event under these conditions. At higher concentrations, the drug causes gross morphological changes.

In any analysis of junctional function using junctional inhibitors, the inhibition must be specific or it will be impossible to distinguish changes in cell behaviour caused by loss of junctional communication from changes resulting from other effects of the inhibitor. From our observations, we therefore decided that cytochalasin B is not a suitable drug.

Loewenstein (1975) has made an extensive examination of the role of Ca^{2+} ions in the formation, maintainance and permeability of intercellular junctions. High intracellular levels of Ca^{2+} block junctional communication and more recent work (Rose *et al.*, 1977) shows that varying levels of intracellular Ca^{2+} modulates the effective diameter of the junctional channels from fully open to fully closed, allowing progressively smaller molecules to pass through as the Ca^{2+} concentration is increased. If this proves to be correct it will have important implications which will have to be taken into account when considering the functions of junctional communication. However, these sophisticated experiments have only been carried out in the one system (the *Chironomus* salivary gland) and it remains to be seen how general the conclusions will prove to be. Sheridan discusses the techniques and some of the difficulties in interpreting the results in Chapter 3.

The experimental manipulations which are necessary to alter the intracellular Ca^{2+} concentration in a defined way are complex and it is possible that disturbing the ion content of the cell, even transiently (Ca^{2+} is rapidly sequestered in the cell), will have other consequences which affect cell behaviour, so at the moment this form of inhibition seems an unlikely tool for studying function.

Another approach to the specific inhibition of junctional communication involves the preparation of antibodies to gap junctional proteins. As yet, despite attempts in several laboratories, there is no published account of such an antibody preparation. The failure to obtain an antiserum could be due to the incorrect methods of antigen preparation or presentation or to the similarity between (vertebrate) species of the junctional subunits (or at least the sites which are involved in cell—cell recognition and junction formation, e.g. human, chick and toad cells can form junctions as well between species as they can within species, Pitts *et al.,* 1977). This could cause tolerance in, for example, rabbits of at least the functionally important sites of mouse junctional proteins.

Another problem may arise from the conformational changes which presumably take place when a junctional subunit precursor becomes incorporated into a junction and forms an intercellular channel. It seems likely that the precursor will have hydrophilic groups on the outside surface of the cell and that the channel, when formed, is leak-proof (i.e. does not allow movement of ions and molecules from inside the channel to the extracellular spaces and vice versa) because of the continuity of hydrophobic groups between the coupled cells. The antigenic sites on the mature junction in isolated preparations (which are used to raise antisera) may not be available to antibodies in the medium surrounding coupled cells and perhaps the most interesting sites from a functional standpoint, the surface recognition sites which initiate junction formation, may be masked or lost during junction assembly.

4.2 CELL MUTANTS DEFICIENT IN JUNCTIONAL COMMUNICATION

The ready availability of tissue culture systems for studying intercellular communication through junctions offers the attractive possibility of genetic analysis, The discovery of 'metabolic co-operation' (Subak-Sharpe *et al.,* 1966; 1969) provided a ready made selection system for the isolation of mutants defective in junction formation. The analysis of the behaviour and properties of one-step mutants and their revertants might throw considerable light on the functions of junctional communication.

There are several possible variations of the selection procedure which we first used some years ago and subsequently these have been tried in other laboratories. However, to date, all these attempts have proved surprisingly unsuccessful.

Our selection procedure used mutant hamster fibroblasts lacking the enzyme hypoxanthine: guanine phosphoribosyl transferase (E.C. 2.4.2.8.; HGPRTase).

These cells are unable to convert hypoxanthine to inosine $5'$-monophosphate (IMP) and are resistant to the toxic hypoxanthine analogue, thioguanine. If a 1:1 mixture of HGPRTase-deficient and wild-type cells is cultured in the presence of thioguanine (50 μg ml^{-1}) all the cells in the mixture are killed if (and only if) junctions are formed between the two cell types. The wild-type cells convert the thioguanine to its nucleotide which they further incorporate and as a consequence are killed. The nucleotides, which pass freely through the intercellular junctions, enter the coupled HGPRTase-deficient cells and kill them too. The only survivors should be HGPRTase-deficient cells which are also deficient in junction formation. The survival rate is between 1 in 10^6 and 1 in 10^8, but in our hands all surviving clones formed junctions as effectively as the original cells. It is difficult to understand why the procedure has not been successful. Perhaps the junction-forming phenotype is very stable (e.g. multiple alleles) or perhaps the mutation is lethal. However, both these suggestions are hard to reconcile with the fact that cell lines are known (e.g. the mouse L line, Pitts, 1971) which appear to be genetically incapable of forming junctions (McCargow and Pitts, 1971; Pitts, 1972) yet which grow and divide as well as junction-forming cell lines.

There is one report (Wright *et al.*, 1976a) of a modified cell type (mec$^-$, derived from a polyoma virus-transformed hamster fibroblast) which has been obtained with a selection procedure based on an analogous rationale but using a cell line deficient in thymidine kinase (E.C. 2.7.1.21; TKase) and hence resistant to the thymidine analogue 5-bromodeoxyuridine (BUdR). The initial results suggested an incomplete loss of junction-forming ability (Goldfarb *et al.*, 1975). Pyrimidine nucleotides appeared not to pass through the intercellular junctions formed by the mec$^-$ cells (explaining their survival in the selection procedure) but purine nucleotides did pass through. One explanation put forward by Goldfarb *et al.* (1975) was that the permeability mechanism has some form of specificity built into it. However, this seems unlikely for a number of reasons. The analysis of junctional proteins suggests that there are very few (only one or two, see Chapter 1) different components (based on SDS gel analysis) and it is difficult to think of a wide variety of 'permeases' all of indistinguishable size. Also, the free intercellular movement of all the small synthetic probes used to analyse junctional permeability (Loewenstein, 1975) must mean that the 'permeases', while distinguishing pyrimidine and purine nucleotides, accept the various fluorescent dyes (such as fluorescein and Procion yellow) and other probes as analogues of naturally occuring cell components.

Further analysis (Wright *et al.*, 1976b) of the mec$^-$ cells showed that the data were also consistent with the alternative explanation that they have a generally reduced level of intercellular communication and that the differences in transfer rates between the two types of nucleotides are only apparent differences caused by differences in the nucleotide pool sizes. Whether the reduced rate of transfer might be due to a reduced number of channels (caused by decreased formation, increased breakdown or a reduced number of junctional subunit precursors) or to a general reduction in the permeability of all the channels, is not yet clear. Further work on mec⁻ cells might provide important insights into the mechanisms and functions of junctional communication but, to date, the complexity of the system has precluded any simple correlation of changes in communication ability with changes in other cell properties.

There are known cell lines which do not form junctions (Pitts, 1971; Finbow and Pitts, 1977). However, these are so unrelated to other cell types which do form junctions that any comparison of other properties (such as topoinhibition, contact inhibition of cell movement, tumour formation etc) would say nothing about their relation to junctional communication.

However, these cell types which cannot form junctions can be fused with junction-forming cells to form hybrids (McCargow and Pitts, 1971; Pitts, 1972; Azarnia et al., 1974; Azarnia and Loewenstein, 1977). Such hybrids contain both sets of chromosomes and form junctions. When a hybrid is formed from a junction-deficient mouse cell (e.g. L cell) and a junction-competent human cell, it will lose human chromosomes during subsequent culture (see Ruddle, 1973). Segregants will therefore arise which have lost the human genes necessary for junction formation and in principle, it is possible to analyse such segregation to determine which other cell properties segregate concordantly and which segregate separately. Unfortunately, the rate of chromosome loss is such that it is difficult to analyse the segregants without further chromosomal loss occuring during analysis.

Loewenstein and his co-workers (Azarnia and Loewenstein, 1977; Larsen et al., 1977) have attempted an analysis of this type and have shown concordant segregation of ability to form junctions, normal growth in culture and failure to grow in soft agar or as tumours *in vivo*. However, between the hybrid which has the dominant human properties of junction formation and growth control and the segregants which have lost all these human properties, there is a reduction in human genetic content of at least 16 human chromosomes and possibly as many as 27. Clearly this does not prove a closely linked relation between junction formation and growth properties, although more than 20 different segregants have been examined and in none of these have the properties segregated separately.

Further analysis of this system might provide the information that Loewenstein set out to obtain (i.e. the loss of ability to form junctions causes loss of growth control in the systems he examined). Relatively stable cell clones containing one or a very few human chromosomes (or even only a part of a human chromosome; Boone et al., 1972) may be produced after prolonged culture of the original hybrid population. Concordant segregation even in these cells does not prove that the phenotypes are the products of the same gene (unless only a single human gene remains), but separation by segregation does show that they are products of different genes.

4.3 JUNCTIONAL PERMEABILITY

Various electrophysiological and biochemical methods have been used to establish the permeability properties of junctions. Some of these are described in Chapter 2 and others have been reviewed elsewhere (Loewenstein, 1975; Pitts and Finbow, 1977). The different approaches have different advantages.

Electrophysiological methods (Loewenstein, 1966; Furshpan and Potter, 1968) have been used in a wide variety of cell and tissue systems. However, the quantitative interpretation, and on occasion the qualitative interpretation, of this kind of data can be difficult when the cells do not have simple and clearly defined spatial relationships. Some of the problems have been outlined by Sheridan (1976) and the particular problems of measuring electrical coupling in early amphibian embryos have been analysed in detail by de Laat *et al.* (1976).

The modification of the electrophysiological methods to allow injection, either by iontophoresis or by pressure, of fluorescent or labelled compounds into specific cells has made a major contribution to our knowledge of junctional permeability. This approach, coupled with the chemical synthesis of a series of fluorescent peptide probes has allowed Simpson *et al.* (1977) to estimate the size limit above which the probes are unable to pass through the junctional channels. This turns out to be somewhat different for different types of molecules (Loewenstein, personal communication) when estimated in terms of molecular weight. However, this probably underlines the rather obvious fact that molecular weight is not the correct criterion to use when defining permeability limits. Instead, molecular size (of the solvated molecule) should be used, but as this is generally not known it is expedient to use molecular weight.

The quite different biochemical approaches which have been developed concurrently give a similar picture of permeability (Bürk *et al.*, 1968; Subak-Sharpe *et al.*, 1969; Cox *et al.*, 1970; Pitts, 1971; 1976; Pitts and Simms, 1977; Pitts and Finbow, 1977; Finbow and Pitts, 1977). These methods have the advantage that they are based on observations made with large numbers of cells (rather than on the results of injecting a few particular cells) and they follow the movement (or lack or movement) of naturally occuring cellular molecules rather than of synthetic probes. A range of different molecular types has been examined and it has been shown that all the small cell components (molecular weight less than 1000) pass freely through the junctions while all macromolecules (and membrane components, presumably because they do not occur in free solution in the cytoplasm) do not pass through.

These are general conclusions and it is possible that other mechanisms exist for the intercellular transfer of small amounts of particular macromolecules which are not detected by the methods so far developed. However, these other mechanisms, if they exist, must be very inefficient as their rate of transfer must be 10^3 to 10^4 times slower (in terms of mass, not molecules, per unit time) than that of junction-mediated transfer for small molecules.

These biochemical methods allow a number of other properties of junctional communication to be described. The rate of movement of nucleotides (and presumably all other small molecules are moving at the same time at a similar rate) between cells is about 10^6 nucleotides per second per cell pair (Pitts, 1976). This is a huge traffic which allows very rapid equilibration of small molecules through complete cell populations. Detectable and measureable concentration gradients are formed between small number of cells only minutes after contacts are established and gradients spreading over distances of a millimetre are established in only hours (Pitts, 1976 and unpublished; Michalke, 1977). More work is required on these systems to determine rates of movement and diffusion coefficients of molecules moving through cell sheets so that the values can be compared with estimates made by Crick (1970), Wolpert (Chapter 5) and others of the required rates of movement of developmentally important signalling substances.

This knowledge of junctional permeability has already allowed a number of predictions to be made about the consequences of junctional communication (Pitts and Finbow, 1977). These predictions, which have been tested in model culture systems as described below, have so far proved correct and they form a valuable basis for further thoughts on function *in vivo*.

4.4 PATTERNS OF COMMUNICATION

If the patterns of intercellular communication were known *in vivo*, in embryos and in adults, and it was also known how these changed during development and differentiation, some insights into function might be provided. Unfortunately, as yet, there are no simple methods for establishing these patterns. If some probe could be found which is modified *in situ* by cellular enzymes so that it cannot recross the cytoplasmic membrane and escape from the cell, but which is small enough to pass freely through junctions, and which could be easily fixed and readily detected on subsequent examination of tissue sections, then it would be possible to detect if all the cells in a tissue are coupled or if there are coupled sub-populations which are not interconnected by junctions. It would be possible to distinguish and map boundaries between coupled sub-populations (if they exist).

However, until such methods are available, the less suitable techniques of electro-physiology and electron microscopy have to be used.

These methods have been used in an attempt to decide whether separate developmental compartments in insects are coupled or not. There are reasons to believe that concentration gradients of diffusible compounds (morphogens) are set up within compartments (groups of cells with an initially common developmental fate) and that there are abrupt changes in concentration at compartmental boundaries (Lawrence *et al.*, 1972). If the morphogen passed through a compartment by junctional transfer then it would not cross compartmental boundaries if the compartments were not coupled. This would provide a simple explanation of the observations. However, it turns out that cells in different compartments in insects are electrically coupled across the boundary (Caveney, 1974) and gap junctions have been observed between cells known to be in different compartments (Lawrence and Green, 1975). These observations suggest that, at least in insect development, junctions provide a general communication network linking all cells and not just local systems operating only within compartments.

4.5 COMMUNICATION SPECIFICITY

Until recently it was reasonable to conclude from the available data that cells could be divided into two categories. The first, which was by far the most common, was represented by a cell type which formed junctions readily with itself and with all other junction-forming cells regardless of which tissue or species (at least within vertebrates) the cells were derived from (Michalke and Loewenstein, 1971; Pitts, 1972; Pitts, Kukulska and Ferry in preparation). The second type did not form junctions with themselves or with any other cell type (Pitts, 1971; Finbow and Pitts, 1977). In hybrids formed from the two cell types (as described above) junction formation is dominant (Pitts, 1972). This is consistent with the suggestion that cells which do not form junctions lack some essential gene product which is necessary in both cells of a coupled pair.

Recent work (Pitts and Bürk, 1976; Fentiman *et al.*, 1976; 1977; Shaw and Pitts, in preparation) has changed the picture and it now appears that several forms of communication specificity can operate, at least in culture systems.

The first form of specificity to be observed involved certain epithelial cell types which rapidly and efficiently form junctions between themselves but not with fibroblasts (which in turn rapidly and efficiently form junctions between themselves). The specificity is not absolute and in about 5% of the situations where epithelial cells are in contact with fibroblasts junctions are formed between the heterologous cell types (Pitts and Bürk, 1976). It is thought that the junctions formed between heterologous cells are the same as those formed between homologous ones but the frequency with which cell membranes come sufficiently close together to permit junction formation is much lower in the heterologous situations. That is, the specificity does not lie in the junctions themselves but in some other characteristic of the membranes (Pitts and Bürk, 1976).

This epithelial—fibroblast specificity has been observed between lines of epithelial cells (e.g. rat liver BRL cells; Coon, 1968) and all lines of fibroblasts so far examined (Pitts and Bürk, 1976; Shaw and Pitts, unpublished observations), between human mammary duct epithelial cells and mammary fibroblasts (or cell line fibroblasts, Fentiman *et al.*, 1976) and between kidney epithelial cells, kidney fibroblasts, BRL cells and fibroblast cell lines (Shaw and Pitts, unpublished results). It appears that this type of specificity is a common property of epithelial cells from a variety of tissues.

This raises the obvious question of what is the role, if any, of junctional communication between epithelial cells and mesenchyme (or tissues derived from mesenchyme). On the surface, it suggests that such communication may not take place, or take place only to a very minor extent. This would agree with the limited morphological data which suggest that contacts between epithelial cells and underlying fibroblasts across basement membranes are rare. However, the culture systems do show an increased heterologous interaction on prolonged coculture (18 h). Furthermore, cell—cell presentation may be important and may depend on the nature of the substratum and the matrix in which the cells are growing and it may to be unreasonable to assume that a coupled cell pair will always have the ability to reform intercellular junctions after these have been disrupted (as happens when tissues are disrupted and the communication properties of the cells examined in culture).

Yet another form of specificity (or this time, lack of it) was first noticed with cultures of lens epithelial cells (Fentiman *et al.*, 1976). These cells form junctions equally well with themselves, with mammary epithelial cells and with fibroblasts. In the context of epithelial-fibroblast specificity they appear to be universal couplers. A number of other universal couplers have subsequently been discovered, including several virus-transformed fibroblast lines (though the parental untransformed cells behave as normal fibrobalsts; Shaw and Pitts, in preparation, a number of cells from breast tumours (primary cultures and an established line, Fentiman *et al.*, 1977), pigmented retinal epithelial cells from chick embryo tissue (Shaw, Parkinson, Edwards and Pitts, unpublished observations) and ketatinocytes from guinea-pig ear (Hunter and Pitts, unpublished observations).

Certain other tumour cells, apparently derived from cell types which form junctions normally, are found not to form junctions in culture. It is often difficult to be certain of the cell type from which a tumour is derived, and tumour may in some cases arise from normal cells which cannot form junctions, but if so, these junction-incompetent normal cells have still to be discovered. However, whatever their origin, such tumour cell types have been described both in primary cultures (Fentiman *et al.*, 1977) and as cell lines (Borek *et al.*, 1969; Fentiman *et al.*, 1977).

At the present time it must be admitted that we do not know the ground rules for communication specificity and what the different forms of specificity mean in functional terms is still obscure. However, further observations may reveal patterns of behaviour which will suggest some simple explanation.

4.6 CONTROL OF CELL PROLIFERATION AND ACTIVITY IN MODEL SYSTEMS

The discovery of 'metabolic co-operation' (Subak-Sharpe *et al.*, 1966; 1969) and its explanation in terms of intercellular nucleotide exchange (Cox *et al.*, 1970; Pitts, 1971; Pitts and Simms, 1977) and the later work (Pitts and Finbow, 1977; Finbow and Pitts, 1977), showing that many (probably all) small molecular weight cellular components freely equilibrate between all the cells in a coupled population, has made it possible to make a number of simple predications about the behaviour of mixed cell populations in culture.

Mutant cells (HGPRTase-deficient, TKase-deficient), as described above, are resistant to toxic base or nucleotide analogues when cultured alone, but are killed by nucleotide exchange in mixed culture with wild-type cells (if junctions are formed between the mutant and wild-type cells). This junction-mediated cell killing has been termed the 'kiss of death' by Subak-Sharpe (Fujimoto *et al.,* 1971). The opposite effect, the 'kiss of life' can be predicted and has been observed experimentally (Pitts, 1971) when the same mutant and wild-type mixtures are cultured in HAT medium (medium containing hypoxanthine, thymidine and aminopterin, a drug which blocks *de novo* purine and thymine nucleotide biosynthesis; Littlefield, 1964; see Fig. 4.1). The wild-type cells synthesize IMP and deoxythymidine 5'-monophosphate (dTMP) from hypoxanthine and thymidine by the enzymes HGPRTase and

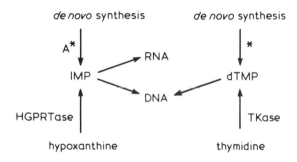

*pathway blocked by aminopterin

Fig. 4.1 Nucleotide biosynthesis.

TKase respectively, and supply not only their own requirements, but also the requirements of the mutant cells (which alone cannot grow in HAT medium).

The most dramatic demonstration of this type of metabolic rescue through junctional communication is the joint, interdependent growth of a mixed culture of HGPRTase- and TKase-deficient cells in HAT medium (Pitts, 1971). Neither cell type alone can survive but they both grow in mixed culture if (and only if) they form intercellular junctions, by mutual nucleotide exchange. The HGPRTase-deficient cells produce all the dTMP for both cell types and the TKase-deficient cells produce all the IMP (Fig. 4.1). All the cells in the mixed population are phenotypically wild-type and the culture grows at the wild-type rate.

This simple experiment in culture may illustrate an important general concept. Marked differences in gene expression in tissue cells *in vivo* may be masked by junction-mediated cell interactions and an apparently uniform phenotype may arise from cells with quite different enzyme activities.

A modification of this type of experiment leads to further observations which may be functionally significant. When unequal mixtures of the two cell types (95% of one and 5% of the other) are co-cultured, there is initial cell death but continued culture of the survivors produces a growing population which contains approximately 50% of each cell type. Because of the metabolic interdependence of the HGPRTase- and TKase-deficient cells, the population is self-regulating. This experiment may illustrate a regulatory mechanism which maintains the different proportions of different cells in tissues *in vivo*.

There are several other cell systems which can be devised where the growth of one or more of the cell types in a mixed culture depends on metabolite exchange. For example, amino acid auxotrophs of Chinese hamster ovary cells (CHO cells) which cannot grow in unsupplemented medium, do grow if co-cultured with wild-type cells, and their growth rate is faster if the two cell types form intercellular junctions (Finbow and Pitts, 1977). The auxotrophs will grow if they do not form junctions with the wild-type cells because amino acids (unlike nucleotides and other intermediate metabolites) can cross the cytoplasmic membrane and move from cell to cell via the medium. However, the cells grow much faster if junctions are formed, which shows that the extracellular pathway is much less efficient than the junctional one.

One other system of this type which is worth mentioning makes use of the natural variation in ouabain resistance between human cells and rodent cells (Baker, 1976). Ouabain inhibits the sodium-potassium ATPase in human cells at concentration 10^3 to 10^4 times lower than those necessary to inhibit the enzyme in rodent cells. So if ^{3}H-thymidine incorporation into acid-insoluble material is followed in human cells (HeLa cells), in TKase-deficient rodent cells (hamster fibroblasts) and in mixtures of the two cell types after treatment with 3×10^{-5} M ouabain for 24 h, it is found that neither the human cells (which are inhibited by the ouabain) nor the hamster cells (which lack TKase) incorporate radioactivity, but the mixed cell culture does incorporate and at a rate similar to that in the absence of the drug. (Pitts and Shaw, 1977). The hamster cells maintain the intracellular ion concentrations in the sodium-potassium ATPase-inhibited human cells and the thus rescued human cells provide dTMP for both cell types. This is a simple biochemical method of showing intercellular ion transfer as well as providing a quite different example of interdependent cellular growth.

A different type of junction-mediated cell interaction is illustrated in a model system developed by Sheridan *et al.*, (1975; 1977). Wild-type cells incorporate hypoxanthine at a rate which varies according to the extracellular concentration of the base. At high concentrations of hypoxanthine the HGPRTase pathway (Fig. 4.1) is more active and consequently the *de novo* pathway of IMP synthesis is inhibited. HGPRTase-deficient cells, on the other hand, make all their IMP by the *de novo* pathway and are unaffected by extracellular hypoxanthine. In mixtures of the two cell types, if (and only if) they form intercellular junctions, the activity of the wild-type cell HGPRTase is further increased (several-fold under optimum conditions) and the *de novo* pathway is inhibited in both the wild-type *and* the mutant cells.

There is intercellular regulation of metabolic activity — the balancing-out of metabolic effort between two cell types of different capabilities.

4.7 JUNCTIONAL COMMUNICATION AND GROWTH CONTROL

Considerable effort has been directed in recent years towards understanding the mechanisms which control gene expression in animal cells. However, a detailed knowledge of these mechanisms will not be sufficient to fully explain the control of cell growth and cell differentiation during embryogenesis and in adult tissues. These control processes also involve intercellular communication and overall they can be divided into three stages, (i) signal initiation, (ii) signal transfer between cells, and (iii) signal interpretation in the cells which divide or differentiate.

The mechanisms which initiate growth control signals are unknown (e.g. the mechanisms which initiate liver regeneration after partial hepatectomy are unknown). The chemical nature of the signal substances themselves is unknown (there are several growth-promoting factors which have been isolated and characterized through their action in tissue culture, but their relevance to growth control *in vivo* is unknown) and it is unclear by which pathways the signals move from cell to cell.

Extracellular signalling substances like hormones or molecules with properties like those attributed to chalones may be involved or the communication network provided by intercellular junctions may be involved, in which case the signalling substances will be intracellular and probably more difficult to detect.

There is no direct evidence to show that junctional communication is involved in growth control, but there are a number of circumstantial reasons for believing that it may play some role.

The structure of the gap junction and junctional permeability appear to be the same *in vivo* as they are in culture (see Pitts and Finbow, 1977) and these junctions are a common feature in most tissues. It is not yet possible to decide, because of the limitations of the methods of investigation (mostly morphological studies), whether all the cells in a given tissue form junctions, but it is clear that the tissues contain populations (and perhaps a single population of all the cells) of coupled cells where metabolite exchange and the intercellular movement of other small ions and molecules must occur. It is therefore inevitable that metabolic activity is shared and co-ordinated in these cell populations in the same way that metabolic co-operation occurs in cell cultures.

Metabolite exchange can lead to intercellular regulation of growth and activity as described above, but as yet there is no evidence to suggest that this form of growth control operates *in vivo*. However, in a study of a number of hepatoma cell lines (each presumably derived from a single normal liver cell) Pitot *et al.* (1964) showed that the enzymic capabilities of these cells were often markedly different from normal liver and from each other. The authors concluded that the hepatoma cells had a range of defects in the control of enzyme synthesis, when compared to normal liver. However, it is conceivable that the variations seen in at least some of these cell lines represent differentiated variations in the individual liver cells from which the tumours were derived. If this is so, then the metabolic interdependence and intercellular growth control of the types studied in culture could be a general property of normal liver.

Yee and Revel (1977) have made the interesting observation from a morphological freeze—cleave study that, after partial hepatectomy of weanling rats, there is a relatively well-synchronized cycle of liver gap junction disappearance (28 h after operation) and reappearance (40—46 h). They comment that there is a striking correspondence between the time gap junctions are lost and the appearance of the first wave of mitoses. Dividing cells can remain coupled during mitosis (O'Lague *et al.*, 1970; Merk and McNutt, 1972) so it is tempting to speculate that there is some functional reason for these changes in communication. Perhaps it is necessary to eliminate metabolic interactions (or the exchange of small control molecules) to allow some other form of cell interaction or some preprogrammed pattern of proliferation and differentiation to take place in temporarily isolated cells. Alternatively, the changes seen in the gap junctions may be caused by general disturbances in tissue structure resulting from mass cell division, but the cells may remain effectively coupled by smaller and less frequent junctions which are difficult to detect morphologically. Further studies, using electrophysiological and biochemical techniques to detect junctions and their permeability, are required before the significance of these findings can be properly assessed.

The loss of growth control by tumour cells is sometimes, but not always, associated with the loss of ability to form permeable intercellular junctions (Borek *et al.*, 1969; Fentiman *et al.*, 1977). Some years ago, Loewenstein (1966) suggested that cancer cells could not form junctions inferring that this was the cause of their abnormal behaviour. However, further work showed that many tumour cells do form junctions but it is still true to say that cells which do not form junctions (if derived from tissues where junctions are normally found) are tumour cells. Further work may show that this statement is also incorrect, but it is consistent with the hypothesis that growth control is mediated by signal substances which pass through intercellular junctions. An inability to form junctions would prevent the control signals reaching the tumour cell and if the tumour cell forms junctions the mechanisms which interpret the signals are presumably defective.

The genetic analysis of junction formation and growth control (as described above) should eventually show whether or not this idea is correct.

The mechanism of topoinhibition (Dulbecco, 1970) in tissue culture is not understood. This form of cellular growth control which is a consequence of high cell density in monolayer cultures of certain cell types, could be mediated by junctional communication. Stoker (1975) has shown that it is unlikely that topostimulation (the release from topoinhibition in wounded cultures) is the result of the breakdown of intercellular junctions but this does not mean that the inhibitory signals are not junction mediated.

Sheridan (1976) has put forward a model to explain the density-dependence of cell proliferation in culture. If the initiation of the cell cycle (and consequent division) depends on fluctuations in cyclic nucleotide concentrations in early G1 phase, then the concentration changes which occur in isolated cells will be damped out at high cell density by loss (or gain) of cyclic nucleotides through junctions with surrounding asynchronous cells. This is a simple idea based on the known permeability of intercellular junctions and observed variations in cAMP and cGMP concentrations during the cell cycle. However, whether the cyclic nucleotide concentration changes are causitive, and whether the changes due to junctional leakage are sufficient to account for the changes in growth behaviour with cell density, are still open questions which require experimental investigation.

Permeable intercellular junctions occur widely in animal tissues and it seems reasonable to believe that they are involved in some form of intercellular communication which is essential for normal tissue function. It seems inevitable that they are involved in intercellular regulation of metabolic activity but their role in intercellular growth control is as yet nothing more (except in model culture systems) than an attractive possibility. Hopefully this review, written at an very early stage in the development of the subject, will stimulate further investigations.

REFERENCES

Azarnia, R., Larsen, W. and Loewenstein, W.R. (1974), *Proc. natn. Acad. Sci., U.S.A.,* **71**, 880.

Azarnia, R. and Loewenstein, W.R. (1977), *J. Memb. Biol.,* **34**, 39.

Baker, R.M. (1976), In: *Biogenesis and Turnover of Membrane Macromolecules* (Cook, J.S. ed.), p. 93, Raven Press, New York.

Boone, C.M., Chen, T.R. and Ruddle, F.H. (1972), *Proc. natn. Acad. Sci., U.S.A.,* **69**, 510.

Borek, C.S., Higashino, S. and Loewenstein, W.R. (1969), *J. Memb. Biol.,* **1**, 274.

Brownstein, B.L., Rozengurt, E., Jimenez de Asua, L. and Stoker, M. (1975), *J. Cell Physiol.,* **85**, 579.

Bürk, R.R., Pitts, J.D. and Subak-Sharpe, J.H. (1968), *Exp. Cell Res.,* **53**, 297.

Caveney, S. (1974), *Dev. Biol.,* **40**, 311.

Coon, H.G. (1968), *J. Cell Biol.,* **39**, 29a.

Cox, R.P., Krauss, M.J., Balis, M.E. and Dancis, J. (1970), *Proc. natn. Acad. Sci., U.S.A.,* **67**, 1573.

Cox, R.P., Krauss, M.R., Balis, M.E. and Dancis, J. (1974), In: *Cell Communication* (Cox, R.P. ed.), p. 67, Wiley, London.

Crick, F.H.C. (1970), *Nature,* **225**, 420.

DeHaan, R.L. and Sachs, H.G. (1972), In: *Current topics in developmental biology* (Moscona, A.A. and Monray, A. eds.), p. 193, Academic Press, New York.

Dulbecco. R. (1970), *Nature,* **227**, 802.

Fentiman, I.S., Taylor-Papadimitriou, J. and Stoker, M. (1976), *Nature,* **264**, 760.

Fentiman, I.S. and Taylor-Papadimitriou, J. (1977), *Nature,* (In press).

Finbow, M.E. and Pitts, J.D. (1977), (In press).

Furshpan, E.J. and Potter, D.D. (1968), In: *Current Topics* in *Developmental Biology* (Moscona, A.A. and Monroy, A., eds.), p. 95, Academic Press, New York.

Fujimoto, W.Y., Subak-Sharpe, J.H. and Seegmiller, J.E. (1971), *Proc. natn. Acad. Sci., U.S.A.,* **68**, 1516.

Goldfarb, P.S.G., Slack, C., Subak-Sharp, J.H. and Wright, E.D. (1975), *Soc. exp. Biol. Symp.,* **28**, 463.

Goodenough, D. (1975), *Cold Spring Harbor Symp. Quant. Biol.,* **40**, 37.

Ito, S., Sato, E. and Loewenstein, W.R. (1974), *J. Memb. Biol.,* **19**, 305.

Laat, S.W., de, Barts, P.W.J.A. and Bakker, M.I. (1976), *J. Memb. Biol.,* **27**, 109.

Larsen, W.J., Azarnia, R. and Loewenstein, W.R. (1977), *J. Memb. Biol.,* **34**, 39.

Lawrence, P.A., Crick, F.H.C. and Munro, M. (1972), *J. Cell Sci.,* **11**, 815.

Lawrence, P.A. and Green, S.M. (1975), *J. Cell Biol.,* **65**, 373.

Littlefield, J.W. (1964), *Science,* **145**, 709.

Loewenstein, W.R. (1966), *Ann. N.Y. Acad. Sci.,* **137**, 441.

Loewenstein, W.R. (1973), *Fedn. Proc., Fedn Am. Socs. exp. Biol.,* **32**, 60.

Loewenstein, W.R. (1975), *Cold Spring Harbor Symp. Quant. Biol.,* **40**, 49.

McCargow, J. and Pitts, J.D. (1971), *Biochem. J.,* **124**, 48P.

Merk, F.B. and McNutt, N.S. (1972), *J. Cell Biol.,* **55**, 511.

Michalke, W. (1977), *J. Memb. Biol.,* **33**, 1.

Michalke, W. and Loewenstein, W.R. (1971), *Nature,* **232**, 121.

O'Lague, P., Dalen, H., Rubin, H. and Tobias, C. (1970), *Science,* **170**, 464.

Pitot, H.C., Peraino, C., Morse, P.A. and Potter, van R. (1964), *Natn. Cancer Inst. Monograph,* **13**, 229.

Pitts, J.D. (1971), In: Ciba Found. Symp. *Growth Control in Cell Cultures* (Wolstenholme, G.E.W. and Knight, J., eds), p. 89, Churchill-Livingstone, London.

Pitts, J.D. (1972), In: 3rd Lepetit Colloquium *Cell interaction*, (Silvestri, L.G. ed), p. 277, North-Holland, Amsterdam.

Pitts, J.D. (1976), In: *Developmental Biology of Plants and Animals* (Graham, C.F. and Wareing, P.F. eds), p. 96, Blackwell, Oxford.

Pitts, J.D. (1977), In: International Cell Biology (Brinkley, B.R. and Potter, K.R., eds) Rockefeller University Press.

Pitts, J.D. and Bürk, R.R. (1976), *Nature,* **264,** 762.

Pitts, J.D. and Finbow, M.E. (1977), In: *Intercellular communication* (DeMello, W.C. ed), p. 61, Plenum, New York.

Pitts, J.D. and Shaw, (1977), (In press).

Pitts, J.D. and Simms, J.W. (1977), *Exp. Cell Res.,* **104**, 153.

Rose, B., Simpson, I. and Loewenstein, W.R. (1977), *Nature,* **267**, 625.

Ruddle, F.H. (1973), *Nature,* **242**, 165.

Saxen, L., Lehtonen, E., Jaarskelainen, M.K., Nording, S. and Wartiovaara, J. (1976), *Nature,* **259**, 662.

Sheridan, J.D. (1974), In: *The Cell Surface in Development,* (Moscona, A.A. ed), p. 187, Wiley, New York.

Sheridan, J.D. (1976), In: *The Cell Surface in Animal Embryogenesis and Development* (Poste, G. and Nicholson, G.L. eds), p. 409, Elsevier-North Holland, New York.

Sheridan, J.D., Finbow, M.E. and Pitts, J.D. (1975), *J. Cell Biol.,* **67**, 396a.

Sheridan, J.D., Finbow, M.E. and Pitts, J.D. (1977), *Exp. Cell Res.,* (In press).

Simpson, I., Rose, R. and Loewenstein, W.R. (1977), *Science,* **195**, 294.

Stoker, M. (1975), *Cell,* **6**, 253.

Subak-Sharpe, J.H., Bürk, R.R. and Pitts, J.D. (1966), *Heredity,* **21**, 342.

Subak-Sharpe, J.H., Bürk, R.R. and Pitts, J.D. (1969), *J. Cell Sci.,* **4**, 353.

Wright, E.D., Goldfarb, P.S.G. and Subak-Sharpe, J.H. (1976a), *Exp. Cell Res.,* **103**, 63.

Wright, E.D., Slack, C., Goldfarb, P.S.G. and Subak-Sharpe, J.H. (1976b), *Exp. Cell Res.,* **103**, 79.

Yee, A.G. and Revel, J.P. (1977), *Science,* (In press).

5 Gap Junctions: Channels for Communication in Development

L. WOLPERT

Acknowledgements
I am indebted to Dr A. Warner for both her critical and constructive comments.
This work is supported by the Medical Research Council.

Intercellular Junctions and Synapses
(*Receptors and Recognition,* Series B, Volume 2)
Edited by J. Feldman, N.B. Gilula and J.D. Pitts
Published in 1978 by Chapman and Hall, 11 New Fetter Lane, London EC4P 4EE
© Chapman and Hall

INTRODUCTION

Cell-to-cell interactions play a role in a variety of processes in development such as cell migration, pattern formation, and induction. The interactions that occur between cells when they are in contact necessarily involve the cell membrane and it is convenient to distinguish between three main classes of interaction (Wolpert and Gingell 1969). In one class the cell membrane acts as a sensor in a mechanical sense: the cells can respond to physical differences in the environment such as mechanical barriers or variations in adhesiveness. For example, if a cell moves by pseudopod extension and retraction and if there is a variation in its adhesiveness with the substratum over which it moves, it is very plausible that it will move towards the region where the adhesiveness is greatest (Gustafson and Wolpert, 1967). There is, in this case, no real communication between the cell and its environment and the interactions are largely external to the cell membrane. In the second class of interactions the membrane acts as a transducer, converting some signal external to the cell into a change in the cell interior. There are numerous examples of this: a classical one would be acetylcholine arriving at the motor end plate, causing a permeability change which leads to action potential production, which in turn leads to calcium release and muscle contraction. Another example would be the activation of adenyl cyclase in the membrane by an external agent resulting in the increase of cyclic AMP internally. The third class involves the cell membrane acting as a channel. The general case would be where the external signal simply traverses the membrane unchanged and alters cell behaviour as with the steroid hormones or glucose. But the more important case is where a special or localized channel is formed between two cells as in the case of gap junction formation.

It is now generally accepted that the low resistance pathways that can be formed between cells, and which are detected by electrophysiological methods, can be correlated with the presence of gap junctions: such junctions appear to provide channels for the movement of small molecules up to a molecular weight of about 1000 from cell to cell in adult tissues and differentiated cells in culture (Sheridan, 1974; McNutt and Weinstein, 1974; Loewenstein, 1977; and see Pitts and Gilula, this volume). Gap junctions have been found in a variety of developmental systems but it must be recognized that no functional role has yet been demonstrated in development. We are thus faced with the question as to what role channels between cells, allowing the passage of small molecules, could play in development.

Three general features of obvious potential value to a developing system should be noted: (a) Gap junctions provide a channel for direct cell-to-cell communication such that the molecules moving from one cell to another do not enter the extracellular space. This could be a great advantage in situations where the maintenance of particular concentrations of small molecules was important. (b) As a consequence of gap junctions providing a channel, channels of communication could be specified by the distribution of gap junctions. The disappearance of gap junctions could effectively block one type of communication between cells. (c) A most important feature of gap junctions is that they provide a channel for interaction between the internal contents of cells and thus interactions need not involve the cell membrane acting as a transducer. Thus the interaction can occur between the internal contents of the cell, and any specificity might involve this interaction rather than that between membranes.

The presence of gap and low resistance junctions in a variety of embryonic systems is shown in Table 5.1. From this it is probably not unreasonable to conclude that the presence of gap and low resistance junctions is the rule rather than the exception in embryonic systems. For example they are present in the early embryos of chick, amphibia, squid and echinoderms. This view is strenthened by the finding that in tissue culture a wide variety of cells can make junctions with each other (Gilula, 1977).

5.1 PATTERN FORMATION

The most likely situation where gap junctions would be expected to play a role is in the cellular interactions involved in pattern formation in early development. Pattern formation is the process of specifying the spatial pattern of cellular differentiation. In general terms it may be viewed as assigning states to cells in an ensemble such that, when they undergo cytodifferentiation, they form the required spatial pattern. One means of specifying spatial patterns of cellular differentiation is by mechanisms based on positional information (Wolpert, 1971). The basic idea of positional information is that pattern formation may result from a two-step process. The cells first have their position specified and then interpret this according to their genome and developmental history. That the behaviour of a cell is largely specified by its position within a developing field is a very old idea going back to Driesch in 1890. Much of the evidence for this comes from operations on early sea-urchin and amphibian embryos which have remarkable capacities for regulation when parts are removed or placed in new positions (Cooke, 1975). This regulation clearly requires cell-to-cell interaction and thus the presence of low resistance junctions in such embryos is suggestive.

It is not known how positional information is specified but several models have been put forward. A very simple one which has been applied to hydra is based on the concentration of a diffusible morphogen which is produced by a localized group of cells − a source − which keeps the concentration constant there. If the substance diffuses and is broken down, then an exponential gradient will be set up; if, however, there is a localized sink a straight line gradient will be established. In principle, the concentration of the morphogen can provide the cell with its position with respect to boundary regions, such as the source. A particularly interesting model for gradients which could provide the basis for positional information has been proposed by Gierer and Meinhardt (1972). The model is based on defined molecular kinetics and does not rely on localized sources. Their mechanism is based on the interaction of an auto-catalytic substance — the activator — with short range diffusion, and a more rapidly diffusing antagonist, the inhibitor. Appropriate reaction schemes can result in a localized high concentration of the activator, which causes inhibitor production, and this results in a monotonic gradient in inhibitor. This concentration gradient could provide a positional signal.

There are other means for specifying positional information which do not make use of a diffusible positional signal. The phase-shift model of Goodwin and Cohen (1969) is based upon a periodic event being propagated from a pacemaker region, together with a second, more slowly propagated, wave. Positional information is specified by the phase difference between the two events. The propagation of the waves requires cell-to-cell interaction which could be mediated by small molecules, even ions, diffusing across gap junctions. Another model is based on the time cells spend in a region, and has been used to account for the specification of positional information along the proximo-distal axis in the chick limb (Summerbell *et al.,* 1973). In principle this does not require cell-to-cell interaction.

From the point of view of cell-to-cell communication it is very important to realize that models for positional information can be based on the movement of small molecules between cells. The only interactions required are those necessary to set up the system of positional values and there need be no interactions between the differentiating regions as such. This also means that there may be a very restricted number of mechanisms for specifying positional information, the variety of patterns being due to differences in interpretation. There is thus no obvious requirement for complex interactions or for the cell-to-cell transfer of large informational (such as RNA) macromolecules. Conversations between cells may thus be very simple, almost tediously so. It is one of the characteristics of models based on postional information that the complexity of pattern formation lies in the cellular response rather than in cellular interactions.

5.2 DISTRIBUTION OF GAP JUNCTIONS IN DEVELOPMENT

A s pointed out above, gap junctions appear to be the rule rather than the exception in developing systems. We may thus first consider whether the distribution of low resistance junctions could provide a means of restricting channels of communication and thus for example, define the boundaries of embryonic fields. The widespread occurrence of junctions makes this very unlikely and the observation of insect segment boundaries is particularly important in this respect. The segmental bound-aries in insects have a special developmental significance. Studies on the pattern of the cuticle suggest that there is a gradient in positional information running from one boundary to the next and that this gradient is repeated in each segment, Thus, at the

Table 5.1 Gap and low-resistance junctions in developing systems

System	Cells	Gap junctions	Low resistance junctions
Squid embryo	Most cells from stage 10–25		+ Potter et al., 1966
Amphibian embryo (Triturus, Xenopus, Ambystoma)	Cleavage, blastula and gastrula	+ Sanders and Dicaprio, 1976	+ Ito and Loewenstein, 1969; Palmer and Slack, 1970; Warner, 1975
Fish (Fundulus) embryo	Cleavage to midgastrula	+ Bennett and Trinkaus, 1970	+ Bennett and Trinkaus, 1970
Chick embryo	Notochord, mesoderm, ectoderm, epiblast	+ Revel et al., 1973	+ Sheridan, 1968
Echinoderm (Asterias) embryo	Blastomeres after 16 cell stage		+ Tupper and Saunders, 1972
Mouse embryo	Blastomeres	+ Ducibella et al., 1975	
Amphibian (Ambystoma) – neural tube	Neural tube and neural plate and lateral plate ectoderm	+ Decker and Friend, 1974	+ Warner, 1973
Amphibian (Bombina, Xenopus, Ambystoma) embryo	Dermatone Myotome	+ Keeter et al., 1975	+ Blackshaw and Warner, 1976
Amphibian (Xenopus) embryo – eye	Developing retina – neural retina and pigment epithelium	+ Dixon and Cronly-Dillon, 1972, 1974	+ Blackshaw and Warner, 1976
Crustacean (Daphnia) embryo – eye	Neuroblasts of optic cartridge	+ Lopresti et al.,	
Human embryo – limb	Apical ectodermal ridge of limb	+ Kelley and Fallon, 1976	

Table 5.1 Gap and low-resistance junctions in developing systems (*continued*)

System	Cells	Gap junctions	Low resistance junctions
Rabbit embryo	Adrenal gland	+ Joseph *et al.*, 1973	+ Joseph *et al.*, 1973
Locust embryo − eye	Undifferentiated cells of ommatidia	+ Eley and Shelton, 1976	
Insect, *Oncopeltus*, 5th stage larva	Epidermal cells including segment boundary	+ Lawrence and Green, 1975	
Insect, *Rhodnius*	Epidermal cells including segment boundary		+ Warner and Lawrence, 1973
Hydra	Epidermal and gastrodermal cells	+ Hand and Gobel, 1972	
Presumptive muscle cells in culture	Myoblasts prior to fusion	+ Rash and Staehelin, 1974	
Tunicate embryo	Blastula and gastrula		+ Miyazahi *et al.*, 1974

segment boundary, there must be a sharp discontinuity as the gradient switches from a low point to a high point (Lawrence *et al.*, 1972). There is also evidence that the boundary forms a sharp discontinuity with respect to other cell properties and in *Oncopeltus*, the segment boundary is a compartment border (Lawrence, 1973). Compartments define a group of cells, usually small in number, whose progeny never subsequently give rise to cells in an adjacent compartment (Crick and Lawrence, 1975). Within a compartment marked clones never cross into an adjacent compartment. The boundary between compartments may reflect differences in adhesiveness between the cells of the two compartments.

In spite of the presumed discontinuity at the segment border Lawrence and Green (1975) have, in *Oncopeltus*, found no difference in specialized cell attachments, such as gap junctions, at the segment border. Even more striking, Warner and Lawrence (1973) have not found any difference in the degree of electrical coupling at the border segment in *Rhodnius*. It is of course recognized that the electrophysiological technique measures the resistance to the passage of small ions, and the possibility remains that the gap junctions may provide the channel for other molecules whose passage could be selectively blocked at the segment boundary (see below).

Since low resistance and gap junctions are common features of embryonic systms, then the exceptions must be treasured for this could give us some insight into the role they play. We must particularly look at situations where, contrary to expectation, gap junctions are absent, and situations where gap junctions disappear. There are thus far only a few cases where these have been described

(a) Blackshaw and Warner (1976) found that in *Xenopus* the dermatome and myotomic layers of the mesoderm were not electrically coupled to each other either before or after somite formation. In *Bombina* and *Ambystoma,* the dermatone and myotome layers were uncoupled once the somites had formed. During somite formation in these amphibians, there are important changes in the distribution of low resistance junctions. In three species the somitic mesoderm is initially coupled and the position of the intersomite border in the unsegmented mesoderm is marked by breaking of low resistance junctions between those cells destined to form the next somite, and the rest of the unsegmented mesoderm. The developmental significance of these events is not clear but Backshaw and Warner suggest that the trigger for the re-orientation of the cells for somite formation could be the loss of low resistance junctions. They also suggest that the electrical recoupling that occurs after somite formation in *Xenopus* and *Bombina*, may be related to the transmission of a depolarizing stimulus prior to the completion of somite innervation, allowing synchronous muscular contraction. In *Ambystoma*, by contrast with the other two species, the somites remain insulated from each other.

(b) At the time of closure of the neural tube in the axolotl, Warner (1973) has found that ectoderm and neural cells lose their low resistance connections with each other at the same time that opposing ectoderm cells establish new connections across the mid-line. Again, the developmental significance is not known. However, it should be noted that in both this and the preceding example dealing with somite formation, uncoupling of low resistance precedes mechanical separation. One must thus recognize the possibility that the loss of gap junctions may not be related to information transfer, but rather reflects changes in cell surface properties associated with the morphogenetic movements.

(c) In the early starfish embryo Tupper and Saunders (1972) found no low-resistance junctions until the 16-cell stage. There is however no reason to believe that cell-to-cell communication occurs during this early period.

(d) Kelley and Fallon (1976) found a decrease in the number of gap junctions in the human apical ectodermal ridge of the developing limb, when the ridge begins to disappear. Gap junctions were not observed between cells of dorsal and ventral limb ectoderm. The apical ectodermal ridge plays a key role in determining limb outgrowth and the specification of the proximo-distal axis. It also may be involved in the specification of antero-posterior axis. There is the possibility that the signal from the mesodermal cell from the zone of polarizing activity (ZPA) which can specify positional information along the antero-posterior axis (Tickle, Summerbell and Wolpert, 1975), is transmitted through the apical ridge. A grafted ZPA is only effective when grafted adjacent to the ridge.

(e) Dixon and Cronly-Dillon (1972, 1974) have reported that in the developing amphibian retina, gap junctions between the cells disappear from the central portion after stage 32, which is the time of specification of the axial polarity of the retina. After this time, gap junctions are only found at the periphery where the retina is growing. In the case of the development of the locust eyes, gap junctions are present between undifferentiated cells, but are absent at the first recognizable stage in the development, when the cells group to form distinctive clusters. Eley and Shelton (1976) suggest that this may correlate with the time of cell determination.

5.3 TIME FOR POSITIONAL SIGNALLING

It is now clear that positional fields are small at the time when they are being specified, less than about 1 mm or 100 in maximum linear dimension. The time to set up such fields is quite long, of the order of hours. Crick (1970) has shown that a gradient of a diffusible morphogen would fit these requirements. He took the effective diffusion constant of the morphogen at 2×10^{-7} $cm^2 s^{-1}$ this was based on the diffusion of a small molecule (mol. wt. 300) which moved across the membrane from cell to cell by facilitated transfer. He showed that a gradient across a line of cells 1 mm long could be set up in a few hours.

One of the few situations where information is available on the time/distance relationship for a signal is in hydra. The situation studied is the transmission of an inhibitory signal from the head end. This inhibitory signal prevents the formation of other heads and is one of the reasons hydra can regenerate a head, when the head is removed. Wilby and Webster (1970) showed that a head can inhibit the formation of another head over quite long distances (0.5 mm) and that this inhibition can be propagated in a proximo-distal direction; that is from the foot end towards the head end. We have investigated the time/distance relationships by grafting an additional head to the proximal end of the gastric region of the hydra, and determining how long it was necessary to wait before removing the host head, so that head regeneration there would be inhibited (Wolpert *et al.*, 1972). The results showed that the times were very dependent on the distance and they could be interpreted in terms of diffusion of an inhibitor, the source of which was at the head end, and which had a diffusion constant of 2×10^{-7} cm^{2}s^{-1}. There was also evidence that signalling would not occur unless cell contact was established (Hicklin *et al.*, 1973). Following grafting, gap junctions are established within a few hours and could provide the channel for the signal (Wakeford, 1975).

Crick's calculations are based on facilitated transfer across the whole of the region where cells are in contact. It is important to consider the effect on the diffusion constant if gap junctions provided the channel for diffusion; that is, if the morphogen has the same diffusion constant across the junction as in the cytoplasm. If the gap junction were present over the whole area of contact between cells, and the cells were of constant cross section, the effective diffusion constant would be unaltered. If however, the gap junction is confined to only a small region of the membrane in the area of contact, the situation is more complex and the effective diffusion constant will be much reduced. Dr J. Lewis has estimated that if the area of contact is much smaller than the cell diameter then, to a first approximation, the effective diffusion constant will be reduced by the ratio of the area of the gap junction to the diameter of the cell. This ratio is not easy to determine. Using isolated amphibian cells Slack and Warner (1975) estimated that free movement of ions across a junctional area of 0.1 μm diameter could account for the electrical coupling. The cells had a diameter of 150 μm and this means that the effective diffusive constant would be 1000 times less than that in the cytoplasm. If, following Crick, we take the diffusion constant of a small molecule such as cyclic AMP, as 10^{-6} cm^2 s^{-1} then the effective diffusion constant will be 10^{-9} cm^2 s^{-1} which is almost certainly too small to account for the observations. If the ratio of the area of gap junction to contact areas is 100 then the effective constant will be 10^{-8} which is probably just plausible.

5.4 PERMEABILITY OF GAP JUNCTIONS IN EMBRYOS

The permeability properties of gap junctions have been studied mainly using differentiated cells *in vivo*, such as the insect salivary gland, or cells in culture. Thus, the conclusion that junctions can pass molecules up to molecular weight of about 1000 cannot be extrapolated directly to early embryos. In fact, while low resistance junctions have clearly been demonstrated in embryo, the morphological evidence for gap junctions is rather poor, and is usually restricted to a few points of cell contact.

The possibility of low resistance junctions having different permeability properties is suggested by studies on the permeability of such junctions to fluorescein. In general, as Sheridan (1974) points out, movement of tracers goes hand in hand with electrical coupling and cells with low resistance junctions between them can readily exchange small tracers such as fluorescein. However, in the case of the early embryos of echinoderms (Tupper and Saunders, 1972) and amphibians (Slack and Palmer, 1969), electrical coupling occurs, but movement of fluorescein cannot be detected: a particularly striking example is Bennett's observation on *Fundulus* (Bennett *et al.,* 1972). Very recent studies by Turin and Warner (1977) have confirmed the absence of fluorescein transfer across low resistance junctions in the amphibian blastula. More important, they have evidence for selectivity in the inorganic anion range, and that small molecules, such as nucleotides, cannot cross the junction. Such studies clearly have very important implications for models requiring molecules larger than ions transversing the junctions: either they must be excluded, or selective transport mechanisms must be invoked.

It is particularly interesting that Slack and Warner (1975) have found rectification between early amphibian cells *in vitro*. Also, Warner (1973) has found that the cells of the neural plate of amphibia have a different membrane potential from the lateral plate ectoderm even though they are connected by low resistance junctions. As Warner points out 'the maintenance of different membrane potentials of cells in the two areas and the different voltage dependence of the conductances implies that cell-to-cell junctional membranes can be selective in their permeability properties, allowing variation, in intracellular potential to be generated across them.

5.5 CELLULAR INTERACTIONS IN DEVELOPMENT IN THE ABSENCE OF CELL CONTACT

In drawing attention to the possible role of gap junctions in cellular interactions, it is important to draw attention to interactions where cell-to-cell contact does not seem to be required. Such situations would naturally exclude gap junctions from playing a role.

It seems in several cases of embryonic induction, cell contact is not required (Hay, 1977). Induction may be defined as developmentally significant interaction between closely associated but dissimilarly derived tissue masses (Grobstein, 1955). Included within such a definition would be primarily embryonic induction as well as the large class of epithelial mesenchymal interactions. Studies on primary embryonic induction *in vitro* with amphibian tissues has suggested that neural development, as judged by morphological criteria, can be initiated in a competent early gastrula ectoderm by a stimulus from the underlying mesoderm without cell contact between the two tissues (Toivonen *et al.,* 1976). However, only initiation can be brought about without contact, and regionalization probably does require contact. Again, epithelial— mesenchymal interactions appear to occur without cell-to-cell contact since the interacting tissues are separated by a basement membrane. For example, early mesoderm can specify the nature of the overlying epidermis in development even though the tissues are separated by a basement membrane (Sengel, 1976). Attention in these situations is now being focussed on the role of the cell matrix (Hay, 1977). It should nevertheless be pointed out that in one case, the induction of kidney tubules by spinal cord tissue, which was previously thought to be mediated by an extracellular matrix, has now been shown by Saxén and his colleagues to require cell contact (Saxén *et al.*, 1976).

There are also several situations where cell contact — an obvious requirement for gap junctions — does not appear to be required, even though cell-to-cell communication within a tissue takes place. Saunders and Gasseling (1963) have found that the antero-posterior discs of the chick limb bud can be repolarized by more posterior tissue probably the zone of polarizing activity even when a Millipore filter is placed between the tissues and cell contact is prevented, and Rose (1970) has presented evidence that substances controlling regeneration in Tubularia can be moved under the influence of an electric field from one tissue to another, even when they are not in contact. Both merit re-investigation, particularly the former, in view of recent studies showing the ability of cell processes to penetrate the Millipore filter (Saxén *et al.*, 1976).

5.6 THRESHOLDS AND PRECISION

All models of development require that cells change their state whether characterized by determination or cytodifferentiation. Irrespective of the type of mechanism by which this cell state is specified — concentration gradient or time differences between wave fronts or cytoplasmic differences — it seems reasonable to assume that ultimately the change of cell state will be governed by the concentration of one or more chemical compounds. If the cell states are discrete there will be thresholds in the cells' response. For concentrations just above a threshold, the cells will adopt one state, and for concentrations just below it, another. This might be applicable not only to the specification of positional values in positional fields, but also to considerations of the cell cycle and the transition from G_o into the cycle: Pardee's restriction point might be regarded as a threshold (Pardee, 1971).

We (Lewis *et al.*, 1977) have recently analysed the problem of thresholds in relation to pattern formation, the first step in the interpretation of a gradient in positional information being considered in terms of thresholds in cell response to a concentration of a chemical. It is possible to base a threshold mechanism on co-operative binding of control molecules to an allosteric enzyme. We have found such a mechanism to be unlikely since for a sharp threshold response, either the gradient would have to be implausibly steep, or the co-operativity implausibly high. We have, instead, put forward a kinetic threshold model which has some implications of cell-to-cell interactions.

The essence of the model is that the transcription of a gene may be promoted by increasing the concentration of a signal substance S, and that there is positive feed-back by the gene product. This results in a situation where increasing the concentra-tion of S results in the system 'flipping' to a new stable state with the gene turned on, even when the signal substance S is removed. This kinetic model is an example of the type of bistable control circuit postulated by Kauffman (1975) to explain determin-ation and transdetermination in the imaginal discs of *Drosophila*. The change in state can be brought about by means which do not involve a change in the signal substance. The system will be affected particularly by the value of the constants which determine the reaction rates and which, in turn, will be determined by enzyme concentration and other metabolites. Fluctuations in other molecules could thus also cause transition from one steady state to another. If such a transition were caused by a fluctuation in the concentration of a small molecule, which might pass from cell-to-cell through gap junctions, one might account for the simulataneous transdetermination of a group of cells as observed by Gehring (1972).

An analysis of the problem of the precision of the specification of a spatial pattern using thresholds and a concentration gradient, indicates that the most important parameter is the variation in the thesholds of individual cells. The level of the threshold will depend upon concentrations of enzymes and other molecules affecting the rate constants. The variability of this threshold value from cell-to-cell is unknown. What is clear is that fluctuations in the concentrations of small molecules may be reduced by their exchange through low resistance junctions. Gap junctions might thus provide an important means for averaging out differences between cells in a positional field.

5.7 CELL MOVEMENT AND CELL CONTACT

A feature of great importance in cell movement, particularly of fibroblast, is contact inhibition: when one cell makes contact with another, its movement in that direction is inhibited (Abercrombie, 1967). We have argued that contact inhibition is a phenomenon referring to the cell as a whole and can depend on several cellular parameters (Gustafson and Wolpert, 1967). An important feature in this process is contact paralysis which refers to the local inhibition of ruffling or pseudopod activity. A very dramatic example of contact inhibition and contact paralysis comes from Dunn's (1971) studies on nerve cells in culture. When a filopod from one nerve cell touches another cell, that filopod is withdrawn as well as other filopods, and the cell moves off in another direction. The striking feature is that contact by one filopod causes retraction of adjacent filopods. It is hard to avoid the conclusion that the local contact has lead to a propagated influence causing adjacent pseudopods to withdraw. The mechanism involved in unknown but it is possible that if a gap junction was formed between the filopod and the cell it touches, then the channel between the two cells could bring about the observed result. Kauffman (1974) has pointed out that if pseudopod extension and contraction were linked to a cyclic process in the cell, then when cells made contact, the response could depend on the phase difference between the cycle in the two cells. It is of interest that Goodwin and Cohen (1969) have suggested a mechanism whereby the movement of nerve cells and the establishment of appropriate connections could be based on a similar mechanism. The point to be emphasized is that these mechanisms locate specificity in the inside of the cell rather than the cell membrane, which is usually regarded as the site of neuronal specificity (Marchase *et al.*, 1975). In this connection it is important to realize that the requirement for a high degree of specificity for the making of neural connections is still rather weak. Gaze and Hope (1976) for example, reviewing the development of retino-tectal connections, show that it is possible to have models which require rather little specificity in the interaction between retinal and tectal cells.

5.8 CONCLUSIONS

The main conclusion to be drawn is that gap junctions in developing systems are still a structure in search of a function. It is also very clear that the gap junction could play a very important role in cell-to-cell interactions particularly in relation to the specification of positional information, the precision of thresholds, and cell movement and contact. Many cell-to-cell interactions require in principle only simple signals using low molecular weight compounds, and gap junctions could provide the channel. It is because gap junctions offer such attractive possibilities that it is necessary not to be deluded into thinking that their role in this connection is established. The most urgent need is to find a way of specifically blocking or abolishing gap junctions so that the effect of their absence can be determined. Almost as important is the necessity to determine just what sort of selectivity there is in the molecules that can pass through them. It is already clear that the presence of low resistance junctions permitting the passage of ions does not imply that larger molecules can also pass.

REFERENCES

Abercrombie, M. (1967), *Nat. Cancer Inst. Monogr.*, **26**, 249
Bennett, M.V.L., Spira, M.E. and Pappas, G.D. (1972), *Dev. Biol.*, **29**, 419.
Bennett, M.V.L. and Trinkaus, J.P. (1970), *J. Cell Biol.*, **44**, 592.
Blackshaw, S.E. and Warner, A.E. (1976), *J. Physiol.*, **255**, 209.
Cooke, J. (1975), *A. Rev. Biophys. Bioeng.*, **4**, 185.
Crick, F.H.C. (1970), *Nature*, **225**, 420.
Crick, F.H.C. and Lawrence, P.A. (1975), *Science*, **189**, 346.
Decker, R.S. and Friend, D.S. (1974), *J. Cell Biol.*, **62**, 49.
Dixon, J.S. and Cronly-Dillon, J.R. (1972), *J. Embryol. exp. Morph.*, **28**, 659.
Dixon, J.A. and Cronly-Dillon, J.R. (1974), *Nature*, **251**, 505.

Ducibella, T., Albertini, D.F., Anderson, E. and Biggers, J.D. (1975), *Dev. Biol.*, **45**, 231.

Dunn, G.A. (1971), *J. comp. Neurol.*, **143**, 491.

Eley, S. and Shelton, P.M.J. (1976), *J. Embryol. exp. Morph.*, **36**, 409.

Gaze, M. and Hope, A. (1976), *Prog. Brain Res.* (in press).

Gehring, W. (1972), In: *Biology of Imaginal Disks* (Ursprung, H. and Nothiger, R., eds.), Springer-Verlag, Berlin.

Gierer, A. and Meinhardt, H. (1972), *Kybernetik*, **12**, 30.

Gilula, N.B. (1977), In: *Cellular Interactions in Development* (in press).

Goodwin, B.C. and Cohen, M.H. (1969), *J. Theoret. Biol.*, **25**, 49.

Grobstein, C. (1955), In: *Aspects of Synthesis and Order in Growth*, (Rudnick, D., ed.), Princeton University Press, Princeton.

Gustafson, T. and Wolpert, L. (1967), *Biol. Rev.*, **42**, 442.

Hand, A.R. and Gobel, S. (1972), *J. Cell Biol.*, **52**, 397–408.

Hay, E.D. (1977), ICCB Symposia Papers, (Brinkley, B.R. and Porter, K.E., eds.), Rockefeller University Press, New York (in press).

Hicklin, J., Hornbruch, A., Wolpert, L. and Clarke, M.R.B. (1973), *J. Embryol. exp. Morph.*, **30**, 727.

Ito, S. and Loewenstein, W.R. (1969), *Dev. Biol.* **19**, 225.

Joseph, T., Slack, C. and Gould, R.P. (1973), *J. Embryol. exp. Morph.*, **29**, 618.

Kauffman, S. (1974), *Exp. Cell Res.*, **86**, 217.

Kauffman, S. (1975), In: Cell Paterning, *Ciba Foundation Symposium*, **29**, 201, Associated Science Publishers, Amsterdam.

Keeter, J.S., Pappas, G.D. and Model, P.G. (1975), *Dev. Biol.*, **45**, 21.

Kelley, R.O. and Fallon, J.F. (1976), *Dev. Biol.*, **51**, 243.

Lawrence, P.A. (1973), *J. Embryol. exp. Morph.*, **30**, 681.

Lawrence, P.A. and Green, S.M. (1975), *J. Cell Biol.*, **65**, 373.

Lawrence, P., Crick, F.H.C. and Munro, M. (1972), *J. Cell Sci.*, **11**, 815.

Lewis, J., Slack, J.M.W. and Wolpert, L. (1977), *J. Theor. Biol.*, (in press).

Loewenstein, W. (1977), *ICCB Symposia Papers*, (Brinkley, B.R. and Porter, K.R., eds.), Rockefeller University Press, New York (in press).

Lopresti, V., Macagno, E.R. and Levinthal, C. (1974), *Proc. natn. Acad. Sci., U.S.A.*, **71**, 1098.

Marchase, R.M., Barbera, R.J. and Roth, S. (1975), In: Cell Patterning, *Ciba Foundation Symposium.* Associated Science Publishers, Amsterdam.

McNutt, N.S. and Weinstein, R.S. (1974), *Prog. Biophys. molec. Biol.*, **26**, 45.

Miyazahi, S., Takahashi, K., Tsuda, K. and Yoshi, M. (1974), *J. Physiol.* **238**, 55.

Palmer, J.F. and Slack, C. (1970), *J. Embryol. exp. Morphol.*, **24**, 535.

Pardee, A.B. (1974), *Proc. natn. Acad. Sci., U.S.A.*, **71**, 1286.

Potter, D.D., Furshpan, E.J. and Lennox, E.S. (1966), *Proc. natn. Acad. Sci., U.S.A.*, **55**, 328.

Rash, J.E. and Staehelin, L.A. (1974), *Dev. Biol.*, **36**, 455.

Revel, J., Yip, P. and Chang, L.L. (1973), *Dev. Biol.*, **35**, 302.

Rose, S.M. (1970), *Am. Zool.*, **10**, 91.

Sanders, E.J. and Dicaprio, R.A. (1976), *Exp. Zool.*, **197**, 415.

Saunders, J.W. and Gasseling, M.T. (1963), *Dev. Biol.*, **7**, 64.

Saxén, L., Lehtonen, E., Kelainen, M.K., Nordling, S. and Waartiovoaara, L. (1976), *Nature,* **259,** 662.

Sengel, P. (1976), In: *Morphogenesis of Skin,* Cambridge University Press, Cambridge.

Sheridan, J.D. (1968), *J. Cell Biol.,* **37,** 650.

Sheridan, J.D. (1974), In: *The Cell Surface in Development* (Moscona, A.A., ed.), Wiley, New York.

Slack, C. and Palmer, J.P. (1969), *Exp. Cell Res.,* **55,** 416.

Slack, C. and Warner, A.E. (1975), *J. Physiol.,* **248,** 97.

Summerbell, D., Lewis, J.H. and Wolpert, L. (1973), *Nature,* **244,** 492.

Tickle, C., Summerbell, D. and Wolpert, L. (1975), *Nature,* **254,** 199.

Toivonen, S., Tarin, D. and Saxen, L. (1976), *Differentiation,* **5,** 49.

Tupper, J.T. and Saunders, J.W. (1972), *Dev. Biol.,* **27,** 546.

Turin, L. and Warner, A.E. (1977), personal communication.

Wakeford, R.J. (1975), Ph. D. Thesis. University of London.

Warner, A.E. (1973), *J. Physiol.* **235,** 267.

Warner, A.E. (1975), In: *Simple Nervous Systems,* (Newth, D.R. and Usherwood, P.N.R. eds.), Edward Arnold, London.

Warner, A.E. and Lawrence, P.A. (1973), *Nature,* **245,** 42.

Wilby, O.K. and Webster, G. (1970), *J. Embryol. exp. Morph.* **24,** 595.

Wolpert, L. (1971), *Curr. Top. Dev. Biol.,* **6,** 183.

Wolpert, L., Clarke, M.R.B. and Hornbruch, A. (1972), *Nature New Biol.,* **239,** 101.

Wolpert, L. and Gingell, D. (1969), In: Homeostatic Regulators *Ciba Foundation Symposium* (Wolstenholme, C.E.W. and Knight, J. eds.), Churchill, London.

6 The Chemical Synapse: Structure and Function

ANDREW MATUS

Acknowledgements
This essay has greatly benefited from the author's association with Drs D.H. Jones and **B.B.** Walters. Many of the issues raised have received more detailed discussion by them elsewhere (Jones, 1976; Walters, 1976). I am also grateful to the fellow investigators who generously provided material prior to publication.

6.1 INTRODUCTION

The correlation of synaptic structure and function has a venerable history beginning with the synapse itself. As envisaged by Sherrington (1897), the morphological basis of the physiologically defined synapse consisted of '. . . intercellular barriers, delicate transverse membranes'. When the application of electron microscopy to nervous tissue first revealed the details of synaptic morphology, it was immediately apparent that just such an arrangement was responsible for the essentially separate contact between the two synapsing neurons. Successive reviewers of synaptic ultrastructure covering nearly two decades (Palay, 1958; Gray and Guillery, 1966; Bloom, 1970; Pfenninger, 1973) have endorsed the belief that such suggestive modifications of cellular morphology as the synaptic vesicles and the elaborate specialised structures associated with the synaptic junctional membranes are functionally significant.

The progress that has been made during recent years has come mainly from two sources. First there has been the continuing analysis of synaptic ultrastructure by electron microscopic examination. This line of enquiry is now benefitting from the increasing use of new and improved techniques of tissue preparation among which freeze-fracture and the visualisation of uptake and binding sites by the use of marker molecules and autoradiography play an important part.

There has also been continuing refinement of the methodology available for the subcellular fractionation of brain tissue. Isolated intact synapses (synaptosomes) have now been subfractionated to provide enriched preparations of synaptic vesicles, plasma membranes and various junctional fragments each of which is the subject of both ultrastructural and biochemical analysis.

6.2 THE SYNAPTIC PLASMA MEMBRANES

The synaptic plasma membranes are those areas of the neuronal surface membrane which enclose the pre- and postsynaptic components of the synapse. They may be divided on ultrastructural and presumptive functional grounds into two major regions: the junctional and the extra-junctional. The junctional region is the presumed site of membrane-bound molecular mechanisms subserving many of the characteristic synaptic functions. Among these are individual steps in the process of synaptic transmission — the release of transmitter via the pre-synaptic membrane, its detection at the

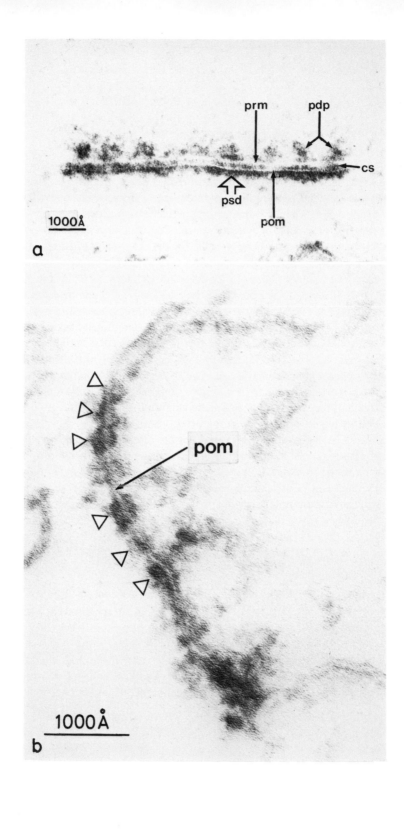

postsynaptic membrane, the subsequent generation of a change in the membrane's electrochemical properties and the final inactivation of the transmitter by enzymic interconversion or cellular re-uptake. Molecules embedded in the pre- and post-synaptic membranes are presumably involved in securing the junctional adhesion. It has often been proposed that surface marker molecules are responsible for encoding the specificity with which neurons in the developing brain establish appropriate synaptic connections (see for example Barondes, 1970) and these too may be present in the junctional membranes, at least during synapse formation.

The presence of macromolecules discharging these functions within the junctional membranes has yet to receive biochemical confirmation. However, the inferred functional complexity of the junctional region is also suggested by the concentration there of specialised membrane-associated structures which are not found elsewhere on the neuronal plasma membrane.

6.2.1 The ultrastructure of the synaptic junction

The specialised junctional structures are revealed as electron-dense elaborations of the apposed pre- and postsynaptic membranes (Gray, 1959; 1961). The exact appearance of these 'junctional densities' depends upon the fixative procedure and the combination of heavy metal stains used in preparing the tissue for electron micro-scopy. Their apparent structure has frequently been described and variously inter-preted (Van der Loos, 1963; De Robertis, 1964; Gray, 1966; Bloom *et al.,* 1970; Pfenninger, 1973).

There is general agreement that the junctional dense-staining material is disposed in three layers. Attached to the cytoplasmic face of the pre-synaptic junctional membrane are the pre-synaptic dense projections which are arranged in a trigonal array making up the pre-synaptic vesicular grid (Akert *et al.,* 1969). The interstices in this arrangement are about the size of synaptic vesicles, and Akert and his colleagues suggest that the whole structure may operate to organise the approach of the vesicles to the pre-synaptic membrane where they discharge their contents via attachment sites situated at the base of each gap between the projections (Pfenninger *et al.,* 1972, further discussed below).

Fig. 6.1 (a) A synaptic junction in the cerebral cortex of an adult rat stained with ethanolic phosphotungstic acid by the method of Bloom and Aghajanian (1966), cs, cleft substance; pdp, pre-synaptic dense projections; pom, post-synaptic unit membrane; prm, pre-synaptic unit membrane; psd, postsynaptic dense material.

Fig. 6.1 (b) A synaptic plasma membrane isolated from rat cerebral cortex. The presumed pre-synaptic side is to the right where wispy remnants of the dense projections remain, although most of this material is removed when the synapto-somes are lysed during subcellular fractionation. The remaining material, com-prising elements of the cleft substance and postsynaptic density, is disposed in discrete aggregations (open triangles) which appear to span the postsynaptic unit membrane (pom).

Attached to the cytoplasmic face of the postsynaptic membrane is another layer of dense-staining material which in thin sections of intact tissue appears as a continuous band. This is the postsynaptic density (Gray, 1959, 1961) which in some cases appears to be in continuity with more diffuse dense-staining material in the underlying cytoplasm which has been referred to as the subsynaptic web (De Robertis, 1964). Finally between the apposed synaptic membranes is the cleft substance whose structural appearance varies considerably after different preparative treatments. In most of the early studies in which simple osmium fixation was employed, a system of fibres crossing between, and presumably joining, the two membranes was described (Van der Loos, 1963; De Robertis, 1964; Gray, 1966). By contrast, fixation with glutaraldehyde and staining with phosphotungstic acid reveals an amorphous and apparently homogeneous material filling the synaptic cleft (Bloom and Aghajanian, 1966; Bloom, 1970). Staining with uranyl salts, particularly in combination with bismuth iodide, shows horizontal lines running parallel to the junctional membranes. There may be either one or two of these depending upon the exact preparative procedure employed (Pfenninger, 1973).

6.2.2 Comparative morphology of excitatory and inhibitory synapses

Gray's original investigation of the synaptic junctional structures with phosphotungstic acid staining revealed two major variations of the basic pattern, which he distinguished as type 1 and type 2 synapses (Gray, 1959). Type 1 synapses (also known as asymmetrical) have a prominent band of postsynaptic dense-staining material which is much less evident at type 2 (or symmetrical) synaptic junctions. Gray's additional suggestion that the synaptic cleft of type 1 junction is wider than that of type 2's has not been found to hold good in all parts of the central nervous system, but the distinction between two major categories of junction based on the appearance of the postsynaptic membrane specialisation has been confirmed by many subsequent studies (e.g. Colonier, 1968; Chan-Palay and Palay, 1970).

An additional distinction between the two classes of synapses which has now attained a convincing status is the morphological differentiation of the synaptic vesicles associated with them. It has been known for some years that vesicle populations at different synapses can be categorised as either spherical or 'flattened' in various ways (Pellegrino de Iraldi *et al.,* 1963; Dennison, 1971). It is now clear that spherical vesicles occur in synapses with asymmetrical junctions while 'flattened' vesicles (whatever the reason for their flattening, Valdivia, 1971) are associated with symmetrical junctions.

The functional significance of these two major categories of synapses has gradually emerged as correlations have been drawn between excitatory and inhibitory synaptic action and synaptic morphology in different parts of the nervous system. The original proposition that type 2 synapses are inhibitory and type 1 excitatory (Gray, 1963; Van der Loos, 1963; Eccles, 1964) was extended by Uchizono (1965) to encompass the distinction of spherical and flattened synaptic

Table 6.1 Comparative properties of type 1 and type 2 synapses

Type 1	Type 2	Reference
Postsynaptic material stained by uranyl and phospho-tungstate	Little stainable postsynaptic material	Gray, 1959, 1961
Stainable postsynaptic material does not bind concanavalin A	Unstained postsynaptic materials binds concanavalin A	Matus and Walters, 1976
Spherical pre-terminal vesicles	'Flattened' pre-terminal vesicles	Uchizono, 1965
80–90 Å particles present in postsynaptic junctional membrane	No junctional membrane particles	Landis *et al.* 1974
Postsynaptic junctional lattice present in isolated synaptic plasma membrane	No lattice structure detectable	Matus *et al.,* 1975a
Junctional adhesion less stable than type 2's	Junctional adhesion more stable than type 1's	Matus and Walters, 1976
Correlates with excitatory synaptic transmission	Correlates with inhibitory synaptic transmission	Gray, 1969

vesicles as further indicators of excitatory and inhibitory synapses respectively. In at least one case, a specific relationship between the high affinity uptake and storage of a known inhibitory transmitter substance (glycine) and pre-synaptic terminals containing flat vesicles has been desmonstrated (Matus and Dennison, 1971; 1972). These distinctions, summarised in Table 6.1, have been corroborated by subsequent studies (Gray, 1969; an extensive compilation may be found in Walters, 1976.

An absolute morphological distinction between physiologically identified excitatory and inhibitory synapses in the olfactory bulb and cerebellar cortex has been found by Landis and his colleagues (Landis *et al.,* 1974; Landis and Reese, 1974). In freeze-etched material from various species they found intramembranous particles associated with the postsynaptic junctional membrane of excitatory synapses which was absent from inhibitory synapses. There are in the region of 150–300 of these excitatory postsynaptic membranous particles in the external leaflet occupying an area co-extensive with the synaptic cleft i.e. they are limited to the junctional region of the postsynaptic membrane. Each of the particles is about 80–90 Å diameter.

Two types of synaptic junctions have also been recognised among synaptosomes (Matus and Walters, 1976). One class of synaptosomes has a junction with prominent postsynaptic dense-staining material and is apparently derived from type 1 synapses. The other type of synaptosome has little if any postsynaptic dense material and this together with the presence of flattened synaptic vesicles within its pre-terminal

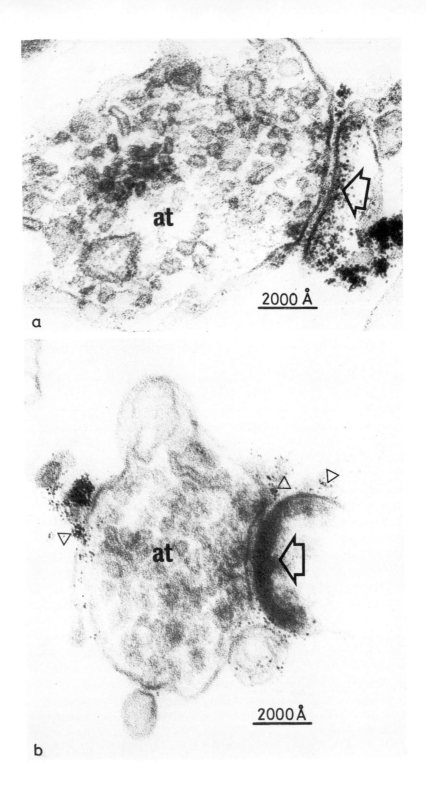

cytoplasm indicates that it originates from type 2 synapses. These two types of synaptosome are clearly distinguishable by the distribution of binding sites for the lectin concanavalin A (which binds to gluco- and mannopyrannoside residues in glycoproteins and glycolipids). The binding sites are revealed by the distribution of electron-opaque ferritin molecules of bound concanavalin A—ferritin conjugate (con A—FT). Con A—FT binding sites on both classes of synaptosomes are present on the external faces of the pre- and postsynaptic junctional and extra-junctional membranes (Matus *et al.*, 1973; Bittiger and Schnebli, 1974; Cotman and Taylor, 1974). Con A is not bound by the postsynaptic density of type 1 synaptosomes (Matus and Walters, 1976). However, subjacent to the postsynaptic membrane of presumptive type 2 synaptosomes (where there is almost no dense-staining material), con A—FT is found in a pattern which suggests that it is bound to a web of material attached to the postsynaptic junctional membrane (Fig. 6.2). As with the morphological data this also suggests that there are two distinct classes of synaptic junctions in the brain. Furthermore, the strikingly different distribution of membrane-bound carbohydrate residues between the two types strongly suggests that they differ significantly in their macromolecular structural components.

6.2.3 The postsynaptic junctional lattice

As will be evident from the foregoing discussion, brain subcellular fractions containing components of the synaptic structure provide a useful accessory method for analysing the ultrastructure of the synaptic membranes and junction (as well as their chemical composition). Most of the observations in this field have been made on type 1 synaptic fragments, for without the benefit of a marker ligand such as Con A—FT, type 2 synaptosomes are morphologically rather dull. Indeed it is difficult to be certain by straightforward electron microscopic examination that they are present in brain subcellular fractions (Matus *et al.*, 1975a).

Synaptic membranes derived from type 1 synapses are readily recognised by their postsynaptic dense material (Fig. 6.3). Close examination reveals that their junctional structure is different in several respects from that of type 1 junctions in intact tissue (Matus *et al.*, 1975a). In the isolated membranes the presynaptic dense projections are missing. This is best appreciated after fixation with glutaraldehyde

Fig. 6.2 Synaptosomes in the same 200 sq. μm field of a subcellular preparation from rat forebrain incubated for 30 minutes with ferritin-conjugated concanavalin A. The tissue was block stained with uranyl acetate; at, pre-synaptic terminal. (a) A synaptosome with type 2 morphology. Electron-opaque ferritin molecules mark concanavalin A binding sites on material attached to the cytoplasmic surface of the postsynaptic membrane (arrow). The material itself is uranyl acetate negative. (b) A synaptosome with type 1 morphology. The uranyl acetate stained postsynaptic density is devoid of concanavalin A binding sites. Ferritin marks such sites on the extra-junctional synaptic plasma membrane.

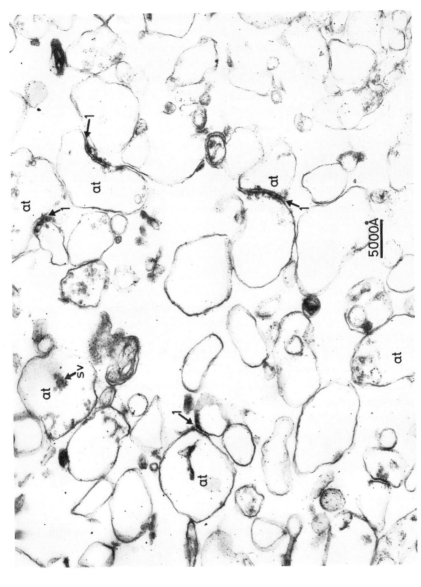

Fig. 6.3 A subcellular fraction enriched in synaptosomal plasma membranes made from rat forebrain. Lysed synaptosomes with type 1 synaptic junctions which lie within the plane of section are readily distinguishable (marked 1 with arrow). Other pre-synaptic terminals (at) are distinguished by residual synaptic vesicles (sv).

and osmium tetroxide (which allows visualisation of the plasma membranes) and staining with phosphotungstic acid which reliably reveals all three layers of junctional densities (Bloom and Aghajanian, 1966). When this is done the pre- and postsynaptic membranes can be identified and it is clear that at least part of both the postsynaptic dense-staining material and the cleft substance have survived the isolation procedure. However most, if not all, of the material attached to the cytoplasmic side of the pre-synaptic junctional membrane in intact tissue is absent from the isolated membranes. The pre-synaptic dense projections have apparently been washed from the membranes by the hypotonic buffer used to lyse the synaptosomes since they are present within intact synaptosomes.

Having established that the junctional structures in isolated synaptic membranes comprise elements of the postsynaptic material and the cleft substance they can be further examined by the glutaraldehyde-ethanolic phosphotungstic acid staining of Bloom and Aghajanian (1966). This has the advantage of providing a 'cleaner' ultrastructural appearance in which more detail may be discerned than when osmium tetroxide fixation is included with PTA staining. Omitting the osmium fixation has the effect of leaving the plasma membranes themselves unstained so that in intact tissue they are seen by negative contrast as electron-lucent lines running between the three electron-opaque bands of junctional structures (Fig. 6.1a). In the isolated membranes there are only two layers of junctional densities and hence only one electron-lucent unstained plasma membrane can be seen running between them (Fig. 6.1b).

Close examination of the cleft substance and postsynaptic material in these isolated membranes reveals that their appearance is not identical to that shown in intact tissue. Rather than appearing as continuous bands they both seem to consist of discrete deposits of PTA-stained material dotted along the postsynaptic plasma membrane (Fig. 6.1b). Furthermore the subunits that make up the cleft substance and the postsynaptic density occupy corresponding positions on either side of the postsynaptic plasma membrane giving a strong impression that each is a subunit which spans the postsynaptic membrane. Each of these subunits is about 200 Å in diameter.

Seen *en face* (Fig. 6.4) the subunits form a roughly regular array which we call the *postsynaptic junctional lattice* (Matus *et al.*, 1975a). The lattice does not seem to represent all the material present in the postsynaptic density and cleft substance at synapses in intact tissue. Much of this material appears to have been eluted from the postsynaptic membrane during the isolation procedure, (as have the pre-synaptic dense projections from the pre-synaptic junctional membrane). This reveals the postsynaptic junctional lattice as an underlying set of subunits tightly bound to the postsynaptic plasma membrane and, if the impression gained from ultrastructural appearances proves to be correct, traversing it.

What relationship the subunits of the postsynaptic junctional lattice bear to the intramembranous particles found in the postsynaptic membrane of excitatory synapses (Sandri *et al.*, 1972; Landis *et al.*, 1974; Landis and Reese, 1974) remains to be determined. The freeze-fracture revealed particles are much smaller (*circa* 80 Å)

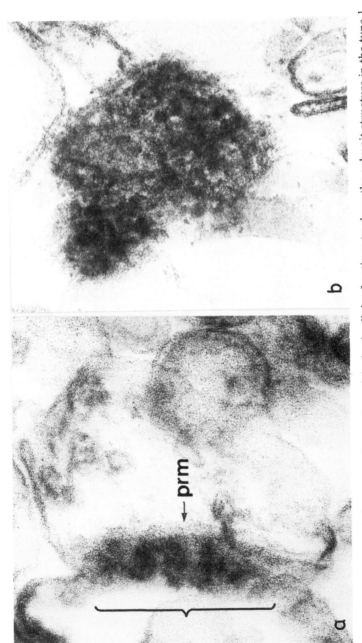

Fig. 6.4 Synaptosomal plasma membranes in enriched subcellular fractions to show the subunit structure in the type 1 postsynaptic junctional lattice. Samples block stained with uranyl acetate and grid stained with lead citrate. (a) A junction cut in cross-section but tilted in the electron beam by means of a goniometer stage to display the cytoplasmic face of the postsynaptic membrane. prm, presynaptic membranes; the bracket indicates the extent of the junctional region. (b) A junction cut *en face*. The junctional region is marked by an overall increase in density within which the denser subunits of the junctional lattice are distinguishable.

than the subunits of the postsynaptic junctional lattice (*circa* 200 Å). They may re-present a core region of the subunits — the portion which actually penetrates the unit membrane — or they may be non-identical laterally intercalated structures. The structure of the postsynaptic membrane as observed with currently available pre-parative techniques is insufficiently regular to allow the optical analysis that established the relationship between the pre-synaptic dense projections and the synaptopores (Pfenninger *et al.*, 1972).

6.2.4 Isolation of the postsynaptic junction lattice

When isolated synaptic plasma membranes are digested with selected ionic detergents their contained junctional dense-staining material is released intact (Cotman *et al.*, 1974; Walters and Matus, 1975a; Matus and Walters, 1975). A variety of features point to the identification of the detergent-insoluble residue with the junctional structures of undigested membranes. The characteristic staining specificity of uranyl salts and phosphotungstic acid is retained. The residue consists of discrete disc-shaped particles of dimensions similar to the overall size of the postsynaptic specialisation in SPM. Viewed *en face* (Fig. 6.5) they display the planar array of subunits which is characteristic of the postsynaptic junctional lattice. These isolated structures are only generated by detergent treatment of SPM— the same treatment applied to other subcellular particles such as mitochondria and myelin fragments does not produce them (Cotman *et al.*, 1974; Matus, unpublished observations). A derivative relationship of the isolated postsynaptic junctional lattices from SPM is also suggested by similarities in the polypeptide components of the two subcellular fractions (see below).

The most interesting feature of the isolated junctional material is the survival of the lattice-like lateral interconnection between the subunit particles after the removal of the plasma unit membrane in which they are embedded. The significance of this interaction will be discussed in combination with evidence presented below regarding the structure of the extra-junctional synaptic membrane and the chemical identity of the major component of the isolated lattice.

6.2.5 Molecular components of the synaptic plasma membranes

The cytochemistry of the synaptic junctional structure
The selective cytochemical staining of the synaptic junctional structures by both anionic (phosphotungstate) and cationic (uranyl) heavy metal species has been thought to indicate the presence of both acidic and basic residues (Bloom *et al.*, 1970, but see Churchill *et al.*, 1976). It also seems that these residues are component parts of proteins since staining of all the junctional structures is markedly reduced by prior treatment of the tissue with proteolytic enzymes (Bloom and Aghajanian, 1968; Barrantes and Lunt, 1970; Pfenninger, 1971, Cotman and Taylor, 1972).

The application of various staining procedures for carbohydrate has shown that it is particularly concentrated within the synaptic cleft (Pease, 1966; Rambourg and

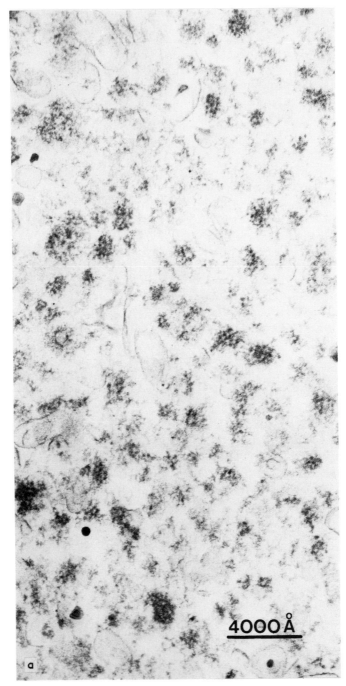

4000 Å

a

Fig. 6.5 Isolated type 1 synaptic junctional lattices in an enriched fraction obtained by digesting a synaptosomal plasma membrane-enriched fraction with sodium deoxycholate. The isolated junctional lattice appear as discrete

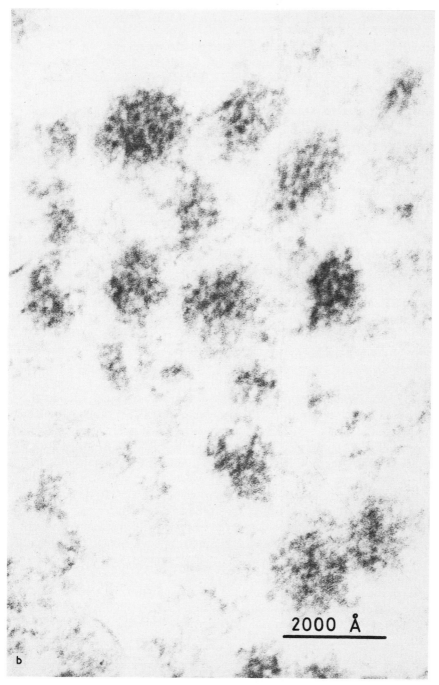

2000 Å

Fig. 6.5 (*continued*) flat rigid discs composed of uranyl acetate stained subunits (compare the appearance of those in (b) to the *en face* view of the
junction shown in Fig. 6.4b).

Leblond, 1967; Rambourg, 1969). A portion of these sugar residues are evidently conjugated to sialic acid since the staining within the cleft by uranyl and lead salts is reduced by prior treatment with neuraminidase. (Bondareff and Sjostrand, 1969).

Chemical analysis of isolated synaptic plasma membranes

As indicated by ultrastructural and cytochemical evidence the isolated synaptic membranes consist of lipids making up the unit membrane, protein which is particularly concentrated in the junctional region, and carbohydrate probably in the form of glycoprotein and glycolipid.

The lipid composition of SPM and isolated synaptic vesicles has been a frequent subject of investigation (Eichberg *et al.*, 1964; Cotman *et al.*, 1969; Brackenridge *et al.*, 1972, 1973; Morgan *et al.*, 1973a). The lipid to protein ratio of synaptic vesicles is higher than that of SPM which is probably a reflection as the latter's content of proteinaceous junctional structures. Vesicles are very low in gangliosides (Breckenridge *et al.*, 1973) whereas these are highly concentrated in the synaptic membranes. The high level of lipid sialic acid in SPM is apparently so characteristic that it is considered an effective marker (Morgan *et al.*, 1973a) as is the intrinsic neuraminindase activity which accompanies it (Tettamanti *et al.*, 1971). A feature of both membranes is their low content of lysolecithin (see also Pearse, 1975) so that the ability of this molecule to induce membrane fusion (Lucy, 1970) is apparently not a potential mechanism subserving presumptive exocytotic fusion of vesicular and synaptic plasma membranes.

Synaptic plasma membrane proteins have been characterised by electrophoretic fractionation in the presence of sodium dodecyl sulphate (SDS) as a solubilising agent. Using proteins of known molecular weights to construct a standard graph this system can be used to obtain reproducible estimates of the molecular weights of unknown proteins (Weber and Osborn, 1969; Neville, 1971). Notable exceptions to this are proteins with substantial carbohydrate moieties which do not bind SDS leading to anomalous electrophoretic behaviour of glycoproteins (Bretscher; 1971; Banker and Cotman, 1972). Nevertheless, molecular weights computed from comparative electrophoretic mobilities have been widely employed to characterise membrane proteins. In the case of synaptic plasma membranes the similar values arrived at by different investigators indicate that the practice is acceptable providing that the molecular weights quoted are regarded as operationally defined.

In general, the proteins of SPM have a higher range of molecular weights than those of either myelin or mitochondria. Most investigators recognise three major SPM proteins (see Table 6.2) whose mean molecular weights from the various estimations are 99 300, 52 300, 43 000. Identities for these polypeptides have been suggested based upon the similarity of their molecular weights to those of protein chains having a known association with plasma membranes. The least well-established identity is that of the 99 300 component which is suggested to be the major subunit of the Na^+/K^+-ATPase (Morgan *et al.*, 1973). These workers also suggest that the 52 300 component is another subunit of this enzyme, but other evidence favours

Table 6.2 Computed molecular weights of major synaptic membrane proteins*

References	Reported molecular weights of 3 major polypeptide components (dalton x 10^{-3})		
Banker and Cotman, 1972 source: rat	99	52.4	41.5
Morgan *et al.*, 1973b source: rat	93	52	39
Wannaker and Kornguth, 1973 source: pig	97	53	43
Karlsson *et al.*, 1973 source: rabbit	95	52	44
Gurd *et al.*, 1974 source: rat	93	52	
Walters and Matus[†], 1975b source: pig	100	53	
Jones, 1976[‡] source: rat	110	54	46
Walters, 1976[†] source: rat	107	50.3	43.8

* Modified from Jones, 1976

[†] The values quoted by Walters (1976) are preferred to those earlier arrived at (Walters and Matus, 1975b) being based on a revised choice of molecular weight markers.

[‡] Differences in values arrived at by Jones (1976) and Walters (1976) reflect choice of molecular weight markers and reproducible procedural variations.

the view that most of the material migrating in this zone is membrane-associated tubulin (see below). This is supported by the co-migration of added microtubule-derived tubulin with this peak. Similarly, added muscle actin co-migrates with the 43 000 dalton peak (co-migration data from Walters and Matus, 1975b). These tentative identifications do not exclude the possibility that other polypeptide species may co-migrate in the same zone as the suggested candidates.

Proteins of the synaptic junction

The treatment of SPM with either sodium *n*-lauroyl sarcosinate or sodium deoxy-cholate results in the solubilisation of about 97% of the synaptic membrane protein (Banker *et al.*, 1974; Walters and Matus, 1975a). The morphological similarity of the two preparations (see above) is further reflected in their contained polypeptides as revealed by electrophoretic separation (compare Fig. 1 in Banker *et al.*, 1974 with Fig. 1c of Walters and Matus, 1975b and Fig. 1b of Walters and Matus, 1975c). Both the deoxycholate- and sarcosinate-derived postsynaptic junctional structures have a major polypeptide whose mobility corresponds to that for microtubule-derived tubulin in the electrophoretic systems employed. The computed molecular weights for the less prominent polypeptide components of the isolated junctional structures in both cases occupy a higher range than do polypeptides in the SPM from which they were derived. However there are appreciable differences in the minor polypeptides of the preparations obtained with the two detergents. The sarcosinate-derived

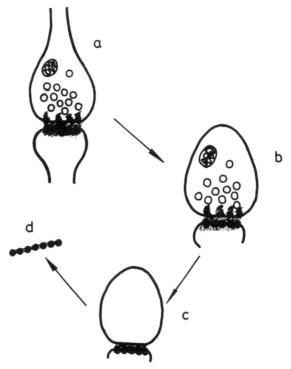

Fig. 6.6 Diagrammatic representation of the successive events in the isolation of the type 1 postsynaptic junctional lattice. (a) Synapse in whole brain tissue. (b) Synaptosome with intact junction. (c) Synaptosomal plasma membrane obtained by hypotonic lysis. The pre-synaptic dense projections and material loosely attached to the post-synaptic specialisation have been removed during this step. (d) The isolated lattice consisting of subunits bound laterally to one another, obtained by digesting the lipid unit membrane of the synaptosomal membranes with detergent.

material contains a prominent component with a computed molecular weight of about 98 000 daltons. In the deoxycholate residue there is only a relatively minor peak at the position corresponding to this apparent molecular weight. On the other hand the deoxycholate-derived postsynaptic junctional lattices contain a prominent component with a computed molecular weight of 62 200 daltons at which position Banker *et al.,* (1974) do not identify a band in the sarcosinate-derived postsynaptic densities.

All of the polypeptides present in the deoxycholate-produced junctional lattice are present in the original SPM further emphasising the derivative relationship of the former to the latter previously inferred from their ultrastructure and cytochemical properties. Some of the SPM proteins are absent from the junctional lattice. The most striking absentees are the prominent SPM polypeptides with apparent molecular weights of 107 000 daltons (? Na$^+$/K$^+$-ATPase) and 43 800 daltons (the actin co-migratory peak). Other components such as those with calculated molecular weights of 183 000 and 62 200 daltons show the same relative abundance in the junctional lattice as in the undigested SPM. At present it is not possible to decide whether this reflects a true evenness of distribution or a fortuitous consequence of the particular preparative procedure employed. Still other proteins of the synaptic plasma membranes are enriched in the isolated lattice structure — the major junctional tubulin-comigrating polypeptide by 3.6-fold on a mol % basis (Walters, 1976).

Tubulin-like properties of the major junctional protein

Both Banker *et al.,* (1974) and Walters and Matus (1975b) recognised the similarity of the electrophoretically determined molecular weight of the major postsynaptic junctional polypeptide to that of tubulin, the major subunit protein of microtubules. Together with J. Lagnado and L.P. Tan we established that the major junctional protein split into two components when electrophoresed in the presence of urea, as does tubulin and that these were phosphorylated in the same manner as tubulin (unpublished results quoted in Walters and Matus, 1975b).

To investigate further this apparent similarity, the tubulin-co-migratory protein from synaptosomal plasma membranes, postsynaptic junctional lattices and electro-phoretically purified microtubular tubulin were compared by peptide mapping. The peptide maps from all three proteins were strikingly similar indicating a close correspondence in their primary structures (Walters and Matus, 1975c). A similar correspondence between the peptide maps of tubulin and the tubulin-co-migratory polypeptide of synaptosomal plasma membranes has also been found by Kornguth and Sunderland (1975). The correspondence between peptide maps of microtubule tubulin and isolated postsynaptic junctional structures has been confirmed for sarcosinate-derived material (Feit *et al.,* 1976).

To obtain a further confirmation of the presence of tubulin-like protein at the synaptic junction an antiserum against electrophoretically purified microtubule tubulin was raised and used to locate tubulin antigen in sections of intact brain tissue by immunoperoxidase histochemistry (Matus *et al.,* 1975b; Walters and Matus, 1975c). The antitubulin serum stained brain microtubules and the post-synaptic densities of brain synapses (Fig. 6.7). There is thus present in the structure of the postsynaptic specialisations of brain synapses a protein which is strikingly similar to microtubular tubulin in both the primary structure of its polypeptide chains and in its antigenicity.

The tryptic digest peptide maps of detergent-derived postsynaptic junctions are very similar but not identical to those of microtubule tubulin (Walters and Matus, 1975c; Feit *et al.,* 1976). This may indicate that they are similar rather than identical proteins — perhaps belonging to a familial group of tubulin-like proteins. On the other hand the dissimilarities may be the result of minor protein components co-migrating along with junctional tubulin during electrophoresis. This possibility also emerges from the results of Feit *et al.,* (1976) who were able to resolve the

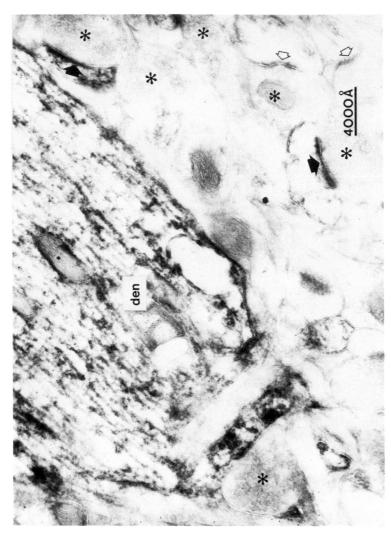

Fig. 6.7 Electron micrograph of rat cerebral cortex tissue immunohistochemically stained by the peroxidase method with an antiserum raised against electrophoretically purified tubulin. Microtubules in a dendrite (den) are stained. The post-synaptic membrane of some synapses are stained by this method (black arrows). Other synaptic junctions are not so stained (open arrows). This material was fixed with glutaraldehyde and formaldehyde followed by osmium tetroxide but was not heavy metal-stained. Asterisks identify pre-synaptic terminals.

tubulin-co-migratory junctional protein into four components by gradient gel electrophoresis. However, their peptide maps were prepared from a combination of the four polypeptides and despite their differing electrophoretic mobilities this produced a peptide map closely similar to that of the two polypeptides of microtubular tubulin. An intriguing possibility suggested by Feit *et al.* is that the subtle differences between the major junctional polypeptides and those of microtubular tubulin are the result of post-translational modification of the polypeptide structure.

6.3 MOLECULAR ORGANISATION IN THE SYNAPTIC PLASMA MEMBRANES

6.3.1 The extrajunctional membrane

Studies on unassociated cells have established that many membrane-bound components are able to move readily within the plane of the membrane. To discover whether this fluid mosaic structure (Singer and Nicolson, 1972) is also apparent in the plasma membranes of cells in complex tissues, we studied the distribution of glycoconjugates which act as receptors for Con A-FT in the surfaces of brain subcellular fractions (Matus *et al.*, 1973). In both the extrajunctional synaptosomal plasma membrane and in myelin membranes Con A-FT binding sites are initially randomly distributed. However they can readily be induced to aggregate into

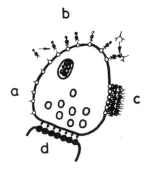

Fig. 6.8 Diagrammatic representation of evidence suggesting the fluidity of the extrajunctional synaptic plasma membrane. (a) Membrane-bound glycoconjugates are randomly distributed in the membrane. (b) A ferritin-conjugated lectin is added which binds to the glycoconjugate. Anti-ferritin serum is added as a bi-functional cross-linking reagent. (c) The ferritin molecules aggregate which indicates that since they were bound via the lectin to the membrane-bound glycoconjugate, the membrane-bound component must be able to move laterally within the plane of the membrane. (d) Junctional lectin-receptors do not aggregate under these circumstances, they are apparently part of a rigid molecular array in the postsynaptic junctional surface.

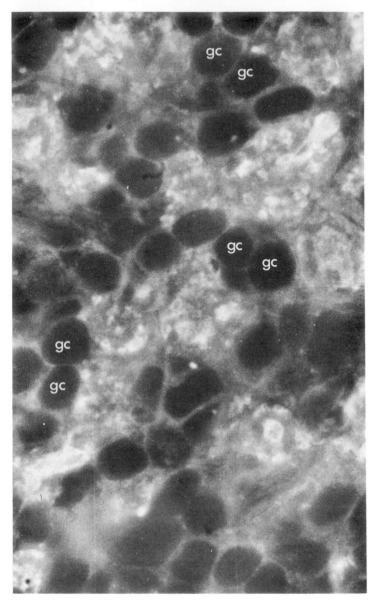

Fig. 6.9 A cryostat section of rat cerebellar cortex treated with an antiserum raised against cerebellar synaptosomal plasma membranes in an immuno-fluorescence procedure. In the granule cell layer shown here, bright fluorescent ring-like structures are distinguishable in the synaptic glomeruli whose size and distribution suggests that they are mossy fibre endings. Pre-terminal axon segments and non-synaptic regions of dendrites within the glomeruli do not appear to have been stained. The neuronal surface membranes of granule cell perikarya (gc) are also unstained.

patches when a bi-functional linkage agent (anti-ferritin) is introduced. Evidently the glycoconjugates to which the Con A-FT binds have a high lateral mobility within the membrane structure.

The aggregation of Con A receptors shows that the extrajunctional membrane is fluid in the sense proposed by Singer and Nicolson (1972) but there is also evidence that other membrane-bound components have restricted mobility (Matus *et al.*, 1975c; Rostas and Jeffery, 1975). Antisera raised against isolated SPM can be used to stain sections of brain tissue immunohistochemically. In adult brain the staining is specifically associated with the synaptic surface membrane – this can be clearly resolved as annular fluorescent rings of synaptic dimensions in brain regions where very large synapses occur such as the mossy fibre endings in the cerebellar cortex (Fig. 6.9; see also Matus *et al.*, 1975c). This shows that some antigens situated in the extrajunctional synaptic surface are limited to the synaptic region of the neuronal membrane in intact tissue.

Thus, although the synaptic membrane is basically constructed on a fluid mosaic plant it is possible to distinguish within it two further levels of supramolecular organisation. One of these is the apparently rigid molecular array of the postsynaptic junctional surface discussed in Section 6.3.2 below. The other is a restraint operating in the extrajunctional region of the synaptic membrane to restrict the movement of certain synaptic surface antigens so that they remain within the area of plasma membrane enclosing the components of the synapse. However this extrajunctional region, although it is partitioned from the rest of the neuronal plasma membrane, does not have the rigid structure characteristic of the junctional region for certain of its surface-bound components enjoy considerable lateral mobility.

The mechanism by which the regionally restricted extrajunctional surface antigens become inserted into the synaptic surface during development is also suggestive of their sequestration from the non-synaptic neuronal surface. The appearance of synaptic surface antigen during development has been studied by using an antiserum against isolated SPM as an immunohistochemical stain. Applied to neonatal rat brain the synaptic surface antigen first appears in the cytoplasm of perikarya and neuronal processes at about the time of onset of the major period of synapse formation (Matus and Jones, 1976). As mature synapses are formed the characteristic pattern of synaptic surface staining gradually emerges while anti-SPM staining disappears from the cytoplasm of neuronal processes. The time course of this process suggests that the synaptic surface antigen which the antiserum reveals is synthesised in the cell body and transported cytoplasmically to the synapse where it is inserted into the surface membrane. It does not appear at any stage to be a component part of the non-synaptic neuronal plasma membrane.

The mechanism by which this restricted distribution of synaptic surface antigen is achieved has yet to be investigated. In a recent review of evidence relating to the restriction of the lateral mobility of surface receptors in various cellular systems Nicolson (1976) distinguished a variety of possible subservient molecular mechanisms. These may be broadly grouped as (a) planar aggregations of protein or lipid (b) lipid domain in formation within which particular proteins may be sequestered or excluded (c) coupling by peripheral membrane components which link together intrinsic membrane components (d) cytoskeletal components, i.e. polymeric molecular forms such as actin filaments and microtubules which are envisaged as anchored in the cytoplasm and bound to membrane components thus restricting their mobility. A succinct diagrammatic exposition of these alternatives is given in Fig. 2 of Nicolson (1976). Any of them singly or in combination appears compatible with present information regarding the structure and molecular components of the synaptic membrane.

Molecular organisation in the synaptic junction
In contrast to the fluidity of the extrajunctional region, components bound within the postsynaptic junctional membrane appear to be part of a rigid molecular array. For example Con A-FT binding sites on the postsynaptic junctional surface do not aggregate, suggesting that the junctional glycoconjugates to which the Con A binds do not possess the lateral mobility evident in their extrajunctional counterparts (Cotman and Taylor, 1974; Bittiger and Schnebli, 1974; Matus and Walters, 1976).

The rigidity of the postsynaptic junctional structure is also suggested by its retention of a recognisable morphology when the lipid unit membrane in which it is embedded is solubilised by detergents (Cotman *et al.,* 1974; Matus and Walters, 1975). It remains to be determined just how specific are the molecular interactions responsible for preserving the structural detail. Since the isolated junctions are soluble in SDS (used to allow their electrophoretic separation, Banker *et al.,* 1974; Walters and Matus, 1975b) covalent bonds between individual macromolecular components are evidently not involved. At the other extreme it is possible that the association of the junctional macromolecules is mediated simply by hydrophobic interaction. However two observations make this seem unlikely: (a) without some specificity of interaction to provide guidance in establishing contiguity relationships it is difficult to envisage how molecular associations implied by functional necessity (e.g. between transmitter receptor and iontophore) could be achieved; (b) the structural differentiation of the postsynaptic junctional structure into lattice subunits suggests that its molecular components do participate in specific interactions.

The role of tubulin in the postsynaptic junctional structure
It is now clear that tubulin-like polypeptides are substantial components of the synaptic plasma membranes (Blitz and Fine, 1974; Kornguth and Sunderland, 1975) and constitute the major protein complement of the type 1 postsynaptic junctional structure (Walters and Matus, 1975c; Feit *et al.,* 1976).

Despite the fact that tubulin-like material makes up so large a part of synaptic membrane and junctional structure, conventional electron microscopic preparations fails to reveal microtubular profiles at either site. However it cannot be lightly concluded from this that microtubules are absent *in vivo.* Using immunohistochemical staining with an antiserum against tubulin we have found tubulin antigen

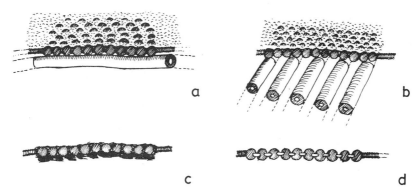

Fig. 6.10 Diagrammatic representation of various possible hypothetical relationships of tubulin molecules to the postsynaptic junctional membrane. The various elements are drawn roughly to scale. (a) Intact microtubules are applied to the cytoplasmic surface of the postsynaptic junctional lattice. This arrangement is not seen by conventional fixation of the synapse and if it exist then the microtubules here must be more susceptible to structural disruption than those in the dendritic cytoplasm. (b) The elements of the postsynaptic lattice act as attachment points for dendritic microtubules. (c) Tubulin is bound to the lattice subunits but is not in a self-assembled discrete structural form. (d) Tubulin molecules, possibly in oligomeric arrays, act as linkage elements forming an intrinsic part of the lattice and binding the subunits one to another.

not only in the postsynaptic 'density' but also as amorphous deposits in the cytoplasm of dendritic spines (Matus *et al.*, 1975b, see Fig. 6.7). This latter material may be derived from inadequately preserved microtubules providing a means of continuity between the microtubular systems of the dendrite and the cytoplasmic face of the postsynaptic junctional membrane. At least part of the postsynaptic junctional tubulin might then represent microtubular attachment points (Matus *et al.*, 1975b).

Such an arrangement has recently been visualised by Westrum and Gray (1976) using Gray's hypotonic albumin fixation technique (further discussed below). Tissue prepared in this way shows microtubules abutting postsynaptic sites in the rat neocortex in precisely the manner suggested to us by the pattern of anti-tubulin staining. Westrum and Gray (1976) themselves suggest that at least part of the postsynaptic thickening is 'derived from the debris of *in vivo* microtubules'.

This kind of relationship between microtubules and the postsynaptic junctional membrane is an accordance with one interpretation of the many observations that a system possessing the pharmacological properties of tubulin is responsible for organising the disposition of membrane-bound components on various cellular surfaces. In this scheme the evidence is interpreted as indicating that cytoplasmic microtubules are linked to the cytoplasmic segment of transmembrane macromolecules whose surface determinants are those which are observed to be under the control of a tubulin-like system, (see review by Nicolson, 1976).

There is however an alternative interpretation of the role of tubulin in organising cell surface determinants. It is contained in the phrase 'molecular linkage element' introduced by Berlin *et al*, (1974) and it implies that the tubulin, while binding to other membrane macromolecules, is not itself extensively polymerised as it is in microtubules. The adoption of this interpretation is favoured by the absence of microtubular profiles in the isolated postsynaptic junctional structures. If tubulin-like molecular linkage elements are involved in directing the disposition of surface components of neurons as they are in other cell types, then they would be expected to be particularly concentrated in highly ordered areas such as the postsynaptic junctional lattice (Walters and Matus, 1975a). It is of course possible that junctional tubulin molecules act both as linkage elements maintaining the organisation of lattice elements within the fluid plasma membrane and as attachment sites for cytoplasmic microtubules.

Molecular components of developing synaptic membranes

During synaptogenesis in the rat neocortex the tubulin-like component of the developing synaptic membranes undergoes an early increase. This ceases quite early in the synaptogenic period whereas other components of the mature membranes continue to undergo a steady increase. We have tentatively suggested that this early insertion of tubulin into the presumptive synaptic membranes may be associated with the establishment of a basic junctional structure such as we have envisaged the postsynaptic junctional lattice to be (Matus and Walters, 1975). The establishment of the lattice-like array of subunits would effectively define a synaptic locus within the neuronal surface and provide a basic molecular framework into which other molecules of the postsynaptic junction could then be inserted.

Possible involvement of carbohydrates in junction formation

The existance of protein and lipid-bound carbohydrate at cell surfaces has been a powerful stimulus to speculation regarding their possible involvement in determining the specificity of cellular relationships within tissues. The concentration of carbohydrate residues within the synaptic cleft, coupled with the exquisite specificity that neurons display in adopting functionally appropriate synaptic connections, provides an additional inducement to search for carbohydrate-mediated interactions subserving the establishment and maintainence of synaptic junctions. Hypothetical schemes which have been proposed implicate enzyme-mediated forging of trans-synaptic oligosaccharide bonds or lectin-like interaction between membrane-bound components (Barondes, 1970; Cotman and Banker, 1974). Little progress has been made in identifying such carbohydrate surface determinants, largely because different populations of synapses, whose connective specificity might involve different surface markers, have not been separately available for comparative analysis.

Recently, two promising approaches have been investigated. Cotman and his colleagues (Churchill *et al.,* 1976) have studied both the carbohydrate composition of glycoprotein components of isolated synaptic junctional preparations, and the binding of isotopically labeled sugars by synaptic junction-enriched fractions. Synaptic plasma membranes, triton X-100-derived junctional complexes, and *n*-lauroyl sarcosinate-derived postsynaptic densities were found to contain mannose, galactose, glucosamine, *N*-acetylneuraminic acid, galactosamine and fucose in addition to glucose. Each of the preparations had about the same level of protein-bound carbohydrate but the synaptic plasma membrane had in addition a substantial glycolipid content, 40% of the membrane carbohydrate being chloroform/methanol extractable. *N*-acetylneuraminic acid was less concentrated in the synaptic junctional complex fraction than in the untreated membranes. This presumably correlates with the extraction of lipid by detergent treatment. Galactose was enriched in the two junctional preparations compared to the original membrane, and mannose was greatly enriched in the postsynaptic junctional density fraction. Glucose was also apparently much enriched in the junctional fractions, although it proved difficult to chose between integral component sugar and binding of hydrolysed sucrose monosaccharide to account for this phenomenon. Certainly the junctional fractions showed progressively higher specific binding of both glucose and sucrose than the synaptic membranes from which they were derived. Other sugars showed different enrichments in binding to the junctional fractions. Fucose binding was markedly enriched in junctions whereas mannose binding was not. Churchill *et al.* point to these differences in binding as possibly indicative of lectin-like interaction involved in the formation and maintenance of synaptic connections. However the practical problem that this approach faces is the heterogeneity of synaptic membrane preparations made from gross brain samples. This means that they contain material from many different classes of synapse and so, by representing an average carbohydrate content, they may mask the carbohydrate specificities which would be expected to occur in individual classes of synapses if the postulated involvement in nerve cell interaction does indeed exist.

A strong indication of the existance of such differences has been obtained by Pfenninger and his colleagues (Pfenninger and Rees, 1976; Pfenninger and Maylie-Pfenninger, 1976). They have grown neurons of different types from rat embryos in culture and studied the binding to their growth cone surfaces of lectins with different carbohydrate specificities. They find that the growth cones of superior cervical ganglion cells bind high levels of wheat germ agglutinin (specific for *N*-acetylglucosamine) and ricin (specific for galactose). Spinal cord growth cones bind concanavalin A (specific for glucose and mannose) most heavily and bind very little ricin. Dorsal root ganglia also bind relatively little ricin but bind wheat germ agglutinin heavily. None of the cultures tested bound fucose-specific lotus seed lectin, so the results of Pfenninger *et al.* and Churchill *et al.* are not at this stage mutually supporting. Nevertheless these studies strongly imply that surface carbohydrate-mediated interactions do occur in the nervous system, and demonstrate the feasibility of their investigation.

6.4   CYTOPLASMIC ORGANELLES

6.4.1 Synaptic vesicles and transmitter release

The small vesicles in the terminal cytoplasm of synapses constitute one of their most striking and characteristic features (Palade, 1954; Palay, 1954; De Robertis and Bennet, 1955). Their discovery coincided with the recognition that transmitter release at the neuromuscular junction is quantised (Fatt and Katz, 1952; del Castillo and Katz, 1954). The correlation between the electrophysiological and ultrastructural observations led in stages to the development of the idea that transmitter is stored in the vesicles (del Castillo and Katz, 1956, 1957). These ideas have become known as the *'vesicle hypothesis'* and a variety of experimental evidence has been produced most, but not all, of which support its conclusions.

Evidence from transmitter storage and release
It is clear from many studies that isolated vesicles obtained by subcellular fractionation do contain bound transmitter substance (Michaelson *et al.*, 1963; De Robertis *et al.*, 1963; Whittaker *et al.*, 1964; Maynert *et al.*, 1964) but it is not agreed that it is this vesicular transmitter which is released when the axon terminal is stimulated. Birks and MacIntosh (1961) distinguished two compartments of releasable acetylcholine at terminals in the superior cervical ganglion. The smaller compartment contains the transmitter in a 'readily releasable' form, while the remainder forms the 'reserve pool' which feeds into the 'readily releasable' compartment to replenish it, maintaining a steady potential release rate. These observations seem to demand either that part of the acetylcholine be within the vesicles and part be in the extravesicular cytoplasm, or that there be two classes of vesicles, one active in transmitter release, the other serving only as a transmitter storage site.

Dunant *et al.*, (1972) studied the release of acetylcholine from *Torpedo* electric tissue, distinguishing between 'bound' and 'free' transmitter, the 'bound' form being apparently equivalent to the vesicular compartment (Marchbanks and Israël, 1971) . Upon stimulation there was an initial fall in the concentration of 'free' acetylcholine while the 'bound' transmitter fell only when stimulation was prolonged. In a variety of tissues (superior cervical ganglion: Collier and MacIntosh, 1969; diaphragm: Potter, 1970; cerebral cortex: Marchbanks, 1969) it has been demonstrated that newly synthesised acetylcholine is preferentially released upon stimulation. Since choline acetyltransferase is a soluble enzyme (Fonnum, 1967) the transmitter is presumably synthesised in the cytoplasm, and so the preferential release of newly synthesised molecules has been taken as suggesting that they originate from an extra-vesicular pool (Marchbanks, 1975). Preferential release of newly synthesised noradrenaline from stimulated splenic nerves has been reported (Kopin *et al.*, 1968), so this phenomenon is not an idiosyncracy of the cholinergic synapse.

The adrenergic system provides at least one item of apparently unshakable pharmacological evidence in favour of the vesicular hypothesis. In adrenergic neurons vesicles contain the soluble proteins chromogranin A and dopamine-β-hydroxylase, and these are released when the nerves are stimulated (Smith, 1971). It is difficult to see how the release of proteins could be accomplished other than by exocytosis and presumably the noradrenaline which is simultaneously released emerges exocytotically.

Evidence from synaptic morphology

Another line of investigation has sought to correlate the stimulated release of transmitter with morphological changes within the pre-synaptic terminal. This type of study has been successful not only in demonstrating dynamic structural changes at stimulated synapses, but also because it has placed an emphasis on understanding hitherto unappreciated details of synaptic ultrastructure. Some of the earliest of these studies utilised agents which when applied to the neuromuscular junction cause cascades of miniature endplate potentials which decay to leave the nerve terminal in a state where transmitter stores are apparently depleted, stimulation often being ineffective in causing transmitter release. Both lanthanum ions (Heuser and Miledi, 1971) and black widow spider venom (Longenecker et al., 1970) produce this effect, and in both cases the morphological consequences of the treatment are a striking loss of synaptic vesicles from the endings (Heuser and Miledi, 1971; Clark et al., 1970).

The physiological effects of these agents are obviously bizarre and later studies have examined the morphological consequences of controlled electrical stimulation at rates comparable to those found *in vivo*. At the neuromuscular junction constant stimulation for periods from one minute upward produces a progressive decrease in the numbers of vesicles per ending which is accompanied by an increase in area of the axon terminal membrane (Cecarelli et al., 1973; Heuser and Reese, 1973). There is some difference of opinion regarding the consequences of this type of treatment in the autonomic nervous system. Stimulation of the sympathetic chain has been reported to produce a reduction of the number of vesicles per ending in the superior cervical ganglion (Pysh and Wyley, 1974; Birks, 1974) but conditions used by Birks produce little or no depletion of transmitter in the ganglion. In fact in a variety of tissue the measured rate of acetylcholine synthesis is sufficient to maintain the store during stimulation at rates much greater than those found physiologically (Birks and MacIntosh, 1961; Potter, 1970). Thus the observation of vesicle depletion by modest stimulus rates would seem to suggest that vesicular volume and stored transmitter levels are uncorrelated.

Recent investigations using the freeze-fracture technique have revealed specialisations of the presynaptic junction membrane which are suggestive of stimulus-coupled exocytosis at this site. The structures concerned are small (*circa* 200 Å) protuberances which appear as invaginations of the plasma membrane directed toward the terminal cytoplasm. They are sometimes open at their uppermost end and these openings can occasionally be seen to communicate with the interior of synaptic vesicles (Pfenninger et al., 1972). Furthermore, the protuberances occupy

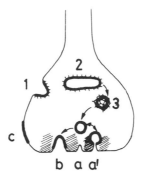

Fig. 6.11 Two alternative views of the vesicle hypothesis of transmitter release, shown diagrammatically. Vesicle membrane is shown as a thick line throughout. (a) The resting state, vesicle in cytoplasm. The cycle begins with the induction of a vesicle attachment site (VAS) as a small invagination in the pre-synaptic membrane. (a') The synaptopore hypothesis suggests that the vesicle fuses transitorily with the VAS and that a channel is formed between vesicle interior and the extracellular space of the synaptic cleft. Following the release of the transmitter the attachment breaks and the vesicle is released directly back into the preterminal cytoplasm as at (a). (b) The recycling hypothesis suggests that transmitter release proceeds by exocytosis, the vesicle completely fusing with the pre-synaptic membrane (c). The vesicle membranes is recovered by micropinocytosis, budding off from the plasma membrane as a coated pit (1), to form a coated *cisterna* (2), which breaks down to form coated vesicles (3), which in turn are released from coats to reform synaptic vesicles (a).

interstices in the pre-synaptic grid of dense projections (see above) where it is known that vesicles approach the pre-synaptic membrane (Akert *et al.*, 1969). On the basis of these observations these structures are now known as vesicle attachment sites, usually abbreviated to VAS. They have been detected in the mammalian and avian nervous systems (Pfenninger *et al.*, 1972) and at the frog neuromuscular junction (Heuser *et al.*, 1974). Their involvement in transmitter release is suggested both by their demonstrated mediation of communication between the vesicle interior and the extracellular space of the synaptic cleft, and by the good correlations which have been found between the numbers of VAS per ending and the state of excitation of the synapse at the time of fixation (Pfenninger and Rovainen, 1974; Heuser *et al.*, 1974). VAS occur with or without the pore-like opening at their innermost end, and it has been reported that there are less of the 'open' variety in tissue fixed during barbiturate anaesthesia (Streit *et al.*, 1972).

The appearance of new VAS during stimulation is dependent upon the presence of calcium ions in the extracellular millieu (Pfenninger and Rovainen, 1974; Heuser *et al.*, 1974) so the characteristics of the process of VAS induction fit well with those known for the stimulus-coupled secretion of transmitter (Katz, 1969). The early parts of the transmitter release process suggested by these observations are straight-forward, but two alternatives have been proposed for the course of events once communication between the vesicular and plasma membranes has been established (see Fig. 6.11). Pfenninger, 1973 (and Pfenninger and Rovainen, 1974) considers that the fusion of the two membranes is transitory. Once the pore between vesicle interior and cleft has been established and the exit of transmitter presumably accomplished, he envisages that the communication between the vesicle and the pre-synaptic membrane is broken so that the vesicle is returned to the cytoplasm without complete-ly fusing with the plasma membrane. This conclusion is based upon the extremely infrequent observation of structures which might represent fusing vesicles in the studies by Pfenninger and his colleagues (see above references). Furthermore Pfenninger and Rovainen (1974) observed very few structures indicative of endocytotic vesicles, which would be necessary for the reformation of vesicles if complete exocytosis occurs.

Quite the opposite conclusion regarding the fate of the discharging vesicle is drawn by Heuser *et al.,* (1974) from their study of the neuromuscular junction. They were able to distinguish between membrane invaginations occurring near the pre-synaptic ridge, which is where synaptic vesicles approach the pre-synaptic membrane, and a second class occurring under Schwann cell processes, where 'coated' vesicles (see below) are found in the process of endocytotic formation. The invaginations at the pre-synaptic ridge (which are induced by calcium-dependent stimulation) are clearly vesicle attachment sites. Heuser *et al.* find them in a range of sizes which they interpret as representing a progressive settling of the vesicle into the pre-synaptic membrane during fusion. The differences in these observations from those of Pfenninger *et al.* may of course turn out to represent real differences in the mechanism of the transmitter release at the neuromuscular junction and at central synapses.

Turnover of synaptic vesicles
Whether or not total exocytotic fusion of vesicles with plasmalemma is part of the normal sequence of events underlying physiological release of transmitter, it is clear that prolonged stimulation of both motor and autonomic nerves causes a depletion of vesicles with a corresponding increase in the area of the terminal membrane. When the stimulus is terminated this sequence of events is reversed, vesicles are reformed and there is a decrease in terminal surface area (Heuser and Reese, 1973; Ceccarelli *et al.,* 1973; Pysh and Wiley, 1974). The retrieval of vesicles is thought to occur by micropinocytosis. This proposition is most strongly supported by the many de-monstrations that extracellular marker molecules which are transported into nerve terminals after depolarisation are present only inside synaptic vesicles, not in the cytoplasm (Douglas *et al.,* 1970; Heuser and Miledi, 1971; Ceccarelli *et al.,* 1973; Heuser and Reese, 1973; Turner and Harris, 1973; Fried and Blaustein, 1976).

The presumed micropinocytotic vesicles have long been associated with the 'coated vesicles' which in conventionally fixed tissue are occasionally observed in all synapses. These were first described by Gray (1961, 1963) as the complex vesicle, which he interpreted as a synaptic vesicle surrounded by a shell of smaller (150–200 Å) vesicles. Shortly afterwards Andres (1964) described what he thought to be pinocytotic vesicles in central synapses which had 'spiky coats'. Westrum (1965) put these observations together with his own in the form of a hypothetical scheme for the production of synaptic vesicles within the pre-synaptic bag.

In Westrum's scheme vesicles 'budded off' from the pre-synaptic membrane to form complex vesicles which ultimately matured into synaptic vesicles, probably via a stage in which they fuse together into membranous sacs. This sequence of events, based upon the observation of central nervous system tissue, is closely similar to that described by Heuser (Heuser and Miledi 1971; Heuser and Reese, 1973) in the recovery of neuromuscular terminals from prolonged stimulation. Here micropinocytotic 'coated' vesicles fuse to form membranous *cisternae* which ultimately disappear to be replaced by synaptic vesicles.

The structural relationship of the complex vesicle to the uncoated synaptic vesicle remained a problem until Kanaseki and Kadota (1969) found a method which preserved both the unit membrane of the synaptic vesicles and the shell of the complex vesicle. Previously available methods had tended to preserve either one or the other so that their relationship could not be established in the same preparation. Kanaseki and Kadota found that the complex shell appeared as a polygonal array of fibres arranged as pentagons and hexagons surrounding synaptic vesicles. The nature of this arrangement is neatly summarised by the title of their paper – the vesicle-in-a-basket.

In the isolated subcellular fractions on which Kanaseki and Kadota performed their study they found both 'basket vesicles' and the empty baskets. They suggest that these represent two stages of vesicle formation. First the nascent vesicle begins as a local deformation of the extra-junctional pre-synaptic membrane induced by the 'crystallisation' of the basket structure on its cytoplasmic surface. The vesicle then buds off from the membrane inside its basket-like shell completing the first stage of formation. In the second stage the pinocytotic vesicle is released from the basket structure as a mature synaptic vesicle.

Taken together the observations described above strongly suggest that recycling of vesicles via the pre-synaptic membrane does occur. Whatever the underlying process is, it will have to accommodate apparent differences of molecular structure between vesicular and synaptic membranes. They differ in lipid content, the most obvious difference being the absence of measurable levels of gangliosides in the vesicles (Breckenridge *et al.*, 1973). Pearse (1975) analysed the lipid composition of coated vesicles and found them to be devoid of lysolecithin. Although electrophoretic analysis of the proteins of synaptosomal membranes and vesicles shows them to contain common polypeptide constituents, there are many others that they do not share (McBride and Van Tassel, 1972; Morgan *et al.*, 1973a).

This lack of biochemical identity between synaptic plasma and vesicular membranes needs to be accounted for but it is by no means an insurmountable objection to the passage of the latter via the former. It is possible that after fusion of the two membranes the vesicular components occupy a restricted domain on the neuronal surface (Nicolson, 1976, see above) so that they are 'prepackaged' ready for reform-ation. Even if vesicular and plasma membrane components form a mixed mosaic after fusion, it is possible that when vesicles are retrieved from the terminal membrane their budding off is preceded by a local molecular restructuring of the membrane. Indeed such molecular rearrangement might be a necessary preamble to the initiation of vesicle formation. The nature of the mechanism could be investigated using marker molecules which bind to surface components of the plasma membrane, rather than the soluble markers which have so far been employed. It has been found that ferritin-concanavalin A bound to the surface of synaptosomes can become incorporated into the interior of synaptic vesicles (Matus *et al.*, 1973). Since the marker was bound to the membrane surface it is difficult to see how it can have arrived inside the vesicle except by endocytosis. It might be possible to reveal the distribution of predestined vesicular (and non-vesicular) plasma membrane components before, during and after stimulation by using marker molecules with binding specificities for different com-ponents of the synaptic surface.

6.4.2 Basket vesicles, the nature of the basket material and the discovery of the cytonet

The *complex* vesicle originally described by Gray (1963) is by morphological criteria identical with the basket vesicle of Kanaseki and Kadota (1969). These have been most often referred to in the literature as coated vesicles (e.g. Heuser and Reese, 1973; Pearse, 1975). The three terms should be regarded as synonymous. The important point to emerge from these observations is that the vesicular coat structure itself appears to be a distinctive organelle with a characterisitic morphology and, in the schemata advanced by Westrum (1965), Kaneski and Kadota (1969), Gray and Willis (1970) and Heuser and Reese (1973), a well-defined functional role.

Gray (1972) produced evidence which brought into question the status of the basket structure as a discrete vesicle-associated organelle, and possibly its hypothesised involvement in pinocytotic vesicle formation. He pointed out that the coat structure could not always be seen to consist of the array of hexagons and pentagons reported by Kanoseki and Kadota. Instead coats often appear to be composed of irregular strands of material which are also found in the interstitial cytoplasm between the vesicles. Gray (1972) observed that there is a clear zone around coated vesicles where this stranded cytoplasmic network is broken. He interpreted this as a retraction zone where an originally continuous network had collapsed onto the vesicle during pre-paration of the tissue for examination. Rupture of the delicate cytoplasmic network would also explain the existence of both coated vesicles and empty coats in Kanoseki and Kadota's subcellular preparations.

In a later paper Gray (1973) summarised these observations and introduced the term cytonet for the synaptic cytoplasmic network he had described. In stressing the continuity of the cytonet Gray had produced a strong argument against its involve-ment in the induction of vesicular pinocytosis.

Gray later revised his conclusions from these observations in the light of other problems of cytoplasmic fine structure and abandoned the cytonet in favour of a pervasive cytoplasmic 'stereoframework'. He stressed the artefactual nature of this structure denying it a definite morphology and suggesting that it best be interpreted as '. . . denatured and fixed protein complex, (which) in itself has no relevant structural meaning'.

While it is true that the cytonet varies in appearance depending upon the details of fixative procedure, there is excellent biochemical evidence attesting to the independent status of the coat (i.e. the cytonet) material. Pearse (1975, 1976) analysed the protein content of coated vesicles by electrophoresis and discovered that they contain essentially one polypeptide of apparent molecular weight 180 000 daltons. She suggests that this unique protein be called 'clathrin', but since it is part of the cytonet rather than merely vesicle coats 'cytonexin' might be a better term (Matus 1976) Pearse's demonstration of a single protein forming a regular supramolecular structure lends weight to Gray's original proposition that the cytonet is a three dimensional cytoplasmic network constituting a diffuse yet distinctive organelle. Pearse's observations are further supported by the demonstration of a specific enzyme activity (a nucleoside diphosphate phosphohydrolase) which Kadota and Kadota (1973) had earlier shown to be associated with the isolated coated vesicles. Accepting the coat as part of the cytonet, this specific association of an enzyme activity with it also suggests a distinctive molecular structure, rather than the artefactually aggregated denatured protein complex of Gray's stereoframework.

6.4.3 Microtubules

Morphology
Electron microscopic examination of brain tissue reveals abundant microtubular structures within neuronal processes. However, as electron microscopists have long known, the same methods of fixation which are excellent for demonstrating microtubules within the axonal cytoplasm fail to reveal them in the pre-synaptic terminal (see for example Peters *et al.,* 1970, p. 151). This is usually interpreted as meaning either that the microtubules do indeed stop short of the synapse as the ultrastructural studies suggest, or that there are special difficulties in fixing the microtubular structure at this site. One way of choosing between these alternatives is to seek better methods of fixation capable of revealing the *in vivo* structure of the axon terminal contents. Alternatively the fixation problem may be circumvented by conducting a biochemical examination to establish whether molecular components of microtubules are present within the synaptic cytoplasm.

Neither type of search can be conducted without considering the evidence which exists implicating microtubules as actively involved in axoplasmic transport (Karlsson and Sjöstrand, 1969; Kreutzberg, 1969; Ochs, 1972). These studies imply that microtubule-mediated distal movement of materials from the perikaryon is directed toward the pre-synaptic terminal. One particular subject of such transport is the synaptic vesicle (Barondes, 1967; Dahlström, 1969, 1971; Banks *et al.*, 1971; Geffen and Livett, 1971; Samson, 1971). Schmitt (1968, 1969; Schmitt and Samson, 1968) has proposed a mechanism for this process in which there are microtubule binding sites around the vesicle circumference which are sequentially made and broken so that the vesicle moves by a kind of rolling adhesion. Ultrastructural evidence of an association between vesicles and microtubules has been obtained by Smith *et al.*, (1970; Smith 1971) in synaptic regions of cyclostome larvae. Here synaptic vesicles are seen lined up along microtubules and apparently attached to them by fibrous sidearms. However the microtubules do not approach the pre-synaptic membrane and synaptic vesicles close to the synaptic apposition are not aligned as they are when associated with microtubules.

The cyclostome larva so far appears to be the sole possessor of microtubules which can be revealed in its synaptic cytoplasm by conventional methods of electron microscopic fixation. However, recently Gray (1975, 1976) has visualised microtubules within the pre-synaptic terminals of vertebrate central nervous system synapses by employing special conditions of fixation. Fresh brain tissue is minced in a solution of serum albumin and after incubation for some minutes is fixed according to the procedure of Kanaseki and Kadota (1969) in which the usual order of fixatives is reversed, osmium tetroxide being applied first followed by glutaraldehyde. The albumin solution used is hypotonic, and tissue prepared this way contains swollen axon terminals from which much of the normal cytoplasmic material is missing but within which microtubular structures are clearly present. Furthermore synaptic vesicles are associated with the microtubules in manner similar to that seen in the cyclostome larva.

The nature of the conditions required to show these microtubules in vertebrate brain synapses gives no obvious clue to explain their obstinate refusal to appear when conventional methods of fixation are employed. The debate which stems from Gray's observations will probably be concerned with how far his fixative procedure is likely to result in a more realistic representation of *in vivo* conditions than the conventional methods which do not show synaptic microtubules. Recently Heuser, *et al.*, (1976) have conducted an investigation of axon terminal ultrastructure at the neuromuscular junction following ultra-rapid freezing followed by freeze substitution fixation. Rapid freezing minimises the metabolic derangement known to occur following cessation of *in vivo* functioning (Lowry *et al.*, 1964). Thus based upon biochemical criteria it would be expected to provide the closest possible indication of *in vivo* structure, provided that the method of subsequent fixation is able to accurately reproduce the immobilised *in vivo* state. In one notable case there is a striking and convincing correlation between the structural implications of biochemical measurements and the results of ultrastructural studies. Biochemical evidence suggested that brain extracellular space should be substantially larger than that shown by conventional electron microscopic fixative techniques (which in fact show virtually nil). Using rapid freezing and freeze-substitution Van Harreveld *et al.* (1965; Van Harreveld, 1972) were able to preserve brain tissue so that it exhibited

extracellular space with a volume of the order of magnitude suggested by the biochemical measurements. It is this promising approach that Heuser *et al.* are now re-
investigating with an emphasis on cytological organisation, and particularly the
dynamic events occurring during synaptic transmission. Tissue fixed by this method
shows excellent preservation of microtubular structure within which subunits are
clearly distinguishable. Furthermore microtubules do appear within the neuromuscular axon terminal occupying a 'core region' of cytoplasm which appears to be
segregated from the synaptic vesicle-packed active zone (Heuser, personal communication).

Biochemical investigations

The results of biochemical studies are usually taken as confirming the presence of
tubulin, the major microtubular subunit protein, within the synapse but a critical
examination of the literature suggests that this conclusion is not absolutely secure. A
major means of detecting the presence of tubulin has been by its ability to bind the
alkaloid colchicine. Colchicine-binding activity provides a rough quantitation of
tubulin levels and it was by this means that brain was found to be extremely rich in
colchicine-binding protein (Borisy and Taylor, 1967; Weisenberg *et al.*, 1968; Dutton
and Barondes, 1971). This evidence of high tubulin levels correlated well with the
known abundance of microtubules in neuronal processes.

Subsequently an indication of the distribution of this colchicine-binding activity
within the brain was sought by assay of subcellular fractions. It was readily established
that synaptosomes contain high levels (Feit and Barondes, 1970; Lagnado *et al.*, 1971).
Feit and Barondes (1970) found that the synaptosomal supernatant obtained after
hypotonic lysis, presumably representing the contents of the synaptic cytoplasm,
was devoid of colchicine-binding activity. Nevertheless a proportion of the protein in
the synaptosomal supernatant was precipitable by vinblastine, a less specific test for
tubulin. On balance though this evidence would seem to confirm the then contemporary
ultrastructural observations in suggesting that tubulin is absent from the synaptic
cytoplasm. However, Feit and Barondes did demonstrate the presence of a protein
component having the appropriate electrophoretic mobility for tubulin (although
their calculation of its apparent molecular weight is unsatisfactory).

In a later publication Feit *et al.* (1971) attribute their inability to detect
colchicine-binding protein in the synaptosomal supernatant to loss of activity during
processing. This is probably true, for using a simpler fractionation procedure
Lagnado *et al.* (1971) were able to detect colchicine-binding protein which correlates
well with the expected distribution of the synaptic cytoplasmic contents during
fractionation. They found 15% of the activity in a crude mitochondrial fraction
(which includes both myelin and synaptosomes in addition to mitochondria). After
lysis, 80% of the recovered activity was associated with the pellet. The supernatant
to the crude mitochondrial fraction contained 15% of the activity and this probably
represents the synaptosomal cytoplasm. However some caution is still necessary
since some of this soluble activity may have originated from sealed myelinated axon

fragments in the mitochondrial pellet whose contents, representing microtubule-rich axonal cytoplasm, may also be released by hypotonic shock. A further caution arising from the paper by Feit *et al.* (1971) is that it does not provide evidence regarding the presence of tubulin in mature synaptosomes although it is often quoted as doing so. Their studies were performed on neonatal mice and, as the published micrograph makes clear, the 'synaptosomal' fraction includes growth cone-like profiles which contain intact microtubular structures. These naturally lead to the detection of tubulin in the 'synaptosomal' supernatant fraction. This study thus still begs the question of whether mature synapses, which do not contain microtubules demonstrable by conventional electron microscopy, contain tubulin.

That there is tubulin associated with synaptosomes was confirmed by Blitz and Fine (1974). They showed that a protein is present in whole synaptosomes which co-migrates with microtubule-derived tubulin during electrophoresis, and has a tryptic-digest peptide map which is closely similar to that of microtubular tubulin. This tubulin-co-migrating protein is also present in the synaptosomal supernatant produced by hypotonic lysis, suggesting that tubulin is indeed present in the synaptic cytoplasm. The only necessary caution (as Blitz and Fine point out) is that the tubulin in the synaptosomal supernatant may have been membrane-associated and have been eluted from the synaptic membranes by the hypotonic buffer. Since structures as substantial as the pre-synaptic dense projections are removed from the pre-synaptic membrane by such treatment (Matus *et al.* 1975a, see above) this is by no means a trivial consideration.

Pharmacological evidence

There is some evidence that tubulin is involved in the calcium-dependent stimulated secretion of certain hormones. This is based on the inhibition of their secretion by the tubulin-binding anti-mitotic drugs colchicine and vinblastine (Lacy *et al.*, 1968. Poisner and Berstein, 1971; Williams and Wolff, 1970). Since the release of neurotransmitter occurs by a calcium-coupled stimulated secretion mechanism with similar characteristics (Katz, 1969), various investigators have searched for evidence of effects of tubulin-related drugs on transmitter release. There appears to date to have been only one clearly positive demonstration (Thoa *et al.*, 1972) but in this case the drugs were used at concentrations much above that usually necessary for their blocking effect upon axoplasmic flow. In other studies the effect of these agents on release was either marginal inhibition (Katz, 1972; Nicklas *et al.*, 1973), marginal enhancement (Turkanis, 1973) or absent (Redburn and Cotman, 1974). The same drugs do have some effect upon transmitter uptake into synaptosomes (Nicklas *et al.*, 1973; Redburn and Cotman, 1974) but this not profound. On balance the evidence is against a tubulin-mediated mechanism of transmitter release or uptake and thus does not provide evidence for the presence of tubulin in the synaptic cytoplasm.

Immunohistochemical evidence

A further criterion for deciding the distribution of a molecule within tissue can be provided by an histochemical localisation. We have studied the distribution of tubulin antigen in perfusion-fixed brain slices by immunoperoxidase histochemistry using an antiserum raised against electrophoretically purified tubulin from microtubules (see above). A good localisation was obtained of anti-tubulin staining associated with axonal and dendritic microtubules and with the postsynaptic junctional specialisation (Matus *et al.,* 1975c). Anti-tubulin staining was also found associated with components in the postsynaptic dendritic spine cytoplasm (Fig. 8). These are not microtubular structures and microtubules are not revealed at this site by conventional electron microscopic fixation. The immunohistochemical localisation of tubulin antigen does not therefore depend upon the presence of an intact microtubular structure. Thus if non-microtubular tubulin is present in the pre-synaptic cytoplasm then the immunohistochemical anti-tubulin staining might be expected to detect it. However in our studies we did not find convincing anti-tubulin staining within the pre-synaptic cytoplasm even though the same synapses showed strong staining of their postsynaptic junctional structure and the underlying postsynaptic cytoplasm. This suggests that either the tubulin antigen is absent from the pre-synaptic cytoplasm or that it is masked at this site. However, it is also possible that because the level of tubulin in the terminal is very low only very weak staining of tubulin antigen will be obtained. There was some indication of weak staining associated with synaptic vesicles which could conceivably indicate an artefactual redistribution of Gray's pre-synaptic tubules.

Is there non-microtubular tubulin at the synapse? It is usually assumed that colchicine-binding protein may in all cases be identified with microtubular tubulin. This same assumption is commonly made of tubulin co-migrating protein in situations where tubulin content is suspected. Now it is beginning to emerge that not all tubulin-like proteins are identical. The major protein component of isolated postsynaptic junctional structures is tubulin-like by various criteria (see Section 6.2.6) but its peptide map, while very similar to that of microtubule-derived tubulin, is not identical to it (Walters and Matus, 1975c; Feit *et al.,* 1976). There may thus be a family of tubulins all with a closely similar primary polypeptide structure in the α and β chains, all possessing binding sites for colchicine, vinca alkaloids, GTP and magnesium ion but varying in the kind of molecular assembly they form. Thus although the tubulin-like protein of the postsynaptic junctional lattice is the major protein constituent of that structure and is evidently present in high concentration within it, careful electron microscopic examination reveals a subunit structure with an absence of microtubular profiles (see above). It may similarly be the case that tubulin in the pre-synaptic bag is a subtle variation of the axonal form which does not form microtubular arrays.

An alternative possibility is that microtubular tubulin may form mixed molecular arrays with other proteins present in the pre-synaptic cytoplasm, and that these arrays are not microtubular in form. In this way the tubulin could be inhibited from forming microtubular structures within the terminal by its participation on a non-tubular mixed molecular structure. Perhaps the importance of Gray's hypotonic fixation conditions are that they leach out of the pre-synaptic cytoplasm proteins associated with tubulin so that it is subsequently enabled to adopt its self-polymerised microtubular form.

Both of these discussion hypotheses involve the idea that the pre-synaptic terminal may contain tubulin which does not form microtubules. Such a phenomenon has recently been found in cultured cell lines. Wiche and Cole (1976) attempted to repolymerise tubulin from supernatants to glioma C_6 and from cells of neuroblastoma clone Neuro-2A. They succeeded with the glioma but failed with the neuroblastoma. They speculate that the neuroblastoma cells may contain tubulin in 'non-ordered' (i.e. non-microtubular) aggregates which do not depolymerise under the conditions in which microtubules do.

REFERENCES

Akert, K., Moor, H., Pfenninger, K. and Sandri, C. (1969), *Prog. Brain Res.,* **31**, 223–240.

Andres, K.H. (1964), *Z. Zellforsch.,* **110**, 559–568.

Banker, G. and Cotman, C.W. (1972), *J. biol. Chem.,* **247**, 5856–5861.

Banker, G., Churchill, L. and Cotman, C.W. (1974), *J. Cell Biol.,* **63**, 456–465.

Banker, G., Crain, B. and Cotman, C.W. (1972), *Brain Res.,* **42**, 508–513.

Banks, P., Mayor, D. and Tomlinson, D.R. (1971), *J. Physiol. (Lond.),* **219**, 755–761.

Barondes, S.H. (1967), *Neurosci. Res. Prog. Bull.,* **5**, 307–419.

Barondes, S.H. (1970), In: *The Neurosciences: 2nd Study Programme.* (F.O. Schmitt ed.), Rockefeller University Press, New York.

Barrantes, F.J. and Lunt, G.G. (1970), *Brain Res.,* **23**, 305–313.

Berl, S., Puszkin, S. and Nicklas, W.J. (1973), *Science,* **174**, 441–446.

Berlin, R.D., Oliver, J.M., Ukena, T.E. and Yin, H.H. (1974), *Nature,* **247**, 45–46.

Birks, R.I. (1974), *J. Neurocytol.,* **3**, 133–160.

Birks, R.I. and MacIntosh, F.C. (1961), *Can. J. Biochem. Physiol.,* **39**, 787–827.

Bittiger, H. and Schnebli, H.P. (1974), *Nature,* **249**, 370–371.

Blitz, A.L. and Fine, R.E. (1974), *Proc. natn. Acad. Sci., U.S.A.,* **71**, 4472–4476.

Bloom, F.E. (1970), In: *The Neurosciences: Second Study Programme.* (F.O. Schmitt, ed.), Rockefeller University Press, New York.

Bloom, F.E. and Aghajanian, G.K. (1966), *Science,* **154**, 1575–1577.

Bloom, F.E. and Aghajanian, G.K. (1968), *J. Ultrastruct. Res.,* **22**, 361–375.

Bloom, F.E., Iversen, L.L. and Schmitt, F.O. (1970), *Neurosci. Res. Prog. Bull.,* **8**, 325–455.

Bondareff, W. and Sjöstrand, J. (1969), *Exp. Neurol.,* **24**, 450–458.

Borisy, G.G. and Taylor, E.W. (1967), *J. Cell. Biol.,* **34**, 525–533.

Breckenridge, W.C., Gombos, G. and Morgan, I.G. (1972), *Biochim. biophys. Acta,* **266**, 695–707.

Breckenridge, W.C., Morgan, I.G., Zanetta, I.P. and Vincendon, G. (1973), *Biochim. biophys. Acta,* **320**, 681–686.

Bretscher, M.S. (1971), *Nature New Biol.,* **231**, 229–232.

Ceccarelli, B., Hurlbut, W.P. and Mauro, A. (1973), *J. Cell Biol.,* **57**, 499—524.
Chan-Palay, V. and Palay, S.L. (1970), *Z.Anat. Entwickgesch.,* **132**, 191—227.
Churchill, L., Cotman, C., Banker, G., Kelly, P. and Shannon, L. (1976), *Biochim. biophys. Acta,* **448**, 57—72.
Clark, A.W., Mauro, A., Longenecker, H.E. Jnr. and Hurlbut, W.P. (1970), *Nature,* **225**, 703—705.
Collier, B. and MacIntosh, F.C. (1969), *Can. J. Physiol. Pharmacol.,* **47**, 127—135.
Colonnier, M. (1968), *Brain Res.,* **9**, 268—287.
Cotman, C.W., Blank, M.L., Moehl, A. and Snyder, F. (1969), *Biochemistry,* **8**, 4606—4612.
Cotman, C.W., Banker, G., Churchill, L. and Taylor, D. (1974), *J. Cell Biol.,* **63**, 441—455.
Cotman, C.W. and Taylor, D.A. (1972), *J. Cell Biol.,* **55**, 696—711.
Cotman, C.W. and Taylor, D.A. (1974), *J. Cell Biol.,* **62**, 236—242.
Dahlström, A. (1969), In: *Cellular Dynamics of the Neuron,* (S.H. Barondes, ed.), Academic Press, New York.
Dahlström, A. (1971), *Phil. Trans. Roy. Soc. B.,* **261**, 325—358.
Davis, G.A. and Bloom, F.E. (1973), *Brain Res.,* **62**, 135—152.
De Robertis, E. (1964), *Histopathology of Synapses and Neurosecretion,* Pergamon Press, New York.
del Castillo, J. and Katz, K. (1954), *J. Physiol. (Lond.).,* **124**, 560—573.
del Castillo, J. and Katz, B. (1956), *Prog. Biophys.,* **6**, 121—170.
del Castillo, J. and Katz, B. (1957), *Collns. Int. C.N.R.S. (Paris),* **67**, 245—258.
Dennison, M.E. (1971), *J. Cell Sci.,* **8**, 525—539.
De Robertis, E. and Bennett, H.S. (1954), *Fed. Proc.,* **13**, 35.
De Robertis, E., Rodriguez de Lores Arnaiz, G., Salganicoff, L., Pellegrino de Iraldi, A. and Zieher, L.M. (1963), *J. Neurochem.,* **10**, 225—235.
Dunant, Y., Gautron, J., Israël, M., Lesbats, B. and Manaranche, R. (1972), *J. Neurochem.,* **19**, 1987—2002.
Eccles, J.C. (1964), *The Physiology of Synapses,* Springer-Verlag, Berlin.
Eichberg, J., Whittaker, V.P. and Dawson, R.M.C. (1964), *Biochem. J.,* **92**, 91—100.
Fatt, P. and Katz, B. (1952), *J. Physiol. (Lond.).,* **117**, 109—128.
Feit, H. and Barondes, S.H. (1970), *J. Neurochem.,* **17**, 1355—1364.
Feit, H., Dutton, G.R., Barondes, S.H. and Shelanski, M.L. (1971), *J. Cell Biol.,* **51**, 138—147.
Feit, H., Kelly, P. and Cotman, C.W. (1976), *Proc. natn. Acad. Sci. U.S.A.,* in press.
Fonnum, F. (1967), *Biochem. J.,* **103**, 262—270.
Fried, R.C. and Blaustein, M.P. (1976), *Nature,* **261**, 255—256.
Geffen, L.B. and Livett, B. (1971), *Physiol. Rev.,* **51**, 98—157.
Gray, E.G. (1959), *J. Anat. (Lond.).,* **93**, 420—433.
Gray, E.G. (1961), *J. Anat. (Lond.).,* **95**, 345—356.
Gray, E.G. (1963), *J. Anat. (Lond.).,* **97**, 101—106.
Gray, E.G. (1966), *Int. Rev. Gen. Exp. Zool.,* **2**, 139—170.
Gray, E.G. (1969), *Prog. Brain Res.,* **31**, 141—155.
Gray, E.G. (1972), *J. Neurocytol.,* **1**, 363—382.
Gray, E.G. (1973), *Brain Res.,* **62**, 329—335.

Gray, E.G. (1975a), *J. Neurocytol.*, **4**, 315–339.

Gray, E.G. (1975b), *Proc. Roy. Soc. (Lond.).*, *Ser. B.*, **190**, 369–372.

Gray, E.G. (1976), *J. Neurocytol.*, **5**, 361–360.

Gray, E.G. and Guillery, R.W. (1966), *Int. Rev. Cytol.*, **19**, 111–182.

Gray, E.G. and Whittaker, V.P. (1960), *J. Physiol. (Lond.).*, **153**, 35–37.

Gray, E.G. and Whittaker, V.P. (1962), *J. Anat. (Lond.)*, **96**, 79–88.

Gray, E.G. and Willis, R.A. (1970), *Brain Res.*, **24**, 149–168.

Gurd, J.W., Jones, L.R., Mahler, H.R. and Moore, W.J. (1974), *J. Neurochem.*, **22**, 281–290.

Heuser, J.E. and Miledi, R. (1971), *Proc. Roy. Soc. (Lond.), Ser. B.* **179**, 247–260.

Heuser, J.E. and Reese, T.S. (1973), *J. Cell Biol.*, **57**, 315–344.

Heuser, J.E., Reese, T.S. and Landis, D.M. (1974), *J. Neurocytol.*, **3**, 109–131.

Heuser, J.E., Reese, T.S. and Landis, D.M. (1976), *Cold. Spring Harbor Symp. Quant. Biol.*, **40**, 17–24.

Jones, D.H. (1976), *Ultrastructure and Molecular Structure of Neuronal Membranes in Developing Rat Brain*, Ph. D. Thesis, University of London.

Jones, D.H. and Matus, D.H. (1975), *Neurosci. Lett.*, **1**, 153–158.

Kadota, K. and Kadota, T. (1973), *Brain Res.*, **56**, 371–376.

Kanaseki, T. and Kadota, K. (1969), *J. Cell Biol.*, **42**, 202–220.

Katz, B. (1969), *The Release of Neural Transmitter Substance*, Liverpool University Press, Liverpool.

Karlsson, J.-O., Hamberger, A. and Henn, F.A. (1973), *Biochim. biophys. Acta*, **298**, 219–229.

Katz, N.L. (1972), *Eur. J. Pharmacol.*, **19**, 88–93.

Kopin, I.J., Breese, G.R., Krauss, K.R. and Weise, V.K. (1968), *J. Pharmac. exp. Ther.*, **161**, 271–278.

Kornguth, S.E. and Sunderland, E. (1975), *Biochim. biophys. Acta*, **393**, 100–114.

Lacy, P.E., Howell, S.L., Young, D.A. and Fink, C.J. (1968), *Nature*, **219**, 1177–1179.

Lagnado, J.R., Lyons, C. and Wickremasinghe, G. (1971), *FEBS Letters.*, **15**, 254–258.

Landis, D.M.D. and Reese, T.S. (1974), *J. comp. Neurol.*, **155**, 93–126.

Landis, D.M.D., Reese, T.S. and Raviola, E. (1974), *J. comp. Neurol.*, **155**, 67–92.

Longenecker, H.E., Jnr., Hurlbut, W.P., Mauro, A. and Clark, A.W. (1970), *Nature*, **225**, 701–703.

Lowry, O.H., Passonneau, J.V., Hasselberger, F.X. and Schulz, D.W. (1964), *J. biol. Chem.*, **239**, 18–30.

Lucy, A. (1970), *Nature*, **227**, 814–817.

Marchbanks, R.M. (1969), In: *Cellular Dynamics of the Neuron*, (S.H. Barondes, ed.), Academic Press, New York, p. 115–135.

Marchbanks, R.M. (1975), *Int. J. Biochem.*, **6**, 303–312.

Marchbanks, R.M. and Israël, M. (1971), *J. Neurochem.*, **18**, 439–448.

Matus, A.I. (1976), *Nature*, **262**, 176.

Matus, A.I. and Dennison, M.E. (1971), *Brain Res.*, **32**, 195–197.

Matus, A.I. and Dennison, M.E. (1972), *J. Neurocytol.*, **1**, 27–34.

Matus, A.I., De Petris, S. and Raff, M.C. (1973), *Nature New Biol.*, **244**, 278–280.

Matus, A.I. and Walters, B.B. (1975), *J. Neurocytol.*, **4**, 369–375.

Matus, A.I. and Walters, B.B. (1976), *Brain Res.*, **108**, 249–256.

Matus, A.I., Walters, B.B. and Jones, D.H. (1975a), *J. Neurocytol.*, **4**, 357–367.

Matus, A.I., Walters, B.B. and Mughal, S. (1975b), *J. Neurocytol.*, **4**, 733–744.

Matus, A.I., Jones, D.H. and Mughal, S. (1975c), *Brain Res.*, **103**, 171–175.

Maynert, E.W., Levi, R. and de Lorenzo, A.J. (1964), *J. Pharmacol. exp. Ther.*, **144**, 385–392.

McBride, W.J. and Van Tassel, J. *Brain Res.*, **44**, 177–187.

Michaelson, I.A., Whittaker, V.P., Laverty, R. and Sharman, D.F. (1963), *Biochem. Pharmacol.*, **12**, 1450–1453.

Morgan, I.G., Vincendon, G. and Gombos, G. (1973), *Biochim. biophys. Acta*, **320**, 671–680.

Morgan, I.G., Zanetta, J.-P., Breckenridge, W.C., Vincendon, G. and Gombos, G. (1973a), *Brain Res.*, **62**, 405–411.

Neville, D.M. (1971), *J. biol. Chem.*, **246**, 6328–6334.

Nicklas, W.J., Puszkin, S. and Berl, S. (1973), *J. Neurochem.*, **20**, 109–121.

Nicolson, G.L. (1976), *Biochim. biophys. Acta*, **457**, 57–108.

Ochs, S. (1972), *Science*, **176**, 252–260.

Palade, G.E. (1954), *Anat. Rec.*, **118**, 335–336.

Palay, S.L. (1954), *Anat. Rec.*, **118**, 336.

Palay, S.L. (1958), *J. Biophys. Biochem. Cytol.*, **2**, (Suppl.) 193–206.

Pearse, B.M.F. (1975), *J. Mol. Biol.*, **97**, 93–98.

Pearse, B. (1976), *Proc. natn. Acad. Sci., U.S.A.*, **73**, 1255–1259.

Pease, D.C. (1966), *J. Ultrastruct. Res.*, **15**, 555–588.

Pellegrino de Iraldi, A., Duggan, H.F. and De Robertis, E. (1963), *Anat. Rec.*, **145**, 521–531.

Peters, A., Palay, S.L. and Webster, H. de F. (1970), *The Fine Structure of the Nervous System*, Harper and Row: New York.

Pfenninger, K.H. (1971), *J. Ultrastruct. Res.*, **35**, 451–475.

Pfenninger, K.H. (1973), *Prog. Histochem. Cytochem.*, **5**, 1–86.

Pfenninger, K.H., Akert, K., Moor, H. and Sandri, C. (1972), *J. Neurocytol.*, **1**, 129–149.

Pfenninger, K.H. and Maylié–Pfenninger, M.F. (1976), *J. Cell Biol.*

Pfenninger, K.H. and Rees, R.P. (1976), In: *Neuronal Recognition*, (F.H. Barondes, ed.), Plenum Press, New York.

Pfenninger, K.H. and Rovainen, C.M. (1974), *Brain Res.*, **72**, 1–23.

Poisner, A.M. and Berstein, J. (1970), In: *Advances in Biochemical Psychopharmacology*, (E. Costa and E. Giacobini, eds.), Raven Press, New York.

Potter, L.T. (1970), *J. Physiol.*, **206**, 145–166.

Pysh, J.J. and Wiley, R.G. (1974), *J. Cell Biol.*, **60**, 365–374.

Rambourg, A. (1969), *J. Microscopie*, **8**, 325–342.

Rambourg, A. and Leblond, C.P. (1967), *J. Cell Biol.*, **32**, 27–53.

Rostas, J.A.P. and Jeffrey, P.L. (1975), *Neurosci. Letts.*, **1**, 47–53.

Redburn, D.A. and Cotman, C.W. (1974), *Brain Res.*, **73**, 550–557.

Schmitt, F.O. (1968), *Proc. natn. Acad. Sci., U.S.A.*, **60**, 1092–1101.

Schmitt, F.O. (1969), *Cellular Dynamics of the Neuron*, (S.H. Barondes, ed.), Academic Press, New York.

Schmitt, F.O. and Samson, F.E., Jnr. (1968), *Neurosci. Res. Prog. Bull.*, **6**, 113–219.

Samson, F.E., Jnr. (1971), *J. Neurobiol.*, **2**, 347–360.

Sandri, C., Akert, K., Livingston, R.B. and Moor, H. (1972), *Brain Res.*, **41**, 1–16.
Sherrington, C.S. (1897), In: *A Text Book of Physiology Vol. 3.* (7th edn.).
   (E.M. Foster, ed.), Macmillan, London.
Singer, G.L. and Nicolson, G.L. (1972), *Science,* **175**, 720–731.
Smith, A.D. (1971), *Phil. Trans. Roy. Soc. (Lond.). Ser. B.*, **261**, 363–370.
Smith, D.S. (1971), *Phil. Trans. Roy. Soc. (Lond.). Ser. B.*, **261**, 395–405.
Smith, D.S., Järlfors, U. and Berànek, R. (1970), *J. Cell Biol.*, **46**, 199–219.
Streit, P., Akert, K., Sandri, C., Livingston, R.B. and Moor, H. (1972), *Brain Res.*,
   48, 11–26.
Tettamanti, G., Morgan, L.G., Gombos, G., Vincendon, G. and Mandel, P. (1972),
   Brain Res., **47**, 515–518.
Thoa, N.B., Wooten, G.F., Axelrod, J. and Kopin, I.J. (1972), *Proc. natn. Acad. Sci.*,
   U.S.A., **69**, 520–522.
Turner, P.T. and Harris, A.B. (1973), *Nature*, **242**, 57–59.
Uchizono, K. (1965), *Nature*, **207**, 642–643.
Valdivia, O. (1971), *J. comp. Neurol.*, **142**, 257–273.
Van der Loos, H. (1963), *Z. Zellforsch*, **60**, 815–825.
Van Harreveld, A., Crowell, J. and Malhorta, S.K. (1965), *J. Cell Biol.*, **25**, 117–137.
Van Harreveld, A. (1972), In: *The Structure and Function of Nervous Tissue*, Vol. 4.,
   (G.H. Bourne, ed.), Academic Press, New York.
Walters, B.B. (1976), *Ultrastructure and Molecular Organisation of Synaptic
   Membranes*, Ph.D. Thesis, University of London.
Walers, B.B. and Matus, A.I. (1975a), *J. Anat. (Lond.)*, **119**, 415.
Walters, B.B. and Matus, A.I. (1975b), *Biochem. Soc. Trans.*, **3**, 109–112.
Walters, B.B. and Matus, A.I. (1975c), *Nature*, **257**, 496–498.
Wannaker, B.B. and Kornguth, S.E. (1973), *Biochim. biophys. Acta*, **303**, 333.
Weber, K. and Osborn, M. (1969), *J. Biol. Chem.*, **244**, 4406–4412.
Weisenberg, R.C., Borisy, G.G. and Taylor, E.W. (1968), *Biochemistry*, **7**, 4466–4479.
Westrum, L.E. (1965), *J. Physiol. (Lond.)*, **179**, 4–6P.
Westrum, L.E. and Gray, E.G. (1976), *Brain Res.*, **105**, 547–550.
Wiche, G. and Cole, R.D. (1976), *Proc. natn. Acad. Sci.*, *U.S.A.*, **73**, 1227–1231.
Whittaker, V.P., Michaelson, I.A. and Kirkland, R.J.A. (1964), *Biochem. J.*, **90**,
   293–303.
Williams, J.A. and Wolff, J. (1970), *Proc. natn, Acad. Sci.*, *U.S.A.*, **67**, 1901–1908.

7 Cholinergic Processes at Synaptic Junctions

R. DINGLEDINE and J.S. KELLY

Acknowledgements
We are grateful to George Marshall for excellent technical assistance. R.D. is a
Fellow of the Pharmaceutical Manufacturers' Association Foundation and of the
Foundations' Fund for Research in Psychiatry.

Intercellular Junctions and Synapses
(*Receptors and Recognition,* Series B, Volume 2)
Edited by J. Feldman, N.B. Gilula and J.D. Pitts
Published in 1978 by Chapman and Hall, 11 New Fetter Lane, London EC4P 4EE
© Chapman and Hall

7.1 INTRODUCTION

Many investigators have been attracted to the study of putative cholinergic pathways in the brain, perhaps by the early successes of biophysicists at the neuromuscular junctions of skeletal and cardiac muscle, and the marked behavioral effects of cholinergic drugs in man.

Very early in this century Dale [1914] recognised that the variability of response to ACh in the peripheral nervous system made it necessary to distinguish two classes of cholinergic effects, which he termed nicotinic and muscarinic. Characteristically, the nicotinic effects of ACh occurred at the skeletal neuromuscular junction and in autonomic ganglia, had a quick onset and short duration, and were easily blocked by excess nicotine or by curare. In contrast, the muscarinic effects were seen only at peripheral targets of the parasympathetic system, were slow in onset and prolonged in duration, and were readily blocked by atropine. Although in the peripheral nervous system it has rarely been necessary to postulate the presence of both responses on the same cell, except in the case of sympathetic ganglia (Eccles and Libet, 1961), most neurons in the central nervous system show mixed responses to the application of cholinergic drugs and cannot be classified simply as either muscarinic or nicotinic (Phillis, 1971; Krnjević, 1974).

All nicotonic responses described to date have been excitatory in nature. The situation is more complicated in the case of muscarinic responses, which can be either excitatory or inhibitory, the nature of the response depending on the location or the type of cell. Furthermore, on occasion, both depolarizing and hyperpolarizing responses to ACh can be elicited on the same cell (Nelson, Peacock and Amano, 1971; cf. Weight and Votava, 1970; Weight and Padjen, 1973).

A central question that remains unanswered is whether nicotinic and muscarinic responses reflect the existence of two distinct molecular species of receptor, or alternatively a single receptor that can be present in different functional states. A number of attempts have been made to characterize cholinergic receptors in the central nervous system by measuring their interaction with slowly reversible cholinergic agents radio-labeled to high specific activity. Most of the earlier attempts however, which depended on nicotinic agents such as d-tubocurarine, hexamethonium and bungarotoxin were inconclusive, and only more recent methods employing muscarinic antagonists have been able to show the presence of ACh binding sites in relatively small regions of the brain. Two muscarinic antagonists have been successfully used to probe the binding properties of central ACh receptors: 3-quinuclidinyl

benzilate (QNB) (Yamamura and Snyder, 1974), and the irreversible nitrogen
mustard analog of propylbenzylcholine (PrBCM) (Burgen, Hiley and Young, 1974).
As might be expected if the binding of these agents reflects a specific interaction
with muscarinic receptors, the relative ability of a wide range of muscarinic
antagonists to displace specifically bound tritiated QNB or PrBCM tends to parallel
their pharmacological activity. By contrast nicotinic antagonists such as *d*-tubocurarine,
pempidine and hexamethonium, and the toxins of the *Naja* venom, have no effect.

The regional distribution of specific ^{3}H-QNB binding in the rat and monkey brain
(Kuhar and Yamamura, 1976) generally parallels that of choline acetyltransferase
and acetylcholinesterase, being highest in the corpus striatum and lowest in the
cerebellar cortex. In many other regions this correlation is less good and may reflect
the presence of mixed populations of nicotinic and muscarinic receptors on central
neurons.

7.2 IONIC MECHANISMS

In a recent review Gage (1976) has very ably summarised the mass of data from the
skeletal neuromuscular junction that has led to the conclusion that the complexing
of ACh with its specific receptor in the post-junctional membrane leads to a conformational change in the receptor, which then causes the formation of an ionic
channel in the receptor complex itself or in an associated region of the cell membrane. The opening and closing of these channels at high frequency caused by the
iontophoretic application of ACh is thought to be responsible for the increased
fluctuation in the membrane potential that can be seen superimposed on the steady
depolarization (Katz and Miledi, 1970 and 1972). Indeed, by the use of statistical
noise analysis, the mean size and duration of these voltage fluctuations can be used to
estimate the approximate size and the half life of individual ionic channels (Katz and
Miledi, 1970, 1972; Anderson and Stevens, 1973). The opening of a single channel
contributes 4×10^{-12} A to the end-plate current and should, therefore, result from
the flow of approximately 10^7 univalent ions per second through a channel. Since
the half life of the channels formed during an iontophoretic application of ACh
appears to be similar to the decay rate of the end plate potentials evoked at the
same junction (Anderson and Stevens, 1973), it has been suggested that the rate-
limiting step in both cases is the same and may be either the relaxation rate of the
open conformation of the ACh receptor complex or perhaps the rate at which ACh
dissociates from the receptor.

At the neuromuscular junction the complexing of ACh with its receptor leads to
an increase in permeability to both sodium and potassium. Although the increase in
membrane permeability to both ions appears to be approximately the same (Takeuchi
and Takeuchi, 1959), the larger disparity between the sodium equilibrium potential
and the membrane potential ensures that the inward flow of sodium ions will be
approximately 18 times greater than the outward flow of potassium ions. It is this

net inward flow of current that leads to the depolarization of the muscle membrane. However, unlike the situation during the action potential where the sodium and potassium channels can be differentiated by the use of tetrodotoxin and tetraethylammonium, it has not yet been possible to determine whether each ion has its own channel at the end plate or whether they share a common channel. On the other hand, there is clear evidence that at several other sites (described below) the actions of ACh can be explained by an alteration in the activation of ion-selective channels.

Although cholinergic synapses can usually be classified as either excitatory or inhibitory, their post-synaptic membranes have now been shown to display a remarkable variety of conductance changes, affecting at different junctions the movement of all three major current-carrying ions, sodium, potassium and chloride. This chapter will, therefore, emphasise the large variety of post-synaptic mechanisms that determine the excitatory or inhibitory nature of cholinergic synapses.

7.2.1 Changes in sodium permeability

As mentioned above, the depolarizing effect of ACh at the neuromuscular junction is associated with an increased conductance to both Na^+ and K^+ (Gage, 1976). Since the only certain nicotinic response to ACh in the CNS is on the Renshaw cell (Curtis and Ryall, 1966), which has not been investigated with intracellular electrodes, we will not discuss this mechanism further. However, it should be mentioned that the fast depolarizing response to ACh in gastropods is predominantly, if not exclusively, dependent on the entry of Na^+ ions (Tauc and Gerschenfeld 1962; Blankenship *et al.*, 1971). Even in this idyllic situation in which several recording and current-passing electrodes can be placed inside the same cell, the absolute value of the reversal potential for the response has not been established (Ascher and Kehoe, 1975). This is in part due to the fact that the agents that block the inhibitory actions of ACh on the same cell also block the Na^+-dependent response. However, hexamethonium selectively blocks the Na^+-dependent response allowing the inhibitory action of ACh to be investigated in a pure form (see below).

In C-cells of the frog sympathetic ganglia, the pharmacological blockade of the fast excitatory response has also revealed the presence of a slow hyperpolarizing response to ACh and a correspondingly slow IPSP (Weight and Padjen, 1973). Both responses are associated with an increase in membrane resistance, and are progessively reduced when the cell is depolarized by current injection (Weight and Padjen, 1973). Although soaking the preparation in 10^{-6} M ouabain reduced the IPSP (Nishi and Kobetsu, 1968) and suggested the possible activation of an electrogenic sodium pump, this mechanism is not consistant with the observed conductance change and voltage dependence of the IPSP and may well be due to a secondary effect on the Na^+ equilibrium potential. Thus, the inhibitory ACh effect was later found to be abolished in Na^+-free Ringer (Weight and Padjen, 1973). It appears therefore, that this cholinergic synapse acts by reducing the resting Na^+ conductance in the postsynaptic element.

Although other workers have also concluded from the effects of ouabain and low temperature that an electrogenic Na^+ pump mediates cholinergic slow IPSPs on identified cells in the abdominal ganglion of *Aplysia* (Pinsker and Kandel, 1969) and in certain snail neurons (Kerkut *et al.,* 1969), a subsequent study by Kehoe and Ascher (1970) showed such slow IPSPs to be the result of an increased K^+ conductance. A misleading secondary effect of both ouabain and low temperature on the K^+ equilibrium potential was later confirmed by direct intracellular measurement of K^+ concentration (Kunze and Brown, 1971).

7.2.2 Changes in potassium permeability

An increase in the resting K^+ conductance is now known to mediate the ACh-evoked hyperpolarization of salivary acinar cells (Petersen, 1970; Schneyer *et al.,* 1972) and certain neurons of gastropods (Ascher and Kehoe, 1975; Ger and Zeimal, 1976), as well as the muscarinic vagal inhibition of vertebrate heart muscle (Trautwein *et al.,* 1956). In all cases the reversal potential is much more negative than the resting potential, and the decrease in membrane resistance elicited by ACh is not altered in Cl^- free bathing solutions, eliminating the possibility of a significant Cl^- flux. The ACh-evoked hyperpolarization of neuroblastoma L-cells is also associated with a fall in membrance resistance and is not affected by changes in extracellular Cl^- concentration, indicating a probable increase in K^+ conductance as the underlying ionic mechanism (Nelson *et al.,* 1971; Nelson and Peacock, 1972).

In addition to these examples of ACh-evoked increase in K^+ conductance there are now two cases in which the action of ACh results in a decrease in the resting membrane K^+ conductance. The muscarinic depolarization of cerebral cortical cells has a very slow time course (Krnjević and Phillis, 1963) and is associated with an increase in membrane input resistance (Krnjević *et al.,* 1971). It is important to note that the membrane resistance of these cortical cells is independent of the membrane potential when the membrane is artificially polarized by current applied by an intracellular electrode, and thus the ACh-evoked resistance changes are not an intrinsic response of the membrane to a depolarization. Since the reversal level for the ACh-evoked depolarization was more negative than the resting potential, it seemed that ACh was inactivating either the K^+ or Cl^- resting conductance. A major role for Cl^- was ruled out when altering the Cl^- equilibrium potential by injecting Cl^- into the cells was shown to have a negligible effect on the ACh reversal potential. The simplest explanation for these observations is that ACh inactivates the resting K^+ conductance and that the depolarization results from a shift away from the K^+ equilibrium potential. ACh also causes a broadening of the spike shape by slowing the repolarization phase of the action potential (Krnjević *et al.,* 1971). This effect could also be caused by a reduction in the outward K^+ current (Hodgkin and Huxley, 1952).

Activation of the cholinergic input to frog sympathetic ganglion cells results in a diphasic depolarization. Blockade of the fast EPSP by nicotinic antagonists allows the study of the muscarinic slow EPSP in isolation. In this situation the slow EPSP was associated with an increased membrane resistance, which was not affected by removal of extra-cellular Cl^- from the bath (Weight and Votava, 1970). Since the EPSP reversal level was very close to that of the spike after hyperpolarization – a measure of the K^+ equilibrium potential in these cells – Weight and Votava (1970) concluded that the slow EPSP is the result of a synaptic inactivation of K^+ conductance.

7.2.3 Changes in chloride permeability

As pointed out by Krnjević (1974) there are no known examples among vertebrates of ACh effecting a change in Cl^- conductance, but there are several quite interesting examples of this in invertebrate neurons. In the land snail *Crymptophallus* there are two types of neurons in which ACh causes an increase in Cl^- conductance, as demonstrated by measuring the ACh reversal potential in solutions of various ionic compositions (Chiarandini and Gerschenfeld, 1967; Chiarandini *et al.*, 1967). However, in one class of cells, the 'D-neurons', this action results in a depolarization, and in the other class, the 'H-neurons', a hyperpolarization. These curious observations were explained by differences in the internal Cl^- concentration in the cells (Kerkut and Meech, 1966): H-neurons have an unusually low internal Cl^- concentration, presumably maintained by an outward Cl^- pump, while D-neurons have an internal Cl^- concentration higher than expected from passive diffusion, presumably maintained by an inward Cl^- pump.

On several *Aplysia* neurons a careful evaluation of the effects of changes in the external ion concentration on the reversal level of the hyperpolarizing response to ACh has shown the presence of two quite separate components (Kehoe, 1972). The first is an early rapid response whose reversal level changes as predicted by the Nernst equation when the external Cl^- is replaced by sulphate or methylsulphate ions and is unaffected by alterations in the external K^+ concentration. Thus this component can be said to be mediated by a selective change in the membrane permeability to Cl^- concentration. The other component behaves as predicted when the equilibrium level for K^+ is altered and is thought to be mediated by a selective increase in ion permeability to K^+ ions. Thus, in the same *Aplysia* neuron one can recognize three responses to ACh, one excitatory and both fast and slow inhibitory, which can be characterized in terms of ion selective channels for Na^+, Cl^- and K^+ respectively.

7.2.4 Comment on multi-receptor systems

Many of the effects of ACh on cells of gastropods described above were obtained by examining the response to local applications of ACh on the somatic membrane, where it is known that there are no synaptic contacts. The synaptic membrane of gastropods is confined to the axon. However, in most instances where an identified cholinergic neurons has been shown to innervate the cell under study, it has been possible to show that the synaptic response is identical to that elicited by the

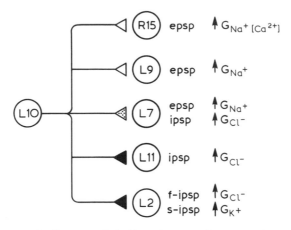

Fig. 7.1 Schematic diagram of cholinergic synaptic connections and ionic mechanisms of cell L-10, an identified cell in the *Aplysia* abdominal ganglion.
  Excitatory and inhibitory synaptic connections are represented by open and closed triangles, respectively. The dotted triangle represents a biphasic synapse, whose sign (excitatory or inhibitory) depends on the frequency of the presynaptic impulse train. Although these synapses are axo-axonic, they are represented as axo-somatic for convenience. The inhibitory synapse made on cell L-2 has both fast and slow components. The arrows indicate a selective increase in ionic conductance to either Na^+, K^+, Ca^{2+}, or Cl^-. From Kandel *et al.,* 1967; Wachtel and Kandel, 1967, 1971; Blankenship *et al.,* 1971.

application of ACh to the somatic membrane. Indeed, in one case a diphasic response to iontophoretic ACh is associated with a synaptic response consisting of a depolarizing and hyperpolarizing element (Wachtel and Kandel, 1971).
  However, perhaps the most interesting aspect of multi-receptor systems is the demonstration that a single cholinergic neuron can produce different effects on several follower cells, depending on the ion permeability affected (Wachtel and Kandel, 1967; Kandel *et al.,* 1967). This is illustrated in Fig. 7.1: a single action potential in cell L-10 in the abdominal ganglion of *Aplysia* gives rise to inhibition or excitation in at least five identified follower cells by generating conductance changes to Na^+, K^+ or Cl^- in the different cells. There is no *a priori* reason why this situation could not be operant in the vertebrate CNS.
  It is also of interest to consider the possible physiological consequences of slow synaptic events. Slow synaptic excitation such as occurs in the frog sympathetic ganglion (Weight and Votava, 1970) and the mammalian cerebral cortex (Krnjević *et al.,* 1971) is clearly unsuited for the fast transmission of digital nerve signals. On the other hand, a slow EPSP or IPSP combined with an increase in membrane resistance can serve to sensitize the cell to other inputs, both excitatory and inhibitory, as pointed out by Weight (1974) and Krnjević (1974). Such a specialized synaptic process might have the effect of raising the over-all level of activity of a

population of neurons. In contrast, therefore, to short-term interactions between neurons, which seem to be associated with conductance increases to ions, the slow potentials generated as a result of conductance decreases may reflect more long-term synaptic interactions that are related to metabolic relationships. Indeed, in some cases cholinergic slow potentials are associated with metabolic events in the post-synaptic cell that may have functions unrelated to the electrical events occurring at the cell membrane. This possibility is discussed more fully in the next section.

7.3 METABOLIC MECHANISMS

In contrast to the quick nicotinic actions of ACh, the long latency and long duration of most muscarinic slow potentials is suggestive of an underlying metabolic event. The hypothesis has been advanced that guanosine 3', 5'-monophosphate (cGMP) is causally related to muscarinic slow potentials (Stone *et al.*, 1975; Greengard, 1976), similar to the mediation of some hormonal (Robison *et al.*, 1971), and probably neuronal (Bloom *et al.*, 1975) adrenergic effects by cAMP. According to this scheme (Greengard, 1976) the activation of muscarinic receptors results in the accumulation of intracellular cGMP by stimulation of guanylate cyclase. A significant role for cGMP phospho-diesterase has apparently been ruled out since the muscarinic effect can be seen in the presence of phosphodiesterase inhibitors. The suggestion is that the cGMP so formed stimulates a specific membrane bound protein kinase, which in turn phosphorylates another membrane-bound 'substrate protein' that controls the permeability of the postsynaptic membrane. Phosphorylation of the substrate protein is thought to lead to a change in passive ion conductance or in the activity of an electrogenic pump, and so to produce the observed slow potential. The details of this very attractive theory are based mainly on the well-known example of cAMP-mediated glycogenolysis, and so far there is only tenuous evidence to support it: activation of muscarinic receptors is associated with a rise in cGMP content in several tissues (George *et al.*, 1970; Kuo *et al.*, 1972; Lee *et al.*, 1972; Kebabian *et al.*, 1975; Weight *et al.*, 1974, extracellularly applied cGMP mimics the muscarinic effects of ACh on neurons of the sympathetic ganglion (McAfee and Greengard, 1972) and cerebral cortex (Stone *et al.*, 1975; but see Phillis *et al.*, 1974), and a cGMP-dependent protein kinase has been described in a membrane preparation from ACh-sensitive mammalian smooth muscle (Casnellie and Greengard, 1974).

This theory has since been expanded to include roles for calcium and phosphati-dylinositol. A role for calcium has been proposed from the observations that Ca^{2+} stimulates cytoplasmic guanylate cyclase (albeit at high concentrations) but inhibits the membrane-bound enzyme (Schultz *et al.*, 1973; Kimura and Murad, 1975; Ferrendelli *et al.*, 1976; Olson *et al.*, 1976), and that in a variety of tissues the ACh-evoked increase in intracellular cGMP is dependent on the extracellular calcium concentration (Schultz *et al.*, 1973; Kebabian *et al.*, 1975; Ferrendelli *et al.*, 1976). Michell (1975) has summarized the evidence that an early consequence of muscarinic receptor activation may be the cleavage of the glycerolphosphate bond of plasma-membrane bound phosphatidylinositol: in several tissues ACh increases the rate of phosphatidylinositol breakdown, and interestingly this phenomenon is not dependent on cGMP or calcium. Michell (1975), therefore, suggested that muscarinic receptor activation results in the immediate cleavage of phosphatidylinositol, which then leads to the sudden intracellular appearance of Ca^{2+} and consequent activation of guanylate cyclase. How phosphatidylinositol breakdown could lead to an increase in the intracellular calcium concentration is not clear; perhaps Ca^{2+} channels are opened in the plasma membrane, or possibly the polar cleavage product, phosphoinositide, diffuses from the inner surface of the plasma membrane into the cytoplasm carrying calcium as its counter-ion.

The first step in a slow muscarinic response is receptor activation, and the last step may be a change in cell membrane potential. The challenge lies in determining the sequential relationships among the middle steps, which may or may not involve calcium movements, phosphatidylinositol breakdown and guanylate cyclase activation. On the other hand, the general theory outlined above, which postulates that a specific sequence of biochemical events couples muscarinic receptor activation to the change in membrane potential, is very powerful in that a range of testable predictions can be deduced from it. However, in at least two crucial experiments these predictions do not seem to have stood up to the test, and the theory as stated above may have to be modified.

The cGMP theory predicts that intracellular applications of cGMP should mimic the effects of activating muscarinic receptors, but Krnjević *et al.* (1976) and Krnjević and Van Meter (1976) have recently shown that in the case of the typical muscarinic slow excitation of motoneurons, intracellular injections of cGMP generated an hyperpolarization associated with a fall in membrane resistance, precisely the opposite effect of both extracellular and intracellular iontophoretic applications of ACh on the same cell. If this observation is confirmed the general cGMP theory will have to be modified to include compartmentation; i.e., it might be postulated that the free cytoplasmic pool of cGMP does not have access to the cellular apparatus regulating ionic fluxes across the plasma membrane, and that activation of muscarinic receptors generates a separate pool of cGMP that does have access to this apparatus. Perhaps an even more critical test of the theory was the question: Do the biochemical events occur quickly enough to be the cause of the observed slow potentials? Some muscarinic actions on smooth muscle occur so slowly that the cGMP levels can be shown to be elevated before the response begins (Goldberg *et al.*, 1975). In contrast the minimum latency at most muscarinic synapses is around 100 ms (Purves, 1976), and a significant rise in cGMP levels or phosphatidylinositol breakdown must therefore occur within a few tens of ms of receptor activation. Unfortunately, in most tissues the earliest change in the rate of phosphatidylinositol breakdown appears to occur several minutes after ACh receptor activation (Michell, 1975). Technical considerations have not permitted cGMP levels to be measured until several seconds after the receptor stimulation (Greengard, 1976). In this regard the development of more sensitive assays, or a cGMP sensitive microelectrode, might circumvent this problem.

An interesting problem related to the metabolic theory is the manner in which the ACh receptor is physically linked to the metabolic apparatus. A high percentage of both the phosphatidylinositol breakdown enzyme (probably a phospholipase C) and guanylate cyclase is present as a soluble enzyme in the cytoplasm (Kimura and Murad, 1975; Michell, 1975; White, 1975). Does the activation of muscarinic receptors stimulate the soluble form or the plasma membrane-bound form of guanylate cyclase? If the soluble form is activated, some diffusible factor (calcium?) and a means of selectively releasing it from the inner surface of the plasma membrane must be postulated.

Quite apart from the problem of characterizing the temporal sequence of events that link muscarinic activation to a change in membrane potential, the possibility should also be considered that the slow changes in membrane potential evoked by ACh may be an epiphenomenon of a more primary metabolic or trophic function at some muscarinic synapses (cf. Bloom, 1975). That is, one may conceive that the primary purpose of some cholinergic synapses is to allow a presynaptic influence over the metabolic machinery of the postsynaptic cell. Many agents that depolarize nerve cells can cause an increase in tissue cGMP (Ferrendelli *et al.,* 1973; Schultz and Hardman, 1975), so this effect need not be specific to ACh and may reflect a more general property of neurons. Cyclic GMP has been shown to dramatically inhibit mitochondrial calcium sequestration (Borle, 1974, 1975). The resulting rise in intracellular calcium concentration may alter the activity of several enzymes as well as influence ion flux across the cell membrane (Krnjević and Lisiewicz, 1972; Meech, 1972).

It must be emphasized that not all cholinergic effects need be associated with a rise in cGMP levels or an increased rate of phosphatidylinositol breakdown. The rapid depolarization produced by ACh at the mammalian sympathetic ganglion and neuromuscular junction probably does not involve either metabolic event. Such short latency effects of ACh are usually nicotinic (Purves, 1976), but recently we have described a short latency ACh-evoked inhibition of neurons in the feline nucleus reticularis thalami that has strong muscarinic character but is not mimicked by the iontophoretic application of cGMP (Ben-Ari *et al.,* 1976a). The nature of this ACh-evoked inhibition is discussed more fully below.

7.4 THE NUCLEUS RETICULARIS THALAMI: A CENTRAL SITE OF CHOLINERGIC INHIBITION

Since cells in most regions of the mammalian CNS are either excited or not affected, but only rarely inhibited, by iontophoretically applied ACh (Krnjević, 1974), we think it worthwhile to summarize our own detailed studies (Ben-Ari *et al.,* 1976a, b; Dingledine and Kelly, 1977) of a central mammalian site where ACh is exclusively inhibitory, the nucleus reticularis thalami (nucR).

Clearly the finding that iontophoretic ACh inhibits one group of cells in the thalamus and excites another, both of which can be distinguished on functional and anatomical grounds, raises the possibility that ACh also has a multi-receptor role in the mammalian CNS similar to that in gastropods and the cells of the frog sympathetic ganglia (cf. Section 7.2.2).

The nucR consists of a thin layer of neurons that encapsulates the anterior, dorso-lateral and ventro-lateral aspects of the thalamus, separating them from the internal capsule. Anatomical studies (Schiebel and Schiebel, 1966; Minderhoud, 1971; Jones, 1975) have shown that the cells of the nucR receive afferent collaterals from through-going thalamo-cortical fibres, and that nucR axons project back onto their associated relay nuclei. Interest has centred on a possible role for the nucR in monitoring and regulating thalamo-cortical transmission by an inhibitory feedback mechanism (Schiebel and Schiebel, 1966, 1970; Waszak, 1974). A number of electrophysiological studies appear to support this hypothesis; i.e., under a wide variety of conditions cells in other regions of the thalamus are silent when cells of the nucR are firing in high frequency bursts (Mukhametov *et al.,* 1970; Filion *et al.,* 1971; Lamarre *et al.,* 1971; Schlag and Waszak, 1971; Waszak, 1974). In other words, cells in the nucR are thought to bear the same relationship to thalamo-cortical relay cells as Renshaw cells do to spinal motoneurons.

Since any overall reduction in the firing rate of cells of the nucR should lead to an increased excitability of the thalamo-cortical relay cells and, therefore, facilitate transmission through the thalamus, any inhibitory influences on the cells of the nucR would be of interest.

We have found that iontophoretically applied ACh inhibits cells of the feline nucR and that this inhibition can be distinguished by pharmacological and physiological evidence from similar inhibitions evoked by GABA or glycine. We have also found that the mesencephalic reticular formation (MRF) has an inhibitory influence over the ACh-inhibited cells in the nucR, and the opposite effect on cells of the ventrobasal complex (VBC) that are excited by ACh.

7.4.1 Localization of ACh–inhibited cells to the nucR

Short iontophoretic pulses of ACh were found to inhibit the spontaneous discharge of virtually every cell found to lie within the region bounded by the stereotaxic co-ordinates AP 9.5–11.0, L 7.0–8.5 and H 4.0–7.0 (atlas of Snider and Niemer, 1961). Subsequent histological analysis showed that micro-electrode tracks in which only ACh-inhibited cells were encountered lay solely within the dorso-lateral nucR. On the other hand, in microelectrode tracks in which a region of ACh-excited cells was found to lie deep to the ACh-inhibited cells, histology showed that the micro-electrode had passed through the shoulder of the nucR to penetrate the VBC of the thalamus, a region long known to contain ACh-excited cells (Andersen and Curtis, 1964a, b). When the depth distribution of 200 ACh-inhibited cells found in the dorso-lateral nucR was plotted (Fig. 7.2), the greatest probability of encountering an ACh-inhibited cell was found to occur at the depth where the width of the nucR is greatest. The chance of finding an ACh-excited cell was also shown in Fig. 7.2 to increase at depths below H 4.0, where the nucR thins out to cover the lateral curvature of the VBC.

Our conclusion that the ACh-inhibited cells lay within the nucR was also strengthened by their pattern of discharge. The average firing rate of the ACh-inhibited cells in the dorso-lateral nucR was 22 Hz (SE = 1.4; n = 114) and their ongoing activity was interrupted by characteristic long duration, high frequency bursts in which the maximum frequency often exceeded 400 Hz (Figs. 7.6, 7.7, 7.8, 7.15). The firing pattern of the ACh-inhibited cells was typical of that attributed to cells of the nucR by many other groups of workers (cf. Negishi *et al.,* 1962; Mukhametov *et al.,* 1970; Schlag and Waszak, 1971; Lamarre *et al.,* 1971; Steriade and Wyzinski, 1972; Waszak, 1974). On the other hand the deeper lying cells found to be excited by ACh (Figs. 7.4 F and G, 7.13 D) had a significantly lower average firing frequency of 6.0 Hz (SE = 0.8; n = 46) and the highest frequency obtained by their rather less prominent periods of burst activity rarely exceeded 100 Hz. Very much earlier Andersen and Curtis (1964a) drew attention to the slow firing and the short duration burst activity of the ACh-excited cells in the VBC.

In addition to the ACh-evoked inhibitions in the dorso-lateral nucR, neurons lying in the rostral pole of nucR, between AP 12.0–13.0 and L 3.0–5.5, were also found to be inhibited by short pulses of ACh. Indeed in these experiments no ACh-excited cells were encountered in the rostral pole of nucR. Fig. 7.3 is a photograph of a sagittal section through the rostal thalamus in the region of the head of the caudate and shows a microelectrode track that passed through the rostal nucR. Electrode tracks in which no cells, or only a few, were encountered were later found by histology to lie within the internal capsule rostral to the thalamus. Such micro-electrode tracks served to delineate the rostral border of the thalamus and to ensure we were not recording from cells of the caudate nucleus, which are also known to be ACh-sensitive (McLennan and York, 1966).

These results show the whole of the dorsal thalamus to be surrounded by a sheet of ACh-inhibited cells. Any possible physiological role for the inhibitory action of ACh in the nucR should be very widespread, perhaps encompassing the whole of the dorsal thalamus.

7.4.2 Nature of the ACh-evoked inhibition

In contrast to the rather long latency of onset (4–8 s) for the ACh-evoked excitation of cells in the VBC, the onset of the ACh-evoked inhibition of the spontaneously active cells in nucR was rapid (Figs. 7.4, 7.5, 7.6, 7.9). Indeed on many occasions on the same cell the latency of onset of the ACh-evoked inhibition was as short as that for the onset of a glutamate-evoked excitation or of an inhibition evoked by equally potent doses of GABA (Fig. 7.11) or glycine (Figs. 7.9 and 7.10).

The ACh-evoked inhibitions proved extremely sensitive to iontophoretic

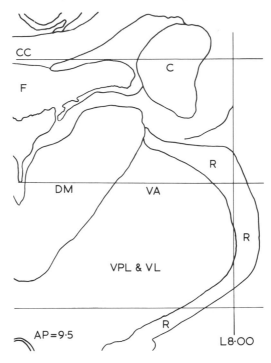

Fig. 7.2(a) The depth distribution of ACh-inhibited and excited cells encountered in the thalamus between the stereotaxic co-ordinates AP 9.5—11.5 and 7.0—8.5.

    The line drawing in A was traced from the photomicrograph designated stereotaxic plane AP 9.5 by Snider and Niemer (1961). NucR is the nucleus reticularis and VBC the ventrobasal complex, comprising the ventral anterior, ventral posterior and ventral lateral nuclei. DM is the dorsal medial nucleus, LD the dorsal lateral nucleus, F the fornix, CC the corpus callosum, Cd the dorsal head of the caudate, s the stria medullaris thalami, and v the fourth ventricle.

applications of atropine (e.g. Figs. 7.5, 7.9, 7.10, 7.11 and Table 7.1), revealing their rather strong muscarinic character. On 12 of 13 cells atropine completely and reversibly blocked the ACh-evoked inhibition. On three of four cells tested the atropine-sensitive ACh-evoked inhibition was also reversibly blocked by an iontophoretic application of dihydro-β-erythroidine, (DHβE) suggesting that the ACh receptor mediating inhibition in the nucR may be of mixed muscarinic-nicotinic character. However, the ratio of the current applied to the DHβE barrel to that applied to the atropine barrel for effective blockade of ACh-evoked inhibitions in the nucR was consistently larger than that for the same microelectrode when antagonizing ACh-evoked excitations in the VBC. In the cortex, Jordan and Phillis (1972) also found ACh-evoked inhibitions to be more readily blocked by atropine than by DHβE.

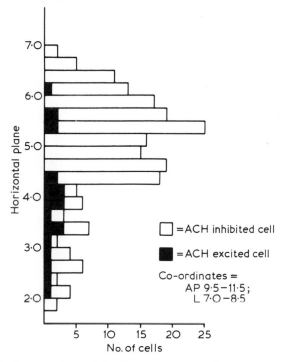

Fig. 7.2(b) In B the open bars of the histogram show the number of ACh-
inhibited cells encountered at each depth and the closed bars the number
of times that the first ACh-excited cell encountered deep to a layer of ACh-
inhibited cells was discovered at that particular depth. In 10 cats, two
hundred ACh-inhibited cells were encountered during 22 microelectrode
tracks (modified from Ben-Ari *et al.*, 1976a).

Earlier suggestions (Randić *et al.*, 1964; Duggan and Hall, 1975) that the
inhibitory action of ACh in the cerebral cortex and the more medial nuclei of the
thalamus might be mediated by an excitatory action of ACh on adjacent inhibitory
interneurons seems unlikely in the nucR in view of the extremely rapid onset for
the ACh-evoked inhibitions and their insensitivity to pharmacological antagonists
of other inhibitory agents (see Section 7.4.4). Our results are also different from
those obtained in the thalamic centromedian nucleus by Duggan and Hall (1975),
who found that ACh had a differential effect whereby it enhanced the glutamate-
evoked excitation of cells while inhibiting their spontaneous firing. We do not
favor their suggestion that the inhibitory action of ACh might be mediated pre-
synaptically. In the nucR, ACh proved to be an even more potent inhibitor of
glutamate-evoked activity than of spontaneous activity. For instance, in one
experiment in which the activity of all 16 cells encountered in one microelectrode
descent was enhanced by the release of glutamate, the current required to release

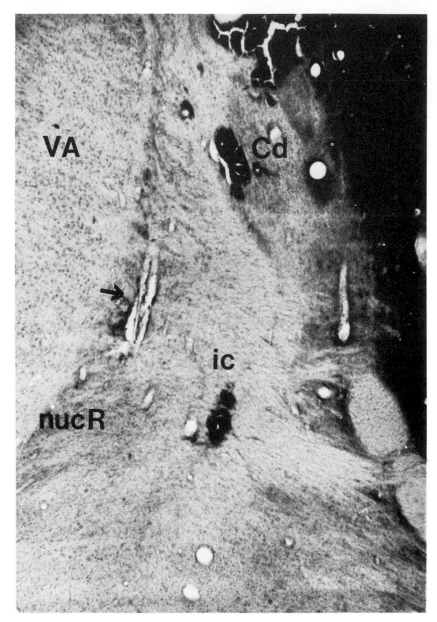

Fig. 7.3 Photomicrograph of a saggital section in which the microelectrode penetrated the rostral nucR in the region of the head of the caudate.

The arrow marks a microelectrode track through the rostral nucR in which all five cells encountered were inhibited by iontophoretic ACh. No vells were encountered in the more rostral track (below ic) which lay solely within the fibres of the internal capsule. NucR is the nucleus reticularis thalami, VA the nucleus ventralis anterior, Cd the head of the candate, and ic the internal capsule.

sufficient ACh to cause 50% inhibition was only 38 ± 5 nA, compared to the 55 ± 7 nA that was required to cause a similar inhibition of 13 spontaneously active cells encountered during an earlier descent by the same microelectrode through the contralateral nucR.

7.4.3 ACh-evoked burst activity

The spontaneous irregular firing of cells in the nucR is periodically interrupted by episodes of high-frequency bursts with relatively long intervening silent periods (Negishi *et al.,* 1962; Mukhametov *et al.,* 1970; Schlag and Waszak, 1971; Steriade and Wysinski, 1972; Waszak, 1974). An interesting property of the inhibitory action of ACh was the way in which it was associated with a dramatic increase in burst activity in neurons of both the dorso-lateral and rostral segments of the nucR. This is clearly shown by the continuous film record and interspike interval histograms (ISIH) of Fig. 7.6, in which increasing doses of ACh are seen to progressively inhibit the interburst spikes while sparing the spikes that occur within bursts. In addition, large doses of ACh caused an absolute increase in the number of spikes that occurred within each of the high frequency bursts.

The increased burst activity that occurred during ACh-evoked inhibition was not merely the result of a reduction in cell firing rate since a similar change in firing pattern was rarely seen during similar degrees of inhibition evoked by GABA or glycine. Similar records from two more cells in which the effect of ACh on the firing pattern of nucR cells was compared with that of an equipotent dose of GABA or glycine are shown in Figs. 7.7 and 7.8. Whereas the ACh-evoked inhibition was associated with a shift in the mode of the ISIH to the left, in each case the reduction in the firing frequency evoked by the amino acid was accompanied by a flattening of the ISIH. An increase in burst activity during ACh-evoked inhibition but not during inhibitions evoked by GABA or glycine was a consistant feature of all 30 cells in which the changes in firing pattern accompanying inhibition by ACh and either GABA or glycine were compared.

The ionic mechanisms responsible for the ACh-evoked inhibition in the nucR will only be revealed by the use of intracellular electrodes. However, the exaggerated burst activity that occurs during the ACh-evoked inhibition, but not during inhibition of the same cells to a similar degree by GABA and glycine, could be regarded as tentative evidence that changes in ionic conductance evoked by ACh must differ from the large increases in Cl^- conductance that are associated with the actions of GABA (Dreifuss *et al.,* 1969) and glycine (Ten Bruggencate and Engberg, 1971). Although the rapid onset of the ACh-evoked inhibition on cells of the nucR is quite unlike the slow onset for the muscarinic inhibition of frog ganglion cells described by Weight and Padjen (1973), the high firing rate of the neurons in the nucR could be the result of an abnormally high Na^+ permeability. In this situation even small reductions in Na^+ permeability could cause the immediate onset of inhibition. Indeed Krnjević (1974) has already suggested that the often-seen initial depressant

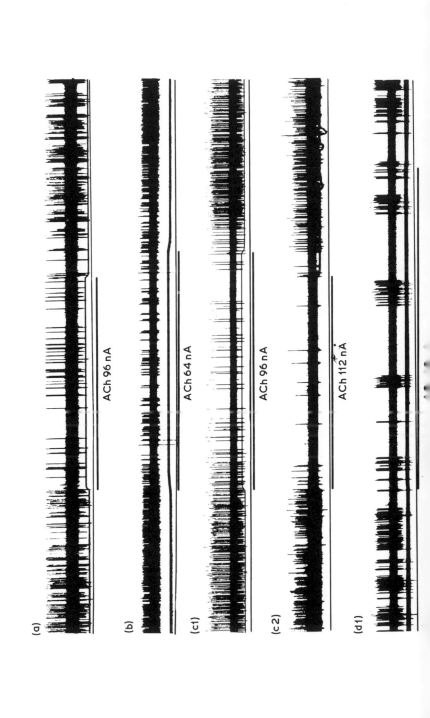

(a)

ACh 96 nA

(b)

ACh 64 nA

(c1)

ACh 96 nA

(c2)

ACh 112 nA

(d1)

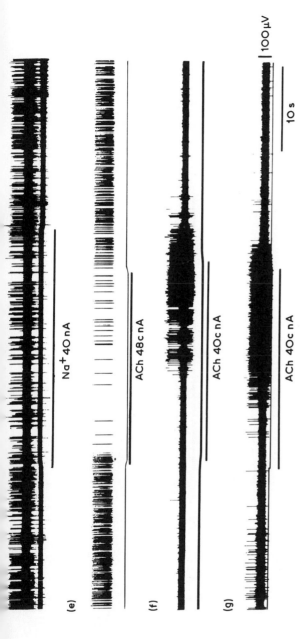

(e)

Na⁺ 40 nA

(f)

ACh 48c nA

ACh 40c nA

(g)

ACh 40c nA

10 s

|100 µV

Fig. 7.4 Moving film records to compare the spontaneous activity and ACh-evoked activity of 5 cells in the nucR and 2 cells in the ventral basal complex of the thalamus (VBC).

Records A–E show the characteristic high firing frequency and periodic burst activity of cells of the nucR. All 5 cells in the nucR were inhibited by iontophoretic ACh and both the onset and the offset of the inhibition occurred within a few seconds of the beginning and end of the ACh application (see also Figs. 7.5 and 7.9). In C, the inhibition is shown to be dose-dependent and in D not to be mimicked by positive current ejected from an adjacent NaCl containing barrel. In contrast, F and G show the spontaneous activity of 2 cells in the VBC to be slow and the onset and offset of the ACh excitation to be greatly delayed in comparison with the inhibition evoked by ACh in records A–E. The letter c that follows the ACh dose in E–G signifies that current compensation was used.

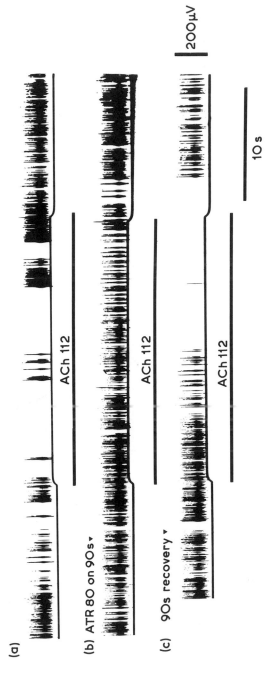

Fig. 7.5 Moving film records to show antagonism of ACh-evoked inhibition of a nucR cell by atropine. A and B show the rapid antagonism by atropine of an inhibition evoked by 112 nA of ACh. Recovery was also rapid and almost complete within 90 s of terminating the atropine application (C).

action of ACh on ACh-excited cells is a special feature of cells with a high spontaneous firing rate. Krnjević *et al.* (1971) have also suggested that ACh promotes bursts on cortical cells by delaying the repolarization of the membrane potential during the falling phase of the action potential. A decrease in the slope of the falling phase of the action potential could lead to an increase in repetitive firing triggered either by spontaneous spikes or by subliminal excitatory synaptic potentials. In this sense the inhibitory action of ACh and the tendency of ACh inhibited cells to fire in bursts could be the result of two independent actions of ACh on neuron of the nucR, an inhibition caused by a decrease in Na^+ conductance and an increased burst activity due to a simultaneous decrease in K^+ conductance.

7.4.4 Pharmacology of the ACh-evoked inhibition

Earlier we mentioned that the ACh-evoked inhibition of the cells in the nucR could be readily antagonized by the anticholinergic agents atropine and DHβE. There have been suggestions that the inhibitions evoked by ACh are artifactual in the sense that they are caused by the spread of ACh to neighboring neurons, the excitation of which leads to inhibition of the neuron under study by release of a transmitter other than ACh (Randić *et al.*, 1964; Phillis and York, 1967a, b, 1968; Jordan and Phillis, 1972; Duggan and Hall, 1975). In much the same way Libet *et al.*, (1975) have suggested that some of the hyperpolarization attributed to ACh and electrical stimulation of the preganglionic trunk in the sympathetic ganglion is the result of dopamine release from SIF cells.

Although both the unique burst-promoting property of ACh and the very rapid onset in the nucR for the ACh-evoked inhibition make this suggestion less attractive, we thought it worthwhile to determine whether the inhibition evoked by ACh could also be distinguished on pharmacological grounds from similar inhibitions evoked on the same cell by GABA and glycine, two putative inhibitory transmitters (Curtis and Crawford, 1969). Indeed, ACh-evoked inhibitions in the cerebral cortex were reported to be blocked by iontophoretic applications of strychnine and could not be differentiated by strychnine from inhibitions caused by either glycine or 5-hydroxy-tryptamine (Phillis and York, 1967a, b; Jordan and Phillis, 1972).

Our pharmacological studies are summarized in Table 7.1. Small iontophoretic applications of strychnine reversibly blocked the inhibitions evoked by glycine without affecting that evoked by ACh on 11 of 12 cells tested. For example in Figs. 7.9 and 7.10 relatively short applications of strychnine are shown on two cells to differentiate between equally effective inhibitions caused by glycine and ACh. In addition in two experiments we also examined the effects of repeated small intravenous doses of strychnine on the ACh-evoked inhibition. On both occasions total infusions of 1.2 mg kg^{-1} of strychnine were without effect on the sensitivity of the cells to ACh, even though current-response curves showed the glycine sensitivity to be reduced by about one half.

As illustrated in Fig. 7.11 a small iontophoretic application of picrotoxin of

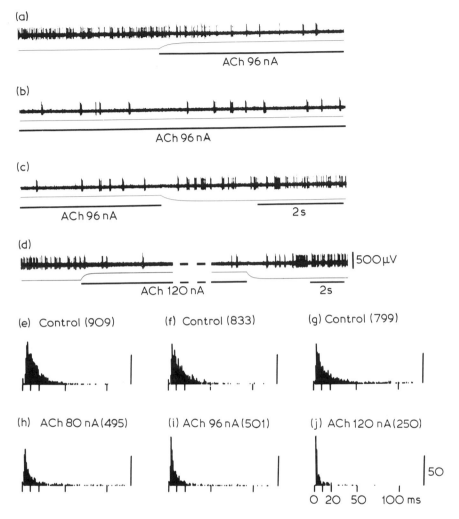

Fig. 7.6 Increased burst activity associated with the ACh-evoked inhibition of two cells in the nucR.

Continuous film records A–C show the enhanced burst activity associated with the ACh-evoked inhibition to consist of both an absolute increase in the number of bursts and an increase in the number of spikes within each burst. Note that the increase in burst activity occurred after the onset of the inhibition. The possibility that burst activity only occurs at higher ACh concentrations is supported by record D, which shows the disappearance of the burst activity at the end of the ACh application to precede that of the inhibition. (E–J) Interspike interval histograms (ISIH) compiled from the same nucR cell. The increased burst activity evoked by ACh 96 nA and 120 nA, which is apparent in

Table 7.1 Pharmacology of ACh-evoked inhibition in the nucR as revealed by specific antagonists

	Atropine	DHβE	Picrotoxin	Methyl bicucculine	Strychnine
Blocks ACh	12/13a	3/4b	2/7	0/5	1/12
Blocks GABA	0/4		9/9c	5/6d	
Blocks GLY	0/6				13/13e
Blocks ACh but not GABA/GLY	8/8				
Blocks GABA but not ACh			4/6	4/4	
Blocks GLY but not ACh					11/12

The denominator of each fraction shows the number of cells on which the antagonist shown at the top of the column was adequately tested, and the numerator the number of cells in which the inhibition evoked by the agonist shown on the left was completely and reversibly blocked. Cells were only included in the analysis if the blockade evoked by the antagonist proved to be reversible.

The mean magnitudes and durations of the currents used to release the antagonists and the time taken from the response of the agonists to recovery were respectively in (a) 52 ± 7 nA, 2.4 ± 0.3 min and 4.6 ± 0.8 min. (b) 100 ± 20 nA, 5.3 ± 0.3 min and 4.4 ± 2.0 min. (c) 45 ± 4 nA, 2.4 ± 0.4 min and 3.3 ± 0.5 min. (d) 46 ± 7 nA, 4.1 ± 0.6 min and 4.0 ± 1.0 min. (e) 51 ± 4 nA, 2.5 ± 0.4 min and 4.8 ± 0.7 min.

sufficient intensity and duration to block the inhibitory action of GABA on all nine cells tested had no effect on an equally effective dose of ACh on four out of six of these cells. In much the same way bicuculline methoiodide proved to be a specific blocker of the inhibition evoked by GABA but not that evoked by an equally effective dose of ACh on all four cells tested (Table 7.1).

In view of the cyclic GMP hypothesis for muscarinic mechanisms described in Section 7.3, we tested whether cGMP or cAMP would mimic the atropine-sensitive ACh-evoked inhibition on cells of the nucR. However, only four out of the

Fig. 7.6 (*continued*)
the film records A–C and D, respectively, is reflected by a shift to the left in the mode of the ISIHs during application of ACh (I, J) as compared with control periods (F, G). Notice that as the dose of ACh is increased the mode of the ISIH shifts progressively further to the left (H, I, J), signifying an increased burst activity during greater degrees of inhibition. The numbers in parentheses above each histogram represent the number of spikes that occurred during the 20 s interval from which the ISIH was compiled.

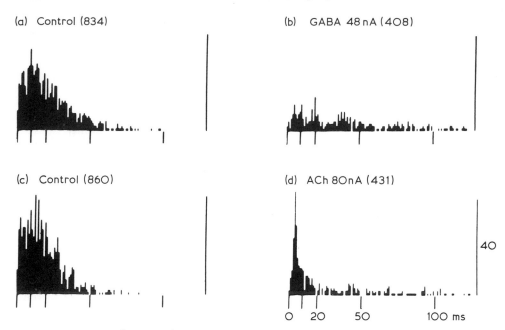

(a) Control (834)

(b)   GABA 48 nA (408)

(c) Control (860)

(d) ACh 80 nA (431)

40

O   20   50   100 ms

Fig. 7.7 ISIH's from a cell in the nucR to show the increase in burst activity
that is associated with inhibitions evoked by ACh but not GABA.

Comparison of ISIH D, compiled during and ACh-evoked inhibition, with
the control C shows an increase to have occured in the number of spikes
with short ISI and a decrease in the number with long ISI. This caused the
mode of D to lie to the left of that in the control C. On the other hand, a similar
degree of inhibition evoked by GABA 28 nA caused a decreased in the number
of spikes with both long and short ISI so that no definite difference exists
between the modes of ISIHs A and B.

48 ACh-inhibited cells tested were inhibited in a dose-dependent manner by one of
these nucleotides, and we are therefore unable to conclude that the ACh-evoked
inhibition of cells in the nucR is mediated by a rise or a fall in one of the cyclic
nucleotide intracellular messengers.

7.4.5 Correlation between effects of ACh and stimulation of the midbrain reticular
formation (MRF)

Electrocortical desynchronisation produced by high-frequency stimulation of the
MRF is accompanied by facilitated transmission through the major thalamic relay
nuclei, including the lateral geniculate (Singer, 1973), medial geniculate (Symmes
and Anderson, 1967), ventro-posteriolateral nucleus (Steriade, 1970) and the ventro-
lateral nucleus (Purpura *et al.*, 1966). In the case of the ventro-lateral and lateral
geniculate nuclei intracellular recordings showed such facilitation to result from an

Table 7.2 Responses of thalamic neurons to iontophoretic ACh and to stimulation of the MRF

Response to ACh	Response to stimulation of the MRF	
	Inhibition	Excitation
Inhibition	52	8
Excitation	6	36

Only neurons of the dorso-lateral nucR and the underlying ventro-basal complex are represented. The response of each cell was tested first to iontophoretic ACh, then to a high frequency train (usually 3 shocks at 200 Hz, repeated at 0.5 Hz) of MRF stimuli. Only data from neurons giving unambiguous responses to both stimuli are presented. A chi-squared analysis of these data confirmed that the responses were not distributed randomly ($P < 0.001$).

attenuation of recurrent inhibitory potentials (Purpura *et al.,* 1966; Singer, 1973), and so the MRF-evoked facilitation was attributed to disinhibition. A disinhibitory mechanism implies the widespread existence of recurrent inhibitory loops that serve to gate sensory transmission through the thalamus. As discussed earlier and reviewed by Waszak (1974), the nucR provides a likely locus for such inhibitory interneurons.

The observation that the MRF evokes disinhibitory potentials in the thalamo-cortical relay cells raises the possibility of an inhibitory pathway from the MRF to the nucR, and indeed there is some evidence that stimulating the MRF can lead to a decrease in unit activity in the rostral pole of nucR (Schlag and Waszak, 1971; Waszak, 1974; Yingling and Skinner, 1975). In addition a direct pathway from the MRF to nucR has been identified (Schiebel and Schiebel, 1958; Edwards and de Olmos, 1976), which may well be cholinergic (Shute and Lewis, 1967).

To determine whether the MRF sends a projection to the nucR or the VBC, we examined the effects of electrical stimulation of the MRF on the ACh-inhibited cells of the nucR and on the ACh-excited cells of the VBC. Concentric bipolar electrodes were placed in two regions of the MRF: the MRF proper (AP 3.0, L 1.5 −3.5, H + 0.5 to −0.5) and the nucleus cuneiformis (AP −1.0 to −1.5, L 3.0 −5.0, H 1.5), which in the rat is the origin of the dorsal tegmental pathway, thought by Shute and Lewis (1967) to be a massive ascending cholinergic tract.

No differences were found between stimulating the MRF or the nucleus cuneiformis, so the information obtained from both will be presented together. Post-stimulus interval histograms (PSIH) showed that most neurons in the dorso-lateral nucR and adjacent VBC responded to repetitive stimulation of the MRF (usually 3 pulses at 200 Hz, repeated every 1 or 2 s) with alternating periods of inhibition and excitation. There was a highly significant correlation between the direction of the *initial* response to MRF stimulation and the response of the cell to ACh, as shown in Table 7.2. 86% of the ACh-inhibited cells in the nucR were intially inhibited by MRF stimulation, and conversely 78% of the ACh-excited cells of the VBC were

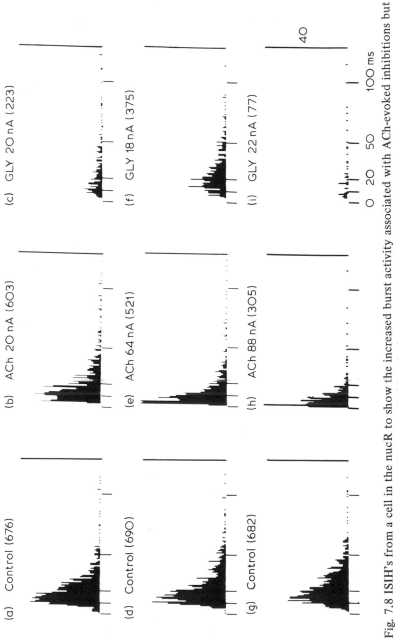

Fig. 7.8 ISIH's from a cell in the nucR to show the increased burst activity associated with ACh-evoked inhibitions but not during similar degrees of inhibition evoked by glycine.

In B, E and H progressively greater inhibitions evoked by increasing doses of ACh are accompanied by increases in the number of spikes with short ISI, signifying an increase in high frequency burst activity. The mode of the ISIHs B, E and H lie to the left of control ISIH A, D and G. The modes of ISIH's C, F and I are no different from those of control ISIH's A, D and G, and show glycine-evoked inhibition of the same cell not to be accompanied by an increase in burst activity.

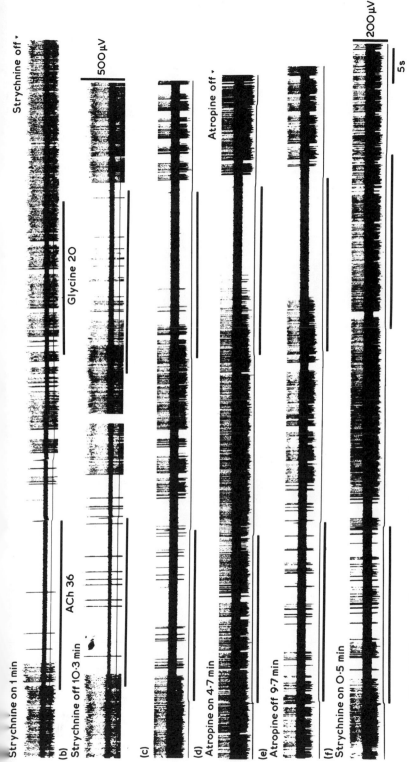

Fig. 7.9 The specific antagonism of glycine and ACh-evoked inhibition by iontophoretic applications of strychnine and atropine respectively.

Alternate ACh and glycine evoked inhibitions of a spontaneously active cell of the nucR recorded on moving film show the inhibition evoked by glycine, but not that by ACh, to be blocked on two occasions (A and F) by short applications of strychnine (40 nA). Recovery from strychnine was complete 10.3 min after the end of the strychnine application (C). (D) 4.7 min after the start of a 40 nA application of atropine, the response to ACh but not that to glycine was blocked. (E) full recovery did not occur for 9.7 min.

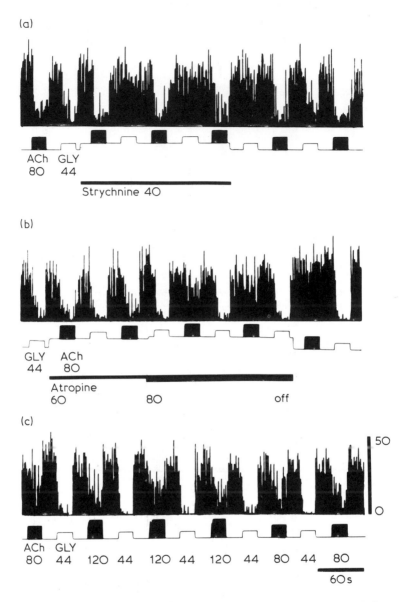

Fig. 7.10 Selective antagonism of inhibitions evoked by glycine and ACh by iontophoretic strychnine and atropine, respectively.

In A a short application of strychnine (40 nA) rapidly blocked the inhibition evoked by a 44 nA application of glycine but not that evoked by an equipotent dose of ACh (80 nA). Recovery was equally rapid. In B a slightly longer application of atropine blocked the inhibition evoked by ACh but did not affect the glycine evoked inhibition. Records B and C are continuous, and show the delayed recovery of the response to ACh from antagonism by atropine.

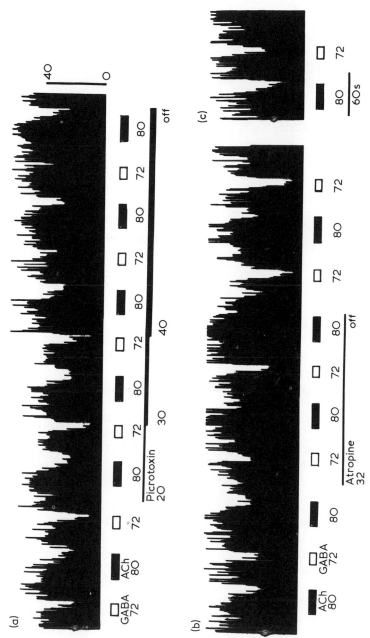

Fig. 7.11 Ratemeter records from a spontaneously active cell of the nucR to show the specific antagonism of GABA and ACh-evoked inhibitions by iontophoretic picrotoxin and atropine respectively.

In A alternate applications of GABA and ACh show the response to GABA but not that to ACh to be blocked reversibly by progressively larger applications of picrotoxin. In contrast the response to ACh but not that to GABA was blocked by a short application of atropine (B). (C) full recovery of the response to ACh occurred after approximately 4 min.

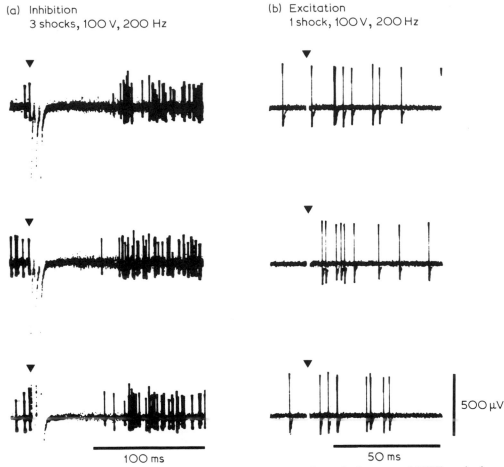

(a) Inhibition
   3 shocks, 100 V, 200 Hz

(b) Excitation
   1 shock, 100 V, 200 Hz

100 ms   50 ms   500 µV

Fig. 7.12 Film records of single unit activity to show the latency of MRF-evoked inhibition and excitation in the nucR and VBC respectively.

In A the 3 records each consist of 5 superimposed sweeps from an ACh-inhibited cell of the nucR, and show the short latency long lasting inhibition evoked by MRF stimulation (3 shocks of 100V delivered at a frequency of 200 Hz every 2 s). In B a single shock of 100V delivered every 2 s is shown to cause a diffuse excitation of an ACh-excited cell in the VBC of the thalamus.

initially excited by the stimulus. The ACh-inhibited neurons in the rostral pole of the nucR responded to MRF stimulation in a similar way to cells in the dorso-lateral nucR: 28 of 35 rostral nucR cells were initially inhibited by MRF stimulation.

The film records of single unit activity in Fig. 7.12 illustrate our finding that the latency of MRF-evoked inhibition in cells of the nucR was often only a few ms, while the MRF-evoked excitation of cells in the VBC was of a more diffuse nature and usually had a longer latency. Typical PSIH illustrating the MRF-evoked responses in a number of ACh-inhibited and excited cells are presented in Fig. 7.13. The duration of the MRF-evoked responses was up to several hundred ms, and often a short burst of spikes would interrupt a period of MRF-evoked inhibition on a nucR cell (e.g., Fig. 7.13 F and G). This type of burst might be due to subsequent activation of the nucR by a pathway that contains an additional synaptic relay.

Since the nucR is thought to inhibit the specific thalamic nuclei, the MRF-evoked excitation in the VBC could result from a combination of disinhibition originating in the nucR and feed-forward excitation mediated by other sites such as the intralaminar thalamic nuclei. These two mechanisms seem sufficient to account for the facilitation of synaptic transmission through the specific thalamic nuclei that accompanies MRF stimulation, but other reticular influences on specific thalamic nuclei are not precluded.

7.4.6 Atropine and the reticular input to the nucR

If the MRF sends a cholinergic projection to the nucR or the VBC one might expect the MRF-evoked responses to be blocked by atropine, since the ACh-evoked responses on the same cells are very sensitive to atropine. Unfortunately, we were unable to consistently and decisively antagonize the MRF-evoked responses with massive iontophoretic (24 cells) or intravenous (4 cells) doses of atropine. The iontophoretic dose of atropine used, 101 ± 11 nA for 12.9 ± 1.8 min (means $\pm$ SE; $n = 24$) was far larger than that needed to completely block the ACh-evoked inhibition of the cells in the nucR, 52 ± 7 nA for 2.4 ± 0.3 min ($n = 13$; see Table 7.1). On the other hand, in 10 cells atropine appeared to slightly reduce the magnitude of a late inhibition occurring in a polyphasic response to stimulation of the MRF, and in four of these cases there was some degree of recovery. Our most striking example of such an atropine antagonism is illustrated in Fig. 7.14, along with a more typical case in which atropine was ineffective.

Do the atropine tests refute the possibility of a cholinergic path from the MRF to the nucR, or could a technical difficulty have prevented an effective atropine blockade? Since the dendrites of cells in the dorso-lateral nucR are extremely long (up to 1–2 mm) and run in densely packed bundles (Schiebel and Schiebel, 1972), it is possible that inhibitory cholinergic synapses present on distant dendrites of nucR cells are relatively inaccessible to atropine. With the notable exception of the nicotinic synapse on the Renshaw cell (Curtis and Ryall, 1966), it has proved very difficult to block other putative cholinergic synapses in the CNS with cholinergic antagonists, even in the habenulo-interpeduncular (Lake, 1973) and septo-hippocampal (Salmoiraghi and Stefanis, 1967) pathways, which are now known to have all the biochemical properties expected of cholinergic tracts (Lewis *et al.*, 1967; Kataoka *et al.*, 1973; Kuhar *et al.*, 1975; Leranth *et al.*, 1975; Storm-Mathisen, 1975).

Acetylcholine

PSIH

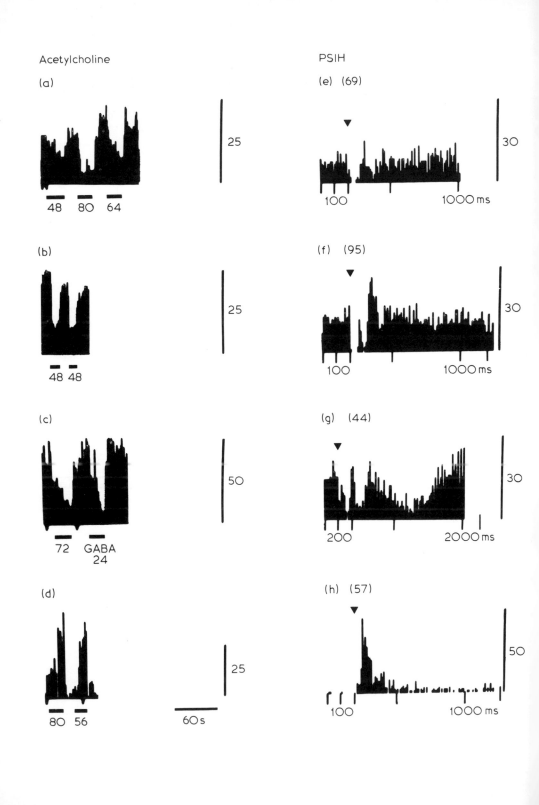

(a)

25

48 80 64

(b)

25

48 48

(c)

50

72 GABA
        24

(d)

25

80 56

60 s

(e) (69)

30

100   1000 ms

(f) (95)

30

100   1000 ms

(g) (44)

30

200   2000 ms

(h) (57)

50

100   1000 ms

The possibility remains that the diencephalic projection of the ascending cholinergic reticular fibers originates lower in the brain stem, or that a small cholinergic component recruited by MRF stimulation was not noticed due to a more prominent non-cholinergic component. It may be that more subtle cholinergic effects evoked by MRF stimulation, or indeed of the two other putative cholinergic pathways mentioned above, are atropine-sensitive but cannot be detected by extracellular recording techniques. It is conceivable that such effects are of a metabolic nature and can only be detected by other techniques.

7.4.7 Possible role for the nucR and ACh in sleep

As described above, ACh seems unique among agents that inhibit the firing of nucR neurons, in that the ACh-evoked inhibition is accompanied by an increase in burst activity. The finding that the spontaneous irregular firing of nucR neurons is intermittently interrupted by high frequency bursts with long intervening silent periods raises the possibility that synaptically released ACh may play a role in the physiological function of the nucR. For instance, it is now firmly established that during 'slow-wave sleep' (i.e., periods of electrocortical synchronisation) the firing pattern of nucR cells is composed almost entirely of burst activity separated by long silent periods, and conversely during periods of wakefulness the same cells discharge continuously in a more regular and evenly spaced manner (Mukhametov *et al.*, 1970; Lamarre *et al.*, 1971). Indeed, interspike interval histograms from a nucR cell, which show the different firing patterns during sleep and wakefulness (Lamarre *et al.*, 1971), are indistinguishable from our own histograms that show the effect of iontophoretic ACh (Fig. 7.15). This comparison suggests the existence of an inhibitory cholinergic input to the nucR that is active during slow-wave sleep. Shute and Lewis (1967) have shown the nucR to contain moderate levels of cholinesterase activity, and the very high choline acetyltransferase activity of this region (Brownstein *et al.*, 1975) also suggests that it is a likely target for cholinergic synapses. Although we have shown that the MRF participates in inhibitory input to the nucR, several considerations make it unlikely that the pathway we stimulated is mainly cholinergic. The MRF-evoked inhibition was usually atropine-insensitive and high frequency stimulation

Fig. 7.13 Typical responses from three neurons in nucR and one in the VBC to ACh and high frequency stimulation of the MRF.

In A–D ratemeter records show the response of the cells to iontophoretic ACh, and in E–H post-stimulus interval histograms (PSIH) show the response of the same cells to MRF stimulation. The typical response of ACh-inhibited cells in the nucR to MRF stimulation was either pure inhibition (E) or an inhibition that was interrupted by a burst (F, G). Occasionally the inhibitory response of an ACh-inhibited cell to stimulation of the MRF was extremely long lasting (G). In D a cell of the VBC is shown to be excited by ACh and in H by MRF stimulation.

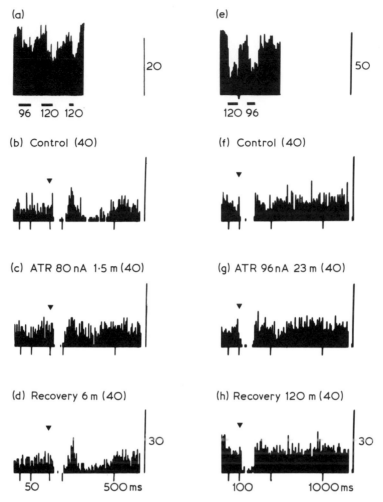

Fig. 7.14 Effects of iontophoretic atropine on MRF-evoked inhibition of 2 cells in the dorso-lateral nucR.

Rate meter record A and PSIH (B–D) show an ACh-inhibited cell that responded to high frequency stimulation of the MRF with an early (8–64 ms) and late (100–240 ms) inhibition (B). In C a small application of atropine, 80 nA for 1.5 min, is shown to have no effect on the early inhibition but to abolish the late inhibition. Recovery (D) occurred after 6 min. In (E–H) another ACh-inhibited cell is shown to respond to stimulation of the MRF with an inhibition of 4 ms latency and 56 ms duration. This cell was more typical in that a very large iontophoretic application of atropine, 96 nA for 23 min, was without effect on the MRF-evoked inhibition. In both cells the ACh-evoked inhibition was abolished near the beginning of the atropine application. On the second cell the iontophoretic application of atropine was so large that recovery of the response to ACh was not complete until 2 hours (H).

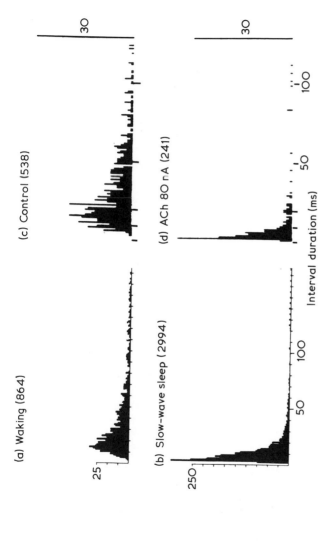

Fig. 7.15 Comparison of the firing pattern of nucR neurons during slow-wave sleep and during ACh-evoked inhibition. ISIH were compiled for a spontaneously active cell in the un-anesthetized feline nucR during a 46 s period of wakefulness (A), characterized by EEG desynchronization, and for the same cell during a 117 s period of slow-wave sleep, marked by EEG synchronisation (modified from Lamarre *et al.*, 1971). For comparison, C and D show ISIH compiled for another cell in the nucR during a 24 s control period (C) and during a 24 s iontophoretic application of ACh (D). Notice that the firing patterns during slow-wave sleep and the ACh-evoked inhibition are similar, and consist largely of ISI less than 10 ms, while the modes of the ISIH in the waking and control conditions are also similar and lie between 15–20 ms. The numbers in parentheses above each ISIH represent the number of spikes from which each ISIH was compiled.

of the MRF in un-anesthetized animals produces electro-cortical desynchronisation and behavioural arousal, precisely the opposite characteristics of slow-wave sleep.

REFERENCES

Andersen, P. and Curtis, D.R. (1964a), *Acta physiol. scand.*, **61**, 85–99.
Andersen, P. and Curtis, D.R. (1964b), *Acta physiol. scand.*, **61**, 100–120.
Anderson, C.R. and Stevens, C.F. (1973), *J. Physiol.*, **235**, 655–691.
Ascher, P. and Kehoe, J.S. (1975), *Handbook of Psychopharmacology*, Vol. 4
    (L.L. Iversen, S.D. Iversen, S.H. Snyder, (eds.), pp. 265–311.
Ben-Ari, Y., Dingledine, R., Kanazawa, I. and Kelly, J.S. (1976a), *J. Physiol.*, **261**, 647–672.
Ben-Ari, Y., Kanazawa, I. and Kelly, J.S. (1976b), *Nature,* **259**, 327–330.
Blankenship, J.E., Wachtel, H. and Kandel, E.R. (1971), *J. Neurophysiol,* **34**, 76–92.
Bloom, F.E. (1975), *Rev. Physiol. Biochem. Pharmacol.,* **74**, 1–21.
Bloom, F.E., Siggins, G.R., Hoffer, B.J., Segal, M. and Oliver, A.P. (1975),
    Adv. Cyclic Nucleotide Res., **5**, 603–618.
Borle, A.B. (1974), *J. Memb. Biol.,* **16**, 207–220.
Borle, A.B. (1975), In: *Calcium Transport in Contraction and Secretion.* (Carafoli, E.,
    Clemented, F., Drabikowski, W. and Margreth, A., eds.), The North Holland
    Publishing Co., New York.
Brownstein, M., Kobayashi, R., Palkovits, M. and Saavedra, J.M. (1975), *J. Neurochem.,*
    24, 35–38.
Burgen, A.S.V., Hiley, C.R. and Young, J.M. (1974), *J. Pharmacol.,* **51**, 279–285.
Casnellie, J.E. and Greengard, P. (1974), *Proc. natn. Acad. Sci., U.S.A.,* **71**,
    1891–1895.
Chiarandini, D.J. and Gerschenfeld, H.M. (1967), *Science,* **156**, 1595–1596.
Chiarandini, D.J., Stefani, E. and Gerschenfeld, H.M. (1967), *Science,* **156**,
    1597–1599.
Curtis, D.R. and Crawford, J.M. (1969), *Ann. Rev. Pharmacol.,* **9**, 209–240.
Curtis, D.R. and Ryall, R.W. (1966), *Exp. Brain Res.,* **2**, 81–96.
Dale, H.H. (1914), *J. Pharmacol. exp. Ther.,* **6**, 147–190.
Dingledine, R. and Kelly, J.S. (1977), *J. Physiol.,* in press.
Dreifuss, J.J., Kelly, J.S. and Krnjević, K. (1969), *Exp. Brain Res.,* **9**, 137–154.
Duggan, A.W. and Hall, J.G. (1975), *Brain Res.,* **100**, 445–449.
Eccles, R.M. and Libet, B. (1961), *J. Physiol.,* **157**, 484–503.
Edwards, S.B. and de Olmos, J.S. (1976), *J. comp. Neurol.,* **165**, 417–432.
Ferrendelli, J.A., Kinscherf, D.A. and Chang, M.M. (1973), *Mol. Pharmacol.,* **9**,
    445–454.
Ferrendelli, J.A., Rubin, E.H. and Kinscherf, D.A. (1976), *J. Neurochem.,* **26**,
    741–748.
Filion, M., Lamarre, Y. and Cordeau, J.P. (1971), *Exp. Brain Res.,* **12**, 499–508.
Gage, P.W. (1976), *Physiol. Rev.,* **56**, 177–247.
George, W.J., Polson, J.B., O'Toole, A.G. and Goldberg, N.D. (1970), *Proc. natn.
    Acad. Sci., U.S.A.,* **66**, 398–403.
Ger, B.A. and Zeimal, E.V. (1976), *Nature,* **259**, 681–684.

Goldberg, N.D., Haddox, M.K., Nicol, S.E., Glass, D.B., Sanford, C.H., Kuehl, F.A. Jr. and Estensen, R. (1975), *Adv. Cyclic Nucleotide Res.*, **5**, 307–330.
Greengard, P. (1976), *Nature*, **260**, 101–108.
Hodgkin, A.L. and Huxley, A.F. (1952), *J. Physiol.*, **117**, 500–544.
Jones, E.G. (1975), *J. comp. Neurol.*, **162**, 285–308.
Jordan, L.M. and Phillis, J.W. (1972), *Br. J. Pharmacol.*, **45**, 584–595.
Kandel, E.R., Frazies, W.T., Waziri, R. and Coggeshall, R. (1967), *J. Neurophysiol.*, **30**, 1352–1376.
Kataoka, K., Nakamura, Y. and Hassler, R. (1973), *Brain Res.*, **62**, 264–267.
Katz, B. and Miledi, R. (1970), *Nature*, **226**, 962–963.
Katz, B. and Miledi, R. (1972), *J. Physiol.*, **224**, 665–699.
Kebabian, J.W., Steiner, A.L. and Greengard, P. (1975), *J. Pharmacol. exp. Ther.*, **193**, 474–488.
Kehoe, J.S. (1972), *J. Physiol.*, **225**, 85–114.
Kehoe, J.S. and Ascher, P. (1970), *Nature*, **225**, 820–823.
Kerkut, G.A., Brown, L.C. and Walker, R.J. (1969), *Nature*, **223**, 864–865.
Kerkut, G.A. and Meech, R.W. (1966), *Life Sci.*, **5**, 453–456.
Kimura, H. and Murad, F. (1975), *J. biol. Chem.*, **250**, 4810–4817.
Krnjević, K. (1974), *Physiol. Rev.*, **54**, 418–540.
Krnjević, K. and Lisiewicz, A. (1972), *J. Physiol.*, **225**, 363–390.
Krnjević, K. and Phillis, J.W. (1963), *J. Physiol.*, **166**, 296–327.
Krnjević, K., Puil, E. and Werman, R. (1976), *Can. J. Physiol. Pharmacol.*, **54**, 172–176.
Krnjević, K., Pumain, R. and Renaud, L. (1971), *J. Physiol.*, **215**, 247–268.
Krnjević, K. and Van Meter, W.G. (1976), *Can. J. Physiol. Pharmacol.*, **54**, 416–421.
Kuhar, M.J., DeHaven, R.N., Yamamura, H.I., Rommelspacher, H. and Simon, J.R. (1975), *Brain Res.*, **97**, 265–275.
Kuhar, M.J. and Yamamura, H.I. (1976), *Brain Res.*, **110**, 229–243.
Kunze, D.L. and Brown, A.M. (1971), *Nature New Biol.*, **229**, 229–231.
Kuo, J.F., Lee, T.P., Peyes, P.C., Walton, K.G., Donnelly, T.E. and Greengard, P. (1972), *J. biol. Chem.*, **247**, 16–22.
Lake, N. (1973), *Exp. Neurol.*, **41**, 113–132.
Lamarre, Y., Filion, M. and Cordeau, J.P. (1971), *Exp. Brain Res.*, **12**, 480–498.
Lee, T.P., Kuo, J.F. and Greengard, P. (1972), *Proc. natn. Acad. Sci., U.S.A.*, **69**. 3287–3291.
Leranth, C.S., Brownstein, M., Zaborszky, L., Jaranyi, Z.S. and Palkovits, M. (1975), *Brain Res.*, **99**, 124–128.
Lewis, P.R., Shute, C.C.D. and Silver, A. (1967), *J. Physiol.*, **191**, 215–224.
Libet, B., Kobayashi, H. and Tanaka, T. (1975), *Nature*, **258**, 155–156.
McAfee, D.A. and Greengard, P. (1972), *Science*, **178**, 310–312.
McLennan, H. and York, D.H. (1966), *J. Physiol.*, **187**, 163–175.
Meech, R.W. (1972), *Comp. Biochem. Physiol.*, **42A**, 493–499.
Michell, R.M. (1975), *Biochim. Biophys. Acta*, **415**, 81–147.
Minderhoud, J.M. (1971), *Exp. Brain Res.*, **12**, 435–446.
Mukhametov, L.M., Rizzolatti, G. and Tradardi, V. (1970), *J. Physiol.*, **210**, 651–667.
Negishi, K., Lu, E.S. and Verzeano, M. (1962), *Vision Res.*, **1**, 343–353.

Nelson, P.G. and Peacock, J.H. (1972), *Science, 177*, 1005–1007.

Nelson, P.G., Peacock, J.H. and Amano, T. (1971), *J. Cellular Physiol., 77*, 353–362.

Nishi, S. and Koketsu, K. (1968), *J. Neurophysiol., 31*, 717–728.

Olson, D.R., Kon, C. and McL. Breckenridge, B. (1976), *Life Sci., 18*, 935–940.

Petersen, O.H. (1970), *J. Physiol., 210*, 205–215.

Philis, J.W. (1971), *Int. Rev. Neurobiol., 14*, 1–48.

Phillis, J.W., Kostopolous, G.K. and Limacher, J.J. (1974), *Can. J. Physiol. Pharmacol., 52*, 1226–1229.

Phillis, J.W. and York, D.H. (1967a), *Brain Res., 5*, 517–520.

Phillis, J.W. and York, D.H. (1967b), *Nature, 216*, 922–923.

Phillis, J.W. and York, D.H. (1968), *Brain Res., 10*, 297–306.

Pinsker, H. and Kandel, E.R. (1969), *Science, 163*, 931–935.

Purpura, D.P., McMurtry, J.G. and Maekawa, K. (1966), *Brain Res., 1*, 63–76.

Purves, R.D. (1976), *Nature, 261*, 149–151.

Randić, M., Siminoff, R. and Straughan, D.W. (1964), *Exp. Neurol., 9*, 236–242.

Robison, G.A., Butcher, F.R.W. and Sutherland, E.W. (1971), *Cyclic AMP*, Academic Press, New York.

Salmoiraghi, G.C. and Stefanis, C.N. (1967), *Int. Rev. Neurobiol., 10*, 1–30.

Schiebel, M.E. and Schiebel, A.B. (1958), In: *Reticular Formation of the Brain* (Jasper, H.H. (ed.), Publ.

Schiebel, M.E. and Schiebel, A.B. (1966), *Brain Res., 1*, 43–62.

Schiebel, M.E. and Schiebel, A.B. (1970), In: *The Neurosciences: Second Study Program*, (F.O. Schmitt (ed.),

Schiebel, M.E. and Schiebel, A.B. (1972), *Exp. Neurol., 34*, 316–322.

Schlag, J. and Waszak, M. (1971), *Exp. Neurol., 32*, 79–97.

Schneyer, L.H., Young, J.A. and Schneyer, C.A. (1972), *Physiol. Rev., 52*, 720–777.

Schultz, G. and Hardman, J.G. (1975), *Adv. Cyclic Nucleotide Res., 5*, 339–351.

Schultz, G., Hardman, J.G., Schultz, K. Baird, C.E. and Sutherland, E.W. (1973), *Proc. natn. Acad. Sci., U.S.A., 70*, 3889–3893.

Shute, C.C.D. and Lewis, P.R. (1967), *Brain, 90*, 497–520.

Singer, W. (1973), *Brain Res., 61*, 35–54.

Snider, R.S. and Niemer, W.T. (1961), *A Stereotoxic Atlas of the Cat Brain*, The Univ. of Chicago Press, Chicago.

Steriade, M. (1970), *Int. J. Neurobiol., 12*, 87–144.

Steriade, M. and Wyzinski, P. (1972), *Brain Res., 42*, 514–520.

Stone, T.W., Taylor, D.A. and Bloom, F.E. (1975), *Science, 187*, 845–847.

Storm-Mathisen, J. (1975), *Brain Res., 80*, 181–197.

Symmes, D. and Anderson, K.V. (1967), *Exp. Neurol., 18*, 161–176.

Takeuchi, A. and Takeuchi, N. (1959), *J. Neurophysiol., 22*, 395–411.

Tauc, L. and Gerschenfeld, H.M. (1962), *J. Neurophysiol., 25*, 236–262.

Ten Bruggencate, G. and Engberg, I. (1971), *Brain Res., 25*, 431–448.

Trautwein, W., Kuffler, S.W. and Edwards, C. (1956), *J. Gen. Physiol., 40*, 135–145.

Wachtel, H. and Kandel, E.R. (1967), *Science, 158*, 1206–1208.

Wachtel, H. and Kandel, E.R. (1971), *J. Neurophysiol., 34*, 56–68.

Waszak, M. (1974), *Exp. Neurol.,* **43**, 38–59.

Weight, F.F. (1974), In: *The Neurosciences: Third Study Program*
 (Schmitt, F.O. (ed.).

Weight, F.F. and Padjen, A. (1973), *Brain Res.,* **55**, 219–224.

Weight, F.F., Petzold, G. and Greengard, P. (1974), *Science,* **186**, 942–944.

Weight, F.F. and Votava, J. (1970), *Science,* **170**, 755–758.

White, A.A. (1975), *Adv. Cyclic Nucleotide Res.,* **5**, 353–373.

Yamamura, H.I., Kuhar, M.J. and Snyder, S.H. (1974), *Brain Res.,* **80**, 170–176.

Yingling, C.F. and Skinner, J.F. (1975), *Electroenceph. Clin. Neurophys.,* **39**,
 635–642.

8 Specific Junction Formation between Neurones and their Target Cells

J. FELDMAN

Intercellular Junctions and Synapses
(*Receptors and Recognition,* Series B, Volume 2)
Edited by J. Feldman, N.B. Gilula and J.D. Pitts
Published in 1977 by Chapman and Hall, 11 New Fetter Lane, London EC4P 4EE
© Chapman and Hall

8.1 INTRODUCTION

Of the many theories for the explanation of specific neuronal connections, two have dominated for over fifty years. The first and earlier was Weiss's. The second was Sperry's. They are outlined in Sections 8.2 and 8.3. Neither theory adequately explains recent data or contains enough detail to interpret what must plainly be a highly complex process. Therefore, this review, after briefly discussing the ideas of Weiss and Sperry, presents a description and analysis of consecutive developmental steps culminating in the establishement of specific neuronal connections.

The essential problem is to know how the spatial contiguity between central nervous system neurones is determined and then transposed by the axonal terminals of these cells to appropriate target cell sites.

In approaching a solution, the first question is whether the patterns of cells within the central nervous system and peripheral target tissues are established independently. If they are, correspondence between matching cells within the two connecting areas could be affected and selective connections then made. Alternatively, the pattern of either the central nervous tissues or peripheral target tissues must be imposed one upon the other via connecting neuronal links which carry information from the modulating tissue to that modulated.

8.2 MODULATION VERSUS SELECTIVE NERVE CONNECTION

The concept of modulation was originally put forward by Paul Weiss in order to explain the phenomenon of the 'homologous' or 'myotopic' response. When an extra limb was grafted onto an animal, both transplanted and normal muscles of the same kind were always seen to contract together (Weiss, 1926, 1936). Weiss explained this by saying that each muscles is uniquely specified; any nerve making effective contact with such a muscle becomes biochemically altered (modulated) by the contact. The axon and cell body of each motoneurone are therefor specified in accordance with the nature of the contacted muscle. In these terms, the establishment of a simple reflex arc (motoneurone linking with interneurone, in turn linking with sensory neurone) can be considered. A dorso-proximal leg muscle, for example, imposes its character upon a motoneurone which contacted the muscle randomly during development. In a retrograde fashion, the motoneurone then imposes this character upon an interneurone, which in turn modulates a sensory neurone such that the latter finally connects with dorso-proximal leg skin. So, a reflex arc could be built which would form the basis for reflex responses in the developed organism.

Evidence to support the concept of modulation has often been presented in the literature. The difficulty in evaluating such evidence lies in the presence of a viable alternative explanation for the results in each case, namely, the possibility that selective reconnection of nerves to the target has occurred. Two examples may be cited: the original work on the development of nerve connections in supernumery limbs of amphibians (Weiss, 1926, 1936) has been superceded by data showing selective innervation of such extra limbs (Grimm, 1971); the innervation of rotated skin grafts by sensory neurones (Miner, 1956; Jacobson and Baker, 1969; Baker, 1976) has been challenged by the work of Bloom and Thompkins (1976) where selective re-innervation of the skin grafts has been inferred.

A strong case can often be made for a selective innervation of target organs by central nervous system neurones during *regeneration* experiments (see reviews by Gaze, 1970; Jacobson, 1970; Chung and Feldman, 1974; Cotman and Banker, 1974; Harris, 1974; Purves, 1976; Landmesser, 1976; Keating and Kennard, 1975; Cotman and Lynch, 1976; Fambrough, 1976; Kuffler and Nicholls, 1976; Keating, 1976; Meyer and Sperry, 1976) and selective re-innervation in *tissue culture* (Olsen and Bunge, 1973; Crain and Petersen, 1975). These experimental studies are taken to provide acceptable analogies for the developmental process itself.

We might usefully take the view at this time that modulation and selective neuronal connection may both operate in development, even although there is no satisfactory evidence for modulation at present. In some parts of the developing nervous system of certain animals, modulation may operate. In many parts of the developing nervous system of other animals, positional patterns of cells within the central nervous system and target organs may equally well develop independently: the subsequent linkage between the two systems would then be effected by selective synapse formation.

The selection process itself may either be active (searching out, recognition of correct target cell, and then stabilization of the linkages) or more passive (axons arrive at the correct loci by such means as pathway guidance and/or a timed sequence of developmental events). Conceivably, a combination of active and passive mechanisms may operate.

Some of these possibilities will now be discussed.

8.3 THE CHEMO-AFFINITY HYPOTHESIS

8.3.1 Sperry's original results

The most powerful model of an active recognition process which might account for selective neuronal connections during development was proposed by R.W. Sperry (1943a,b, 1944, 1945a,b, 1948, 1949, 1950, 1951, 1955, 1958, 1963, 1965; Meyer and Sperry, 1976). The model was developed to explain the pattern of regenerating retino-tectal connections which developed in lower vertebrates, after one eye had been rotated.

A brief introduction to the anatomy of the optic nerve in lower vertebrates is given now, before describing regeneration of the nerve in these animals.

Adult goldfish optic nerves contain about 100 fascicles, each of which comprise 50–100 fibres, most of which are myelinated. At the optic chiasma, the two optic nerves curl round one another, without interlacing their fibres (Gaze, 1970). The fibres then travel up the sides of the diencephalon to reach the contralateral surface of the tectum (visual brain). Adult newts have fewer fibres than goldfish (nearly 30 000). Most of these are unmyelinated. Frogs and toads also have optic nerves with mainly unmyelinated fibres (50 000 in adult *Xenopus*; 500 000 in adult frog). The axons make direct contact with one another, and are contained within compact bundles. At the optic chiasma, fibres from the two eyes mingle with one another before separating into the two tracts (Gaze, 1970). One tract from each eye then passes up the side of the contralateral diencephalon to reach the tectal surface, where fibres peel off in successive rows to reach their terminal sites.

In the early 1940s, two hypotheses were popular as explanations for the basis of selective neuronal connections: contact guidance of axons along oriented substrates (Weiss, 1934, 1939, 1941, 1945, 1956) and experience i.e. repetitive usage of synapses would stabilize the contacts. Sperry cut one optic nerve (which resulted in subsequent scrambling of the half a million optic axons present at the scar site) and rotated the eye connected to the nerve, in several classes of lower vertebrate. The animals consistently behaved as if they saw upside-down and back-to-front, and this behaviour persisted for some months after the operation.

These results excluded the possibilities that contact guidance operated to guide axons to their proper places, since the fibres which grew through the scar site were scrambled there, which can be assumed to disrupt the normal spatial relationships between fibres. This data also ruled out experience as an operative factor since the animals failed to re-learn normal vision. The two hypotheses of Sperry's contempories were thus ruled out. Instead, Sperry proposed that retinal ganglion cells became stamped with markers which in some way related to the particular positions of the cells at a particular time during early development. Cells of the optic tectum (visual brain) became independently and similarly marked, and later, during development, optic cells actively seek out and find their predestined partner cells in the tectum. This process can be repeated during regeneration, and can explain the movements in direction opposite from that in which the lure is presented, and which the experimental animals with one eye rotated and optic nerve cut had shown.

Sperry then presented a fairly comprehensive model of the way in which the retino-tectal cells might become labelled. This time he was able to include the ideas of his contemporaries (embryologists)! The early developing retina and tectum were considered as flat two-dimensional fields for the sake of simplicity (for in fact, each has a third dimension). It was imagined that there might be at least two morphogens, arranged in gradients across the antero-posterior and dorso-ventral axes of the sheets of cells. In this set-up, each cell is unique in that its position is specified by two particular morphogen values. An analogy is each square in a piece of graph paper which can be located by virtue of its position, and particular combination of X and Y values.

Retinal and tectal cells were thought to express this uniqueness in the form of particular cytochemical labels. Corresponding retino-tectal pairs would 'recognize' one another and link, by chemo-affinity.

In 1963, Attardi and Sperry tested for the phenomenon of selective connection by removing one half or the centre or the periphery of an adult goldfish eye. The regenerating axons from the remaining part of the eye were traced back after 20 days to their places on the optic tectum, using a modified Bodian stain. It was found that fibres terminated at their appropriate places, even travelling over inappropriate tectal territory to do so. For example, nasal retinal fibres passed over empty rostral tectum in order to link with caudal tectal surface.

Selective termination of retinal ganglion neurones at appropriate tectal loci has also been demonstrated by other workers in goldfish (Sharma, 1972a,b, Cook and Horder — in the early patterns of regeneration in goldfish retino-tectal projections only, 1974; Meyer, 1975), *Xenopus* (Straznicky, 1973) and chick (Crossland *et al.* 1974). The last-named authors, for example, removed part of the retina from chick embryos on about the third day of incubation. They then studied the projection of the remaining retina onto the developing tectal surface, using ^{3}H-proline to trace axons. The retinal axons always travelled back to that part of the optic tectum with which they would normally synapse, bypassing inappropriate territory where necessary. These authors were able to show the actual sites of termination of retinal ganglion cell axons, since in the chick fibres dip down into the tectum from the *stratum opticum,* running along the tectal surface, at approximately their site of termination. This anatomy is different from that in the lower vertebrates, where axons travel for some distance in the layers in which they finally make synapses, and terminating fibres cannot therefore be easily distinguished from fibres of passage.

It is unfortunate that to date, experiments performed have not provided details as to the numbers cells contacted by one axon. The working out of the exact ways in which axons might select their final targets must depend, to some extent, upon such knowledge.

8.3.2 Mismatching experiments

In 1963, Gaze, Jacobson and Székely made 'compound' eyes in *Xenopus* embryos. For example, they removed the temporal half-eye from each of two embryos placed nose-to-nose in a dissecting dish, and then transplanted the nasal half-eye from one to the other, so creating double-nasal 'compound' eyes in which a correspondence between the dorso-ventral axes of the transplant and the host half-eyes was maintained. Double-temporal eyes were similarly constructed. The retino-tectal projections from each half-eye were mapped, using electro-physiological methods. It was found that the naso-temporal extent of each half-eye mapped to the entire rostro-caudal extent of the dorsal tectal surface. The Sperry hypothesis would have predicted that each half-eye would project to only the appropriate half of the rostro-caudal extent of the dorsal tectum.

Since this time, numerous experiments have been performed (reviewed by Keating, 1976; Keating and Kennard, 1975; Meyer and Sperry, 1976) in which half-retinae are made to connect with whole tecta; whole retinae are made to connect with half-tecta; or, half-retinae and half-tecta are allowed to make connections in embryos or adult animals in which optic regeneration is known to be possible, such as goldfish, frog, toad, salamander and newt. The results of Attardi and Sperry (1963) on the one hand, and of Gaze, Jacobson and Székely (1963) on the other, represent the alternative outcomes between which experiments of this type necessarily discriminate (Chung and Feldman, 1974).

8.3.3 Attempts to conserve Sperry's original hypothesis

Several attempts have been made to conserve the essence of Sperry's hypothesis, already outlined. First, Sperry (1965) proposed that the results of the 'compound' eye experiments of Gaze, Jacobson and Székely (1963) could be explained, if it were assumed that the optic tectum receiving axons from only one type of half-eye (say, nasal half and not temporal half) responded by an overgrowth and differentiation of only the appropriate half-tectum. The overgrown half-tectum would then macroscopically resemble a whole tectum, but the nature of the tectum would be made manifest by virtue of the spread of the retino-tectal projection from the appropriate half-retina.

Straznicky, Gaze and Keating (1971) tested this hypothesis by uncrossing the optic chiasma in animals in which 'compound' eyes had been surgically constructed during embryonic life. They found that the normal eye projected across the entire extent of the dorsal surface of the 'suspect' hypertrophied half-tectum, as did the 'compound' eye across the normal tectum. Sperry's explanation for the 'compound' eye experiments was therefore inadequate.

Secondly, Sperry has suggested that the cytochemical labels on retinal and tectal cells may not be stable as originally stated (Sperry, 1951), but instead, cells may become relabelled within a retinal or tectal field of cells which alters in response to the creation of new boundaries defining the field. New boundaries could be effected by, say, surgical cuts or ablations of part of an organ.

Such a scheme seems more acceptable when applied to a growing embryonic organ such as *Xenopus* 'compound' half-eyes (Straznicky, Gaze and Keating, 1971), especially as such half-eyes can regulate to form whole eyes (Feldman and Gaze, 1975; Berman and Hunt, 1975). However, it becomes harder to accept such a notion when explaining the results in adult animals, which do not show regulation. This explanation has nevertheless been suggested for adult goldfish (Yoon, 1971; 1972a,b,c) and anurans (Meyer and Sperry, 1973; 1974; 1976).

Furthermore, three sets of experimental results appear to argue against the idea that regulation may occur.

In 1972 Sharma (1972a,b) made rectilinear lesions across goldfish tecta, and was subsequently able to record normal maps — even though new boundaries had been created. Meyer and Sperry (1976) argued that the type of incision made, and also the length of post-operative recovery might have allowed the old boundary conditions to be re-established.

Cook and Horder (1974, 1977) showed an initial absence of compression of the retino-tectal projection in adult goldfish with half-tecta. This is to say that the visual map from the whole eye was not squashed in an ordered way onto the remaining half-tectum. The projection subsequently compressed with time. Crushing the optic nerve a second time did not cause an immediate compression either. The latter might have been anticipated, were the tectal fragment to have regulated in terms of cell relabelling.

Feldman, Gaze and Keating (1975) observed, by chance, in one animal of a series of *Xenopus* in which optic fibres had been made to travel to both tecta, that the projection of fibres from half the retina of a known normal retina (which projected across the whole of one tectum) also projected across the whole extent of the (opposite) tectum. In this animal, the fibres from the half-retina belonged to an unregulated eye, and yet they did not go to their proper places, in accordance with the Sperry hypothesis. So, they spread their connections, making the necessity for regulation redundant in this instance, and also possibly redundant in other experimental situations for which the idea has been invoked. This single result was reported since the anatomy of projection achieved by chance, is difficult to repeat by experiment. It is most unusual to be in a position of knowing that part of a retina belongs to a whole retina, and therefore cannot be supposed to have regulated.

Chung and Feldman (1973) have already pointed out that once a general theory about a system does not apply, unamended, when the system is perturbed, then in effect the theory becomes untestable. At the very least, such a theory changes from a strong to a weaker one, and stimulates the search for an alternative general theory.

8.4 A SEQUENCE OF DEVELOPMENTAL FACTORS DETERMINE SPECIFIC NEURONAL CONNECTIONS

The formation of specific neuronal connections is probably best understood as a series of steps in development. Some of the steps have been already suggested by Sperry and others. Some steps have not. They will be described in sequence now in order to give a coherent picture. These are the mechanisms which I think are most important in bringing about selective neuronal connections in development.

8.4.1 Early programming of the genome

In contrast to the predictions made about selective reconnection, Sperry's proposal that retinal cells are programmed early in development has been unequivocally borne out by experiments (Székely, 1954, Jacobson, 1968a). Eyes which are rotated early in development, long before axons have been formed, develop rotated retino-tectal projections later. A correlation of particular steps in the early programming with particular cell division cycles (Jacobson, 1968b; Hunt, 1975; Bergey, Hunt and Holtzer, 1975) and with the presence of gap junctions (Dixon and Cronly-Dillon, 1972, 1974) has been proposed.

8.4.2 Gradients

The assigning of gradients of chemicals to sets of cells contained within a particular part of a developing system, and the interpretation of such information by the cells, are subjects for wide, theoretical debate (Wolpert, 1969, 1971; McMahon and West, 1976).

A particularly interesting suggestion found in Sperry's original model has been put forward by Roth and his colleagues (Marchase, Pierce and Roth, 1977). These workers have proposed that the presynaptic cell may couple with the post-synaptic cell, because the one carries on its membrane an enzyme which binds specifically to a substrate carried on the other. Different pairs of pre- and post-synaptic cells might have different affinities because they have different concentrations of the enzyme and its substrate on their membranes.

Marchase, Pierce and Roth suggest specifically that the membrane-bound enzyme may be GM1 synthetase, and have indeed demonstrated a graded concentration of this enzyme across the retina. The activity per mg protein is highest ventrally, and decreases in a dorsal direction. They have, however, only indirect evidence for a complementary gradient of substrate (the ganglioside GM2) across the tectal surface.

Such gradients could explain the *in vitro* selective adhesion which has been shown to exist between populations of chick embryo dorsal retinal cells and ventral tectal surfaces, or ventral retinal cells and dorsal tectal surfaces (Barbera, Marchase and Roth, 1973; Barbera, 1975; Roth and Marchase, 1976). The gradients might even be invoked to account for the selective adhesion which has been shown to exist, for example, between dissociated *retinal* cells taken from dorsal chick retina and mono-layers of ventral *retinal* cells (Gottlieb, Rock and Glaser, 1976). In other words, the same substrate gradient might be present on both retinal and tectal cells. The substrate on either of the 2 cell populations would react with the gradient of retinal enzyme in an identical way.

The part that gradients of membrane-bound enzymes and their complementary membrane-bound substrates might play in development still remains, however, an open question. If antibodies against putative substrates (for example GM2) could be shown to prevent the formation of retino-tectal projection patterns *in vivo*, then the gradient enzymologists and substratologists would be in business!

8.4.3 Pathway guidance

Given a form of protoplasm with power to extend itself in a definite direction so as to form a fibre, the next step is to determine the influences which may modify the direction of its growth and produce the specific arrangement of nerve tracts found in the mature organism.

Harrison (1910)

Axons may arrive at their correct target zone during development because they have been guided down the correct pathways. Some examples may be cited.

In stage 28–29 chick embryos, spinal nerves destined for the limb muscles reach the muscle masses when these are not yet differentiated into individual muscles (Landmesser and Morris, 1975; Landmesser, 1976). If spinal nerves 1–3 are electrically stimulated at this time, Landmesser and her colleague have found that only the anterior, medial surface of the tigh muscle mass will contract. This part of the undifferentiated muscle mass later forms the sartorius and femerotibialis muscles, which are also supplied by spinal nerves 1–3. Spinal nerves therefore appear to enter the correct part of the target muscle mass, as though they have been previously guided to the right spot.

Retinal axons may be guided towards the optic tectum. The optic stalk provides mechanical guidance for axons leaving the developing eye-cup. Chung and Cooke (in press) have shown that when the pre-optic nucleus and hypothalamus are experimentally induced to form more posteriorly than normal, the optic fibre pathways change their direction, seemingly in a way that keeps constant the distances between the optic chiasma and these nuclei.

Even if the optic fibres are deliberately or accidentally misrouted (Hibbard, 1967; Gaze, 1970) or the timing of entry of optic fibres disrupted (Feldman, Gaze and Keating, 1971), the tectum seems to act as an aligning beacon which orients the retinal population. The spatial contiguity between the incoming retinal axons might be preserved by one mechanism (related to either graded chemical labels or, perhaps, synchrony in discharge of nearest neighbour retinal cells—Hope, Hammond and Gaze, 1976; Willshaw and von der Malsburg, 1976; Gaze and Hope, 1977; Gaze, in press). The alignment of the entire, ordered retinal fibre input may then be achieved by a couple of markers in or on the tectum (Willshaw and von der Malsburg, 1976) or perhaps markers which act like arrows and convey directional properties upon consecutive small areas of tectum (Hope, Hammond and Gaze, 1976).

The mechanisms which might operate to effect pathway guidance in development are now considered.

I want to suggest that, early in vertebrate development, programmed retinal cells send out axons which migrate over virgin terrain to predestined targets in a fashion analogous to migrating birds.

Birds have numerous directional cues available to them, and apparently natural selection has favoured the development of abilities to make use of all available cues, which include the use of sun, stars, the position of the sunset, the directionality of the winds, the direction of the earth's magnetic field, the presence of topographical landmarks and the activity and call notes of birds of the same species (Emlen, 1975).

Some cues may give more accurate information than others, some may be available throughout the flight, some may be available regardless of flight conditions whereas others may be employed at specific geographical conditions only or under optimal meteorological conditions.

It is probable that the cues can be combined in a variety of ways depending on such factors as weather conditions and the age of the bird (Keeton, 1974).

Aeons of selective pressure may equally well have shaped the behaviour of axons as that of birds. Axons have to navigate wide distances of virgin terrain during development, and it is quite likely that they should do so on a basis of responsiveness to multiple cue systems, not all of which will be available to any given cell at one particular time. As with migrating birds, we do not yet know enough to explain how an individual cell finds its way to its destined target. Some suggestions as to directional cues be made, and there is some evidence that suggests a hierarchy of importance of such cues.

Chemo-affinity

Sperry (Attardi and Sperry, 1963; Meyer and Sperry, 1976) has suggested that chemo-affinity factors might operate to determine the patterning of fibres within central fibre tracts and even within the optic nerve itself.

The *in vitro* experiments of Barbera, Marchase and Roth (1973) in chick retino-tectal systems and the pathway selectivity through the tectum observed in chicks in which retinal quadrants have been ablated (Crossland *et al.,* 1974) would support the idea that pathway guidance may depend in part, at least, upon selective adhesion between axons and substrate.

Tissue culture experiments have been exploited to demonstrate that cell–substrate adhesion may determine cell movement (Carter, 1965) and the direction of growth cone elongation (Letourneau, 1975). Elongating growth cones select surfaces to which they adhere most strongly, or, do not choose surfaces from which they detach most readily (Trinkaus, 1976). Thus cell–substrate adhesion may equally well determine the direction of nerve fibre outgrowth *in vivo*.

Toole (1976) has suggested that an increased hyaluronate might play a part in the extensive neuronal migrations that occur during the development of embryonic chick brain.

Chemotaxis
Another 'variation on a theme of chemo-affinity' can be imagined in that some cytochemical labels might become detached from target cells and attract their appropriate neurones by chemotaxis. Ramón y Cajal (1960, in translation) was convinced some fifty years ago that chemotaxis was instrumental in directing fibres towards the source of some diffusible chemical emanating from the target tissue. *In vitro* experiments would seem a potentially productive way of studying candidate factors for chemotaxis. However, reports of selective outgrowth between paired explants are not common, although some have been made (Peterson and Crain, 1970; Levi-Montalcini and Chen, 1971; Chamley, Goller and Burnstock, 1973; Olsen and Bunge, 1973; Coughlin, 1975; Crain and Peterson, 1975; Chamley and Dowel, 1975).

In many of these studies Nerve Growth Factor (NGF) has been implicated as a chemotactic factor, although the evidence is never strongly convincing. NGF has been studied by Levi-Montalcini and her colleagues (reviewed by Levi-Montalcini, 1972; Chamley, Campbell and Burnstock, in press). These studies provide a good example of how a diffusible factor that stimulates directional axonal growth can be produced by a tissue (such as sarcoma 180). Chamley, Goller and Burnstock (1973), for example, showed preferential growth from rat sympathetic ganglia to explants of atrium and vas deferens as compared with explants of kidney, adrenal medulla, uterus and ureter. The authors proposed that the density of ganglionic outgrowth towards any particular explant correlated with the density of the normal innervation of the tissue explanted. They suggested that a diffusing chemical (possibly NGF) from the explants was involved. Later, Chamley and Dowel (1975) showed that there was no preferential growth towards the atrium and vas deferens by neurones that are insensitive to the action of NGF. Ebendal and Jacobson (1977) have found that ganglionic neurones which respond by a directionally preferential outgrowth towards appropriate targets in culture, respond likewise to capillary tubes containing NGF.

Contact guidance and contact inhibition
Harrison (1910) made it clear that solid support is essential for successful axonal outgrowth. Weiss (1934, 1941, 1945) re-affirmed this, but stressed in addition that orientation by extracellular topography (contact guidance) may contribute substantially to the direction of axonal outgrowth. In the embryo, orienting structures might be extracellular matrices (Bard and Elsdale, 1972; Ebendal, 1976a); cells or their processes (Rakič and Sidman, 1973; Henrikson and Vaughn, 1974); or other axons, such as, for example, pioneering nerve fibres (Lopresti, Macagno and Levinthal, 1973; Bate, 1976). Such oriented surfaces direct axons during development. Nornes and Das (1972), for example, examined the possible guiding role that

might be played by oriented surfaces existing in embryonic rat spinal cord at the time of early outgrowth of the axons. Pioneering fibres were seen to extend ventrally and then longitudinally along the surface between the regressed neuro-epithelium and the column of motor neuroblasts, and also along the oriented surface existing between the motor neuroblast column and the external limiting membrane. Later, axonal processes extended along and accumulated upon the initial pathfinder axons, so creating the longitudinal fasciculus.

Ebendal (1977) has used scanning and transmission electron microscopy to study the migration of neural crest cells and scelerotome cells, and also the elongation of ventral root axons, in stage 16–20 chick embryos. His work suggests possible mechanisms which might operate to promote contact guidance *in vivo*. Migrating cells appeared to explore, with pseudopodia, the substrate of matrix fibrils upon which they travelled: the fibrils around the notocord showed spatial arrangements which could direct the pathway of the scelerotome cells. The basis for the influence of spatial arrangements in the matrix upon the directed movements of migrating cells or elongating axons, might relate to corresponding variations in the adhesiveness of the substrate (Letourneau, 1975; Ebendal, 1976c).

It is important to separate the concepts of contact guidance by an oriented substrate from pathway guidance by selective adhesion (a mechanism which has already been discussed above). Two differences are apparent: in contact guidance, orienting structures may actually be observed and mechanical guidance is stressed, whereas in cases where selective adhesion is hypothesized, associated morphological features are not necessary to the postulate and chemical composition of the substrate seems all important. Also, Ebendal (1977) has observed specialized contacts between migrating cells, and filopodia from axonal growth cones were seen to contact both the extracellular space ahead, and mesenchymal cells. He has suggested that the specialized contacts might correlate *in vivo* with the phenomenon of contact inhibition (of cell movement), as has been demonstrated in cultured fibroblasts (Heaysman and Pegrum, 1973).

That contact inhibition might contribute to pathway guidance in the migration of cells and axons has also been considered by other authors (for example, see Nelson and Revel, 1973; Bard, Hay and Meller, 1975; Ebendal, 1976b). What is being emphasized here is the notion that contact guidance *in vivo* may be a phenomenon that relies upon more than one mechanism for its effects.

A possible analogy between axonal pathway guidance and bird migration, relying on two or three directional cues plus the call notes between birds (like signals for contact inhibition) can be usefully accented.

A hierarchy of directional cues
Some of the factors which might operate as directional cues during pathway guidance have now been noted.

It was suggested at the beginning of this section that, amongst the many cues available to growing axons, some might provide more important information to axons than others, depending on prevailing conditions. In order to try and find out which cues might count more to an axon provided with multiple sources of information, it is necessary to test one cue against another, and so construct a hierarchy amongst the cues, from which the relative importance of a cue may easily be deduced.

Some examples of such experimental situations have been chosen to illustrate this idea. Axons are exposed to conditions in which at least 2 cues operate. In certain circumstances one cue will dominate. In other situations, another cue takes precedence. It is assumed that in nature cues will vary in importance in a similar way, given that the conditions remain unaltered. Where conditions change, so the value of cues may also be expected to alter.

Van der Loos (1965) examined 'improperly' oriented pyramidal cells in the cerebral cortex, a subpopulation of some 20% of cells. He was able to show that the dendrites from such cells were always oriented according to the orientation of the cell body. The axons from such cells, however, always corrected their orientation of growth so that they became parallel to the axons from normal cells. In following the direction of outgrowth taken by the normal (80%) population of pyramidal cells, the axons of abnormal cells demonstrate their sensitivity to certain specific directional cues – cues to which the dendrites of the same cells had failed to respond.

Where an explant is growing on an oriented substrate, there may be a conflict between guiding cues from the substrate, and the effect of contact inhibition (that is, the inhibition of further movement in the same direction when two cells contact one another). Under some circumstances the one cue may dominate, and therefore come higher in the hierarchy. In other circumstances the other cue may be higher in the hierarchy.

Thus, Ebendal (1976c) observed that the orientation of outgrowing axons from ganglia explanted on the aligned surface of collagen fibrils was determined by the density of axonal outgrowth. When the latter was low, the axons oriented along the alignment axis of the substratum; when the density was high, the axons formed radial arrays. The author has suggested that when many axons are present, contact inhibition operates maximally, whereas guidance along the aligned collagen fibril surface is minimal. Under conditions of low density, the balance of the above two postulated directional cues is reversed with an ensuing change in axonal orientation resulting.

Dunn (1973) has also shown that contact inhibition may be at least as important as surface orientation in guiding outgrowing axons.

8.4.4 Timing of axonal outgrowth

A variety of directional cues may well play an important part in the determination of pathway guidance of axons, and thereby the eventual establishment of selective connections. It is important to consider, however, that a critical timing of events must also correspond in normal development with the actual outgrowth of fibres and availability of informational cues. In the migration analogy, winds and local vegetation will differ with the seasons.

Nornes and Dal (1972), for example, have stressed the correlation between the systematic release and settling of rat spinal cord neuroblasts and the subsequent direction of axonal growth from these cells within the embryonic cord.

Lopresti, Macagno and Levinthal (1973) have made three-dimensional reconstructions of elongating optic axons in *Daphnia* embryos. They have shown that receptor cells from the eyes (ommatidia) send out axons in a well-defined temporal sequence to optic ganglion neuroblasts. The axons appear to connect randomly with passing, undifferentiated neuroblasts. This contact triggers the further differentiation and migration of the axon-neuroblast units. The authors have concluded that this temporal sequence of the events is sufficient to account for the adult patterns of connections between ommatidia and optic ganglia neurones.

8.4.5 Final selection of target site

Once fibres have reached their target zone, they are still left with the task of finding their exact position within the zone. How this process is achieved is largely unknown. Three important factors may operate at this time of development to determine the final target site: competition between fibres; shrinkage of the initially established axonal territory, probably in association with some competitive principle, and local chemical and electrical effects. Each of these factors will now be considered separately.

Competition

Ideas about how competition between axon terminals may operate to bring about selective connections between the axons and their target sites are based predominantly on the results of nerve regeneration experiments. It is assumed that the same factors which operate in development also act in regeneration, but of course development and regeneration are probably not identical. It is possible that in the adult developmental forces are attenuated. On the other hand, in the adult, guiding pathways might have already been laid down, temporal sequences of events must be different, and target cells could be in relatively advanced stage of differentiation when contacted.

Different attributes may determine the successful innervation of a target by one neuronal population as opposed to another. Four possibilities will be considered: fibres may be (i) more active, (ii) more 'correct', (iii) more capable of making new connections, because they have not yet used up their potential to form synapses, having established relatively few at the time of meeting with the target, (iv) able to travel to the target site more quickly. Each possibility will now be discussed.

More active fibres win

The first example is about the establishment of intertectal connections in *Xenopus*.

The detailed spatial order of the direct retinal projection to its contra-lateral tectum was first successfully shown in adult amphibia by Gaze (1958) and

Maturana, Lettvin, McCulloch and Pitts (1959), and in tadpoles by Gaze, Chung and Keating (1972); that of the ipsilateral projection by Gaze and Jacobson (1963).

The ipsilateral visuo-tectal projection can be broken down into two components: the first is the retinal projection from the central binocular visual field to the contra-lateral tectum; the second is the intertectal projection from the latter to the ipsilateral tectum. Since the contra-lateral and ipsilateral projections are both spatially organized, it must follow that the intertectal connections are also topographically organized (Keating, 1974).

When *Xenopus* larvae were placed in total darkness from stages 58 to 9–12 months after metamorphosis (when the visuo-tectal projections were mapped), the contra-lateral visuo-tectal responses were found to be normal as assayed by electro-physiological methods. The multi-unit ipsilateral responses, however, were seen to be much larger than in normal light-reared animals (Feldman, Gaze and Keating, 1970). These data indicate that the intertectal connections are less precisely organized when animals are dark-reared beyond metamorphosis, than when the same type of animals are light-reared.

The effects of dark-rearing animals with *one rotated eye* provide stronger support than the above results for the notion that function may alter the details of the pattern of retino-tectal connections.

Gaze, Keating, Székely and Beazley (1970) and Keating, Beazley, Feldman and Gaze (1975) have shown that when an eye from a light-reared animal is rotated before stage 63, the intertectal connections are changed. The contra-lateral retino-tectal connections do not alter. The *contra-lateral* visuo-tectal projection from a rotated eye was seen to be rotated, whereas the *ipsilateral* projection was normal. The projections from the normal eye were in reverse: the *contra-lateral* projection was normal, and the ipsilateral projection rotated. Put in another way, congruence of the projections from both eyes to one tectum was observed – from the rotated eye and the normal eye to the tectum contra-lateral to the rotated eye, the congruent projections were rotated; from the rotated eye and the normal eye to the opposite tectum, the congruent projections were both normal. Such congruence can only be explained by assuming that the intertectal connections have been changed so that the invariant direct retino-tectal pathways can become linked in a new way which allows binocular visual patterns at one tectum to coincide.

In sharp contrast, when an eye was rotated either after stage 63 (Keating, Beazley, Feldman and Gaze, 1975) in a light-reared animal; or else, after stage 63 with subsequent dark-rearing (Keating and Feldman, 1975) intertectal connections did not become modified from that to be observed in normal animals. In these animals, the contra-lateral projection from the rotated eye is rotated and the ipsilateral from the same eye to the *opposite* tectum is also rotated. The contra- and ipsilateral projections from the normal eye are both normal. Thus, there is always an angular disparity between the ipsilateral projections of the rotated eye and the contra-lateral projections of its unoperated partner eye. These results mean that the inter-tectal connections have remained invariant when an eye is rotated after metamorphosis, or rotated in an animal that has been brought up in the dark. No congruence has occurred between the projections from the binocular field of the two eyes at one tectum.

Both sets of results are easily explained if it is assumed that intertectal connections are formed just before metamorphosis, by the directed growth of fibres to link neurones in both tecta that were simulataneously activated, i.e. by a visual stimulus in the binocular visual field. The growth of the pathways seems to take place during metamorphosis, when the eyes are gradually moving to their frontal position. After metamorphosis the eyes have stopped moving and the connections seem to have stabilized, so that in the normal animal or the animal with one rotated eye modifications can no longer occur.

Eye rotation in *Rana pipiens* tadpoles does not result in altered intertectal connections (Jacobson, 1971; Jacobson and Hirsch, 1973). This difference in result could 'reflect a species difference, or a difference in either the techniques of rearing the animals or those of recording the visual responses (Keating, 1974). However, if one eye is removed, or covered, in *Rana* before metamorphosis, the long-term monocular deprivation appears to affect the detailed organization of the intertectal connections (Jacobson, 1971). The latter authors have concluded that binocular visual function during metamorphosis is only necessary in order to maintain the already established intertectal connections. This is a quite reasonable alternative to the view proposed by Keating (1974) that visual experience is responsible for the organization of fine detail, converting the already established crude pattern to a precisely organized one.

Wiesel and Hubel (1963, 1965) have reached similar conclusions about the binocular visual connections in area 17 of the cat, as those come to by Jacobson and Hirsch (1973) in *Rana.* On the other hand, Keating's suggestions for *Xenopus*, outlined above, are echoed in other studies on cat visual cortex. Barlow and Pettigrew (1971) and Blakemore (1974) have provided data which suggest that precise disparity tuning of cat cortical cells depends upon visual experience; Schlaer (1971) reared kittens with prisms in front of their eyes, and achieved the same registering of visual maps from the binocular field, as has been obtained in *Xenopus.*

The two mechanisms which may account for an alteration of connections due to functional activity have been termed 'growth' and 'switching' mechanisms (Keating and Feldman, 1975). The former denotes the idea that the mature synapse results from a continuous process of growth and degeneration of axonal endings, modifications being produced by functional activity (J.Z. Young, 1951). The latter idea of switching may be roughly explained as follows. A limited redundancy is thought to be built in to the developing nervous system. A sub-set of all synapses is active at any one time, the remainder are switched off. Synaptic arrangements may be altered by switching off previously active synapses, and/or switching on previously inactive synapses. Such models have been proposed to explain alterations in connections which have been observed in neuromuscular pathways (Cass, Sutton and Mark, 1973); somato-sensory systems (Wall and Werman, 1976; Wall, 1977) and visual systems

(Keating, 1974). This wide range suggests that such a mechanism might be operating universally in developing nervous systems.

A second example may be given which illustrates that the pattern of activity from incoming neurones may determine the formation of synaptic contacts. Chung, Gaze and Stirling (1973) have produced changes in the pattern of connections between *Xenopus* retina and its contra-lateral tectum by exposing animals to continuous stroboscopic illumination. The characteristic depth distribution of optic fibre types in the tectum was completely disrupted by this manoeuvre.

More 'correct' fibres win

If the optic nerve is cut in lower vertebrates, the nerve will regenerate, and connections between the retina and tectum will form in the same order as in normal animals (Section 8.3). It is possible that competition between retinal axons at the tectum controls selective synaptogenesis in these regeneration experiments, and also in the mismatch experiments (Section 8.3.2) where part of the retina or tectum is removed (Keating, 1976).

For competition to play a determining role in the final selection of target sites by regenerating optic nerve terminals, there must be some variation on the theme of retino-tectal matching by means of two complementary gradients of morphogen (Section 8.3.1). The distribution of gradients of morphogens can still be across the antero-posterior and dorso-ventral axes. However, now, the *quantitative* variation of morphogens becomes the key mechanism for determining the outcome of competitions. Cells with more morphogen will win a site with more morphogen-complement.

On this basis, the normal ordered pattern of retino-tectal connections could be determined, since the quantities of morphogen and morphogen-complement will be graded in corresponding ways across corresponding axes of retina and tectum. Matching of half-retinae to whole or half-tecta or half-tecta to whole retinae could also be explained as, in all cases, graded distributions of morphogen are still present, and competitions can still take place between cells with more morphogen for the sites with more morphogen-complement. Matching between the two systems could also be understood in situations where the incoming retinal axons are originally misrouted (Hibbard, 1967). Competition at the tectum would ensue, and this would result in the correct alignment of fibres.

Models of competition on a basis of properties distributed along gradients have also been detailed by Prestige and Willshaw (1975), Cotman and Banker (1974) and Marchase, Barbera and Roth (1976).

The neuro-muscular system of the lower vertebrates offers further examples for considering competition between fibres for final target sites, where more 'correct' fibres appear to win.

During development itself, it has been observed that an excess of neurones appear to travel from the spinal cord to developing muscle masses. Those neurones which do not succeed in making connections at the periphery in amphibia die (Hughes and Prestige, 1967; Lamb, 1976). It is generally assumed that too many neurones travel to a particular muscle site, competition ensues, the winners make connections and the losers die.

That selective reinnervation occurs in fish neuro-muscular systems had been suggested by the regeneration experiments of Sperry and Arora (1965) and Mark (1965). Since, in this system, axons do not connect up in an orderly way within the muscle, competition cannot be inferred from the observation of selective reconnection itself, as in the visual system. However, experiments can be designed in which nerves can be made to compete for particular muscle cell targets.

Hoh (1971) has shown that in toads, selective re-innervation of skeletal muscles by their 'correct' (native, original) axons can be produced experimentally. Two types of skeletal muscle fibres occur in toads — the fast-twitch type which is focally innervated by low-threshold fibres, and the slow-graded type, which is diffusely innervated by high-threshold fibres. Hoh's earlier experiments had demonstrated that when a cross-union is effected between the two types of nerves and muscle fibres, functional innervation of the wrong muscle types is seen. The mechanical properties of the muscles remain the same as in the normal animal and fibre types do not become altered. Hoh therefore went on to design an operative procedure which allowed regenerating high- or low-threshold nerves access to innervate either the sartorius (containing fast-twitch fibres only) or anterior semitendinosus muscles, (which contain fast-twitch and slow-graded fibres). Stimulation of low-threshold nerve fibres was seen to result exclusively in fast-twitch responses in both muscles, and high-threshold fibre stimulation caused only slow-graded responses in anterior semitendinosus muscles. Since great care had been taken to prevent collateral nerve regeneration from intact nerves, and since modulation of these muscle fibre-types does not occur in cross-union experiments, Hoh's results seem to indicate that under suitable experimental conditions selective re-connection occurs between nerve fibres and matching muscle types.

Cass, Sutton and Mark (1973) cut one nerve which supplies the axolotl limb. They observed the takeover of the de-afferented area by the adjacent 'foreign' nerve. This was followed by a recapturing of its original territory by the regenerating 'native' nerve. When the original nerve was cut a second time, foreign takeover was effected so much more quickly than at the time of the first cut, that the authors surmised that mature but functionally silent synapses from the foreign nerve must be present. Yip and Dennis (1976) have substantiated the findings of Cass *et al.* by showing that transmitter release from foreign terminals was reduced when the original nerve regenerated. However, no direct evidence for the presence of silent synapses has been forthcoming.

A final example may be cited from a regeneration experiment in the autonomic nervous system. Here, two types of target cells appear to be re-innervated correctly by two different types of fibres in a regeneration experiment which allows for the alternative of random innervation. Landmesser and Pilar (1972) found that the choroidal and ciliary cells in the avian ganglion were re-innervated by their 'correct' small and large preganglionic fibres respectively.

So far, there is no information about the mechanisms which 'correct' fibres employ to compete successfully against foreign fibres. However, an indication of a putative mechanism is given in the next section.

Fibres supporting fewer synapses win

As originally presented, the experiments of Marotte and Mark (1970a,b) appeared to argue for the recapture of native territory by the original nerve. The latter appeared to regenerate and displace a foreign nerve which had been crossed experimentally into goldfish eye-muscles. The nerve cross first caused incorrect reflex rotations of the eye. Later the original reflexes were restored. However, in 1975, Scott made intracellular recordings for single muscle fibres in goldfish eye muscle preparations similar to those described by Marotte and Mark. More than three months after the nerve cross, she was able to demonstrate simultaneous innervation by foreign and original nerves without physiological repression.

A similar sequence of events has been observed in experiments designed to test the effects of cutting preganglionic fibres to mammalian superior cervical ganglia. Langley (1895, 1897) showed that cutting the preganglionic sympathetic supply to the cervical sympathetic trunk of cats resulted in the re-establishment of the specificity of the original connections. When slightly more than three-quarters of the preganglionic supply was removed, the remaining 10–20% of fibres sprouted and re-innervated the vacated sites after a month, i.e., areas of contact were made which were foreign to these fibres in the normal animal (Murray and Thompson, 1957). After six months, however, normal connections become established once more (Guth and Bernstein, 1961).

The story of recapturing of original territory by a native nerve which emerges from this assembly of experiments has again been somewhat upset by more recent findings (Purves, 1975). This author used intracellular recording methods to show dual re-innervation of some guinea pig superior cervical ganglion (SCG) cells by the vagus nerve and cervical symphathetic trunk. The dual innervation persisted for some ten months. Purves pointed out that the results did not necessarily mean that connections within the SCG are not normally highly specific. The large number of vagal fibres growing into the ganglion could overwhelm some more subtle selective mechanism.

What, then, could be the mechanism which might determine dual innervation, and the parts played by the nerve terminals participating in such innervation? Purves (1976) has suggested a possible mechanism. Those neurones which are supporting a larger number of synapses than normal might be displacable by neurones supporting fewer than their normal complement of synapses. In the experiments of Guth and Bernstein (1961), for example, foreign terminals sprout from neurones which already synapse with their normal complement of sites on target cells. These neurones will lose a competition with native re-innervating nerves which are not supporting any synapses to start with. On the other hand, in the experiments of Purves (1975, 1976) both the foreign and original nerves do not support any synapses when they commence their innervation. This mechanism, then might account for some experiments in which an original nerve is observed to recapture territory from a foreign nerve. It might also account for the displacement of original terminals by a foreign nerve (Freeman, in press) or of one foreign nerve by another (Grinell, Rheuben and Letinsky, 1977). The mechanism is also useful in that it may account for dual innervation of target cells, such as in the examples reported above, or even in mammalian muscle fibres (Frank *et al.*, 1975).

Fibres which arrive first win
The exact timing of arrival of fibres at a target site might in certain instances be sufficient by itself to effect selective connections. Gottlieb and Cowan (1972) for example, have suggested that temporal factors may determine the distribution of afferents from rat hippocampus field CA_3 via crossed and uncrossed pathways to the dentate gyrus. Homologous areas of dentate granule cells from both sides of the brain become innervated by those fibres which arrive first. These are ipsilateral fibres dorsolaterally, and contralateral fibres ventromedially. Gottlieb and Cowan found that labelled axonal terminals yielded consistent grain counts representing the sum of grains due to crossed and uncrossed terminals at consecutive points along the gyrus axis. These findings could mean that only a limited number of sites are available. If two groups of afferents terminate at the same time in any one target area, it can be inferred that they must complete for the limited available sites.

A hierarchy of axonal attributes
Neurones might be classified in a hierarchy according to their ability to form synapses with a given target. The original nerve will make the best sorts of contacts. The ability to make successful contacts will depreciate with a corresponding increase in foreign nature of the innervating neurones. With reference to the last example discussed in the previous section where native preganglionic fibres and foreign vagal fibres were seen to dually innervate sympathetic neurones (Purves, 1975, 1976), it is interesting that in addition to the observations already noted, it has also been shown that ingrowing vagal axons establish far fewer synapses. Since approximately equal numbers of native and foreign fibres re-innervate the sympathetic ganglia, and since, as has been mentioned previously, both nerves are not supporting any synapses upon initial re-entry to the target, it seems that a hierarchy in abilities to form synapses might indeed exist.

Raisman (1977) has accurately counted the number of synapses made by native and foreing nerves as they regenerate back to the superior cervical ganglion of adult rats. His results suggest that regenerating preganglionic fibres form about the same number of synapses as normal nerves. Foreign nerves (vagus and hypoglossal) make far fewer synapses.

When lesions are made in central nervous system tracts, regeneration of injured fibres may be observed as, for example, in lower vertebrates when the optic nerve is cut or crushed. However, two other responses to injury can occur — axonal sprouting by intact neighbouring axons, or, misrouting of fibres which do not normally inner-vate the de-afferented target. It is possible that the mechanisms for pathway guidance may not be adequate along central pathways to align regenerating fibres, especially in mammals, where regeneration of central fibres does not appear to be established under any circumstances. Instead, neighbouring axons may sprout and establish new synapses (Raisman and Field, 1973) or anomalous pathways may be created (Lund, Cunningham and Lund, 1973; Schneider, 1973; Lynch, Deadwyler and Cotman, 1973; Schneider and Jhaveri, 1974; Cotman and Lynch, 1976). It may prove very difficult to distinguish between these alternatives (Stanfield and Cowan, 1976). Nevertheless, the study of such different types of response to injury will probably help delineate hierarchies of axonal attributes which determine more, or less, successful synapse formation, and thereby contribute to future understanding.

Maturation of axons associated with shrinkage of axonal territory

Three examples demonstrate that axons may shrink their terminal territory as part of a maturation process occurring during later development. This process obviously contributes to the process whereby the final target site is achieved.

Rakič (1976) has shown that in prenatal rhesus monkeys, axons from each eye converge on the same target area where their terminals overlap. After a short time, the invading axonal terminals become segregated into columns, each of which receive fibres from the left and right eyes in alternation. Thus the size of a given input from each eye appears to shrink naturally as prenatal development proceeds.

Rakič has gone on to propose that shrinkage — a part of the normal maturation process — fails to occur in the terminals from the *functioning* eye of a monocularly deprived monkey. In these animals the functioning eye projects wider bands of terminals to the cortex than in normal animals. These wider bands form at the expense of the bands of terminals from the closed eye (Hubel, Wiesel and LeVay, 1976). Competition between active and inactive fibres might contribute to the limitation of the territory supplied by each axon.

During the second post-natal week, the number of mammalian muscle fibres innervated by each axon is reduced to about one-fifth of the number present at birth (Redfern, 1970; Bennett and Pettigrew, 1974). The axonal terminals appear to be retracted as part of the normal maturation process. The same retraction occurs when muscle are partially denervated (Brown, Jansen and van Essen, 1976). In this experiment many muscle fibres became completely denervated. This must mean that the retraction of terminals is largely an intrinsic process, which does not involve competition. However, in the normal post-natal mammal, one axon terminates on one muscle fibre. Changeux and Danchin (1976) have drawn up a model for this maturation process. They have suggested that all the motor nerve terminals gathered on an endplate receive similar numbers of impulses, but in a randomly different temporal sequence. All the terminals will share equal areas of membrane, or use up equal quantities of a hypothetical substance produced by the post-synaptic cell.

An increase in impulse traffic will correspondingly increase the amount of space or hypothetical factor taken up by a terminal. If not enough of either remain, the terminal will regress. In this way, some sort of competition might be said to operate. The temporal sequences of activity are seen as the determinant of the stabilization of particular synapses.

A recent report in the New Scientist (31 March, 1977, p. 775) has drawn attention to the work of J. Lichtman, cited by Purves, who has shown that 4 out of 5 axons withdraw from mammalian submandibular ganglion cells.

Effect of local environment
That cells will migrate to a site and only then differentiate has been admirably demonstrated for autonomic neuroblasts by LeDouarin and Teillet (1974). Ramón y Cajal (1960) was impressed by the observation that developing axons will travel for long distances without forming sprouts. This they only do upon arrival at a suitable target site.

Chemical signals
Ramon y Cajal considered that chemotactic substances attracted growing axonal tips to the correct targets. By extending this concept, it could be said that local variations in concentrations of chemicals might equally well attract or influence the siting of a growing terminal.

Diamond *et al.* (1976) have suggested, for example, that the density of nerve sprouting within a given sensory nerve field, in salamander, may be controlled by an interaction between sprouting factors, constantly manufactured by the target field, and, neutralising agents transported down invading nerves. It is especially interesting that Diamond and his colleagues have concluded that nerves will normally sprout only within their 'body space' territory — a target space allotted to them during early development, and relating to the body co-ordinates. This supports the idea put forward here, that chemical signals may act locally.

Electrical influences
Electrical influences have been suggested as a source of guidance to outgrowing axons since pathway guidance was first suggested (Sperry, 1951). However not much work has been done to substantiate this notion.

Berry and his colleagues (Bradley and Berry, 1975; Berry and Bradley, 1975) have used network analysis with Golgi—Cox impregnated sections to assay the development of rat cerebellar Purkinje cells. They were able to compare the influence of the two distinct afferent systems to Purkinje cells (parallel and climbing fibres) upon the dendritic growth of Purkinke cells in normal animals and animals in which one or other afferent had been destroyed. Fluctuations in the prevailing synaptogenesis of climbing and parallel fibres could be correlated with the branching patterns of the Purkinje dendrites. Also, growth of the dendrites seems to be directed to areas of neurophil where ongoing synaptogenesis was most active.

8.5 A PARADIGM FOR FUTURE RESEARCH

I would like to end this review by quoting the conclusions of Chung and Cooke (in press):

We therefore conceive of ordered retino-tectal connections as the final manifestation of a series of developmental steps, each of which is governed by different sets of mechanisms. The organiser in the blastoporal dorsal lip first establishes the primary embryonic field, which later induces the primitive nervous system. Precursor cells within the primitive neural tube acquire a determination to develop into a specific part of the nervous system, the degree of this determination becoming progressively more specific with the advancing stages of the embryo. As the growing axons are guided to the developing tectum, a polarising structure located in the diencephalic regions provides a reference system for the array of incoming axons so that the axes of the retina and the tectum become aligned. Finally, topographically ordered connections between the retina and the tectum evolve gradually as connections are transiently formed and re-formed. If our view is correct, then the quest for the mechanisms underlying initial formation of selective nerve connections lies not so much in establishing the presence or absence of unique labels on each retinal and tectal cell, as in unravelling the processes of dynamic intercellular interactions which are taking place throughout embryonic and larval life.

I think this work of Chung and Cooke, which is summarized in their conclusions, heralds the sort of experiments which will be done. Hopefully, such information will constructively add to the conceptual concertina of complexity and simplicity in ideas, which must surely tread hot on the heels of those who would understand the building of a vertebrate nervous system.

8.6 SUMMARY

The formation of specific synapses should be seen as the last step in a whole series of developmental events.

There are probably four main steps which precede the formation of a synaptic site at a specific locus:

(1) Positional information programmes neuronal genomes early in development.
(2) Pathway guidance operates.
(3) Competition between fibres determines selection of terminal positions of nerve endings.
(4) The local environment of sprouting fibres makes a contribution to the final selection of synapse sites.

At all times, multiple events in development are co-ordinated to the effect of the above four steps. Timing is therefore as important as spatial relationships in embryogenesis.

REFERENCES

Attardi, D.G. and Sperry, R.W. (1963), Preferential selection of central pathways by regenerating optic nerve fibres. *Exp. Neurol.,* **7**, 46–64.

Baker, R.E. (1976), Some comments on central and peripheral plastic changes in nerve connexions. In: *Molecular and Functional Neurobiology.* (Gispeu, W.H. ed.), pp. 47–86, Amsterdam, Elsevier Scientific Publishing Co.

Barbera, A.J. (1975), Adhesive recognition between developing retinal cells and the optic tecta of the chick embryo. *Dev. Biol.,* **46**, 167–191.

Barbera, A.J., Marchase, R.B. and Roth, S. (1973), Adhesive recognition and retinotectal specificity. *Proc. natn. Acad. Sci. U.S.A.,* **70**, 2482–2486.

Bard, J. and Elsdale, T. (1972), Collagen substrata for studies on cell behaviour. *J. Cell Biol.,* **54**, 626–637.

Bard, J.B.L., Hay, E.D. and Meller, S.M. (1975), Formation of the endothelium of the avian cornea: A study of cell movement *in vivo. Dev. Biol.,* **42**, 334–361.

Barlow, H.B. and Pettigrew, J.D. (1971), Lack of specificity of neurons in the visual cortex of young kittens. *J. Physiol.,* **218**, 98–100P.

Bate, C.M. (1976), Pioneer neurons in an insect embryo. *Nature,* **260**, 54–56.

Bennett, M.R. and Pettigrew, A.G. (1974), The formation of synapses in striated muscle during development. *J. Physiol.,* **241**, 547–573.

Bergey, G.K., Hunt, R.K. and Holtzer, H. (1973), Selective effects of bromodeoxuridine on developing *Xenopus laevis* retina. *Anat. Rec.,* **175**, 271.

Berman, N.J. and Hunt, R.K. (1975), Visual projections to the optic tecta in *Xenopus* after partial extripation of the embryonic eye. *J. Comp. Neurol.,* **162**, 23–42.

Berry, M. and Bradley, P. (1975), The growth of the dendritic trees of Purkinje cells in the cerebellum of the rat. *Brain Res.,* **112**, 1–35.

Blakemore, C. (1974), Development of functional connexions in the mammalian visual system. *Br. med. Bull.,* **30**, 152–157.

Bloom, E.M. and Thompkins, R. (1976), Selective reinnervation in skin rotation grafts in *Rana pipiens. J. exp. Zool.,* **195**, 237–245.

Bradley, P. and Berry, M. (1975), The effect of specific deprivation of either the climbing or the parallel fibre input on the development of the dendritic tree Purkinje cells in the cerebellum of the rat. *J. Anat.* **120**, 407–408.

Brown, M.C., Jansen, J.K.S. and Van Essen, D. (1976), Polyneuronal innervation of skeletal muscle in new-born rats and its elimination during maturation. *J. Physiol.,* **261**, 287–422.

Carter, S.B. (1965), Principles of cell motility. The directionality of cell movement and cancer invasion. *Nature,* **208**, 1183–1187.

Cass, D.T., Sutton, T.J. and Mark, R.F. (1973), Competition between nerves for functional connections with axolotl muscles. *Nature,* **243**, 201–203.

Chamley, J.H., Campbell, G.R. and Burnstock, G. Contraction and innervation of smooth muscle cells in culture. In: *Functions and Comparative Anatomy of the Artery.* Vol. (Schwartz, C.J., ed.), Plenum Press, New York. (In press).

Chamley, J.H. and Dowel, J.J., (1975), Specificity of nerve fibre 'attraction' to autonomic effector organs in tissue culture. *Exp. Cell Res.,* **90**, 1–7.

Chamley, J.H., Goller, I. and Burnstock, G. (1973), Selective growth of sympathetic nerve fibres to explants of normally densely innervated antonomic effector organs in tissue culture. *Dev. Biol.,* **31**, 367—379.

Changeux, J.P. and Danchin, A. (1976), Selective stabilisation of developing synapses as a mechanism for the specification of neuronal networks. *Nature*, **264**, 705—712

Chung, S.H. and Cooke, J. (1975), Polarity of structure and of ordered nerve connections in the developing amphibian brain. *Nature,* **258**, 126—132.

Chung, S.H. and Cooke, J. Observations on the formation of the brain and of nerve connections following embryonic manipulation of the amphibian neural tube. *Phil. Trans. R. Soc. B.,* (in press).

Chung, S.H. and Feldman, J.D. (1973), Neurospecificity and retino-tectal connections: thirty years later. In: *Biological Diagnosis of Brain Disorder.* pp. 193—212. (Bogoch, E., ed.), Spectrum Wiley Publications, New York.

Chung, S.H., Gaze, R.M. and Stirling, R.V. (1973), The maturation of visual toad units. *J. Physiol.,* **230**, 57—58.

Cook, J.E. and Horder, T.J. (1974), Interactions between optic fibres in their regeneration to specific sites in the goldfish tectum. *J. Physiol.* **241**, 89—90.

Cook, J.E. and Horder, T.J. (1977), The multiple factors determining retinotopic order in the growth of optic fibres into the optic tectum. *Phil. Trans. R. Soc. Lond. B.,* **278**, 261—276.

Cotman, C.W. and Banker, G.A. (1974), The making of a synapse. In: *Reviews of Neuro-Science.* Vol. I. pp. 1—61. (Ehrenpreis, E. and Kopen, I.J. eds.), Raven Press, New York.

Cotman, C.W. and Lynch, G.S. (1976), Reactive synaptogenesis in the adult nervous system: the effects of partial deafferentation on the synapse formation. In: *Neuronal Recognition.* pp. 69—108, (Barondes, S.H. ed.), Chapman and Hall, London.

Coughlin, M.P. (1975), Target organ stimulation of parasympathetic nerve growth in the developing mouse submandibular gland. *Dev. Biol.,* **43**, 140—158.

Crain, S.M. and Peterson, E.R. (1975), Development of specific sensory evoked synaptic networks in fetal mouse cord-brain stem cultures. *Science,* **188**, 275—278.

Crossland, W.J., Cowan, W.M., Rogers, L.A. and Kelly, J.P. (1974), The specification of the retino-tectal projection in the chick. *J. comp. Neurol.,* **155**, 127—164.

Diamond, J., Cooper, E., Turner, C. and Macintyre, L. (1976), Trophic regulation of nerve sprouting. *Science,* **193**, 371—377.

Dixon, J.S. and Cronly-Dillon, J.R. (1972), The fine structure of the developing retina in *Xenopus laevis. J. Embryol. exp. Morph.,* **28**, 659—666.

Dixon, J.S. and Cronly-Dillon, J.R. (1974), Intercellular gap junctions in pigment epithelium cells during retinal specification in *Xenopus laevis. Nature,* **251**, 505.

Dunn, G.H. (1973), Extension of nerve fibres, their mutual interaction and direction of growth in tissue culture. In: *Locomotion of tissue cells. Ciba Found. Symp.,* **14**, 211—223.

Ebendal, T. (1976a), Experiments *in vitro* on neuron development and axon orientation in the chick embryo. *Abs. Uppsala. Fac. Sci.* **368**, 5—18.

Ebendal, T. (1976b), Migratory mesoblast cells in the young chick embryo examined by scanning electron microscopy. *Zoology*, **4**, 101—108.

Ebendal, T. (1976c), The relative roles of contact inhibition and contact guidance in orientation of axons extending on aligned collagen fibrils *in vitro. Exp. Cell Res.,* **98**, 159–169.

Ebendal, T. (1977), Extracellular matrix fibrils and cell contacts in the chick embryo: possible roles in orientation of cell migration and axon extension. *Cell Tiss. Res.,* **175**, 439–458.

Ebendal, T. and Jacobson, C.O. (1977), Tissue explants affecting extension and orientation of axons in cultured chick embryo ganglia. *Exp. Cell Res.,* **105**, 379–389.

Emlen, S.T. (1975), The stellar-orientation system of a migratory bird. *Sci. Am.,* **233**, 102–111.

Fambrough, D.M. (1976), Specificity of nerve-muscle interactions. In: *Neuronal Recognition.* pp. 25–68, (Barondes, S.H. ed.), Chapman and Hall, London.

Feldman, J.D. and Gaze, R.M. (1975), The development of half-eyes in *Xenopus* tadpoles. *J. comp. Neurol.,* **162**, 13–22.

Feldman, J.D., Gaze, R.M. and Keating, M.J. (1970), The effect on intertectal neuronal connexions of rearing *Xenopus laevis* in total darkness. *J. Physiol.,* **212**, 44–45.

Feldman, J.D., Gaze, R.M. and Keating, M.J. (1971), Delayed innervation of the optic tectum during development in *Xenopus laevis. Exp. Brain Res.,* **14**, 16–23.

Feldman, J.D., Gaze, R.M. and Keating, M.J. (1975), Retinotectal mismatch: A serendipitous result. *Nature.* **253**, 445–446.

Frank, E., Jansen, J.K.S., Lømo, T. and Westgaard, R. (1975), The interaction between foreing and original motor nerves innervating the soleus muscle of rats. *J. Physiol.,* **247**, 725–743.

Freeman, J.A. Possible regulatory function of acetylcholine receptors in maintainance of retino-tectal synapses. *Nature* (In press).

Gaze, R.M. (1958), The representation of the retina on the optic lobe of the frog. *Q. J. exp. Physiol.,* **43**, 209–214.

Gaze, R.M. (1970), *The Formation of Nerve Connections,* Academic Press, New York.

Gaze, R.M. The problems of specificity in the formation of nerve connections. In: *Specificity in Embryonic Development.* (Garrod, D., ed.), Chapman and Hall, London (in press).

Gaze, R.M., Chung, S.H. and Keating, M.J. (1972), Development of the retino-tectal projection in *Xenopus. Nature New Biology,* **236**, 133–135.

Gaze, R.M. and Hope, R.A. (1977), The formation of continuously ordered mappings. *Prog. Brain Res.* **45**, 327–355.

Gaze, R.M. and Jacobson, M. (1963), The path from the retina to the ipsilateral tectum in the frog. *J. Physiol.,* **165**, 73–74.

Gaze, R.M., Jacobson, M. and Székely, G. (1963), The retinotectal projection in *Xenopus* with compound eyes. *J. Physiol.,* **165**, 484–499.

Gaze, R.M. and Keating, M.J. (1972), The visual system and 'neuronal specificity'. *Nature,* **237** (5355) 375–378.

Gaze, R.M., Keating, M.J., Székely, G. and Beazley, L. (1970), Binocular interaction in the formation of specific intertectal neuronal connexions. *Proc. R. Soc. Lond. Ser. B.,* **175**, 107–147.

Gottlieb, D.I. and Cowan, W.M. (1972), Evidence for a temporal factor in the occupation of available synaptic sites during the development of the dentate gyrus. *Brain Res.*, **41**, 452–56.

Gottlieb, D.I., Rock, K. and Glaser, L. (1976), A gradient of adhesive specificity in developing avian retina. *Proc. natn. Acad. Sci. U.S.A.*, **73**, 410–414.

Grimm, L.M. (1971), An evaluation of myotypic respecification in axolotl. *J. exp. Zool.*, **178**, 479–496.

Grinnell, A.D., Rheuben, M.B. and Letinsky, M.S. (1977), Mutual repression of synaptic efficiency by pairs of foreign nerves innervating frog skeletal muscle. *Nature*, **265**, 368–370.

Guth, L. and Bernstein, J.J. (1961), Selectivity in the re-establishment of synapses in the superior cervical sympathetic ganglion of the cat. *Expl. Neurol.*, **4**, 59–69.

Harris, A.J. (1974), Inductive functions of the nervous system. *A. Rev. Physiol.*, **36**, 251–304.

Harrison, R.G. (1910), The outgrowth of the nerve fibre as a mode of protoplasmic movement. *J. exp. Zool.*, **9**, 787–848.

Heaysman, J.E.M. and Pegrum, S.M. (1973), Early contacts between fibroblasts: an ultrastructure study. *Exp. Cell Res.*, **78**, 71–78.

Henrikson, C.K. and Vaughn, J.E. (1974), Fine structural relationships between neurites and radial glial processes in developing mouse spinal cord. *J. Neurocytol.* **3**, 659–675.

Hibbard, B. (1967), Visual recovery following regeneration of the optic nerve through the oculomotor nerve root in *Xenopus*. *Exp. Neurol.*, **19**, 350–356.

Hoh, J.F.Y. (1971), Selective reinnervation of fast-twitch and slow-graded muscle fibres in the toad. *Exp. Neurol.*, **30**, 263–376.

Hope, R.A., Hammond, B.T. and Gaze, R.M. (1976), The arrow model: retinotectal specificity and map formation in the goldfish visual system. *Proc. R. Soc. Lond. Ser. B.* **194**, 447–466.

Hubel, D.H., Wiesel, T.N. and Le Vay, S. (1976), Functional architecture of area 17 in normal and monocularly deprived Macaque monkeys. *Cold Spring Harbor Symp. Quant. Biol.*, **46**, 581–589.

Hughes, A. and Prestige, M.C. (1967), Development of behaviour in the hindlimb of *Xenopus laevis. J. zool. Res.*, **152**, 347–359.

Hunt, R.K. (1975), The cell cycle, cell-lineage and neuronal specificity. In: *Results and Problems in Cell Differentiation*. **7**, pp 43–62. (Reinert, J. and Holtzer, H., eds.), Springer-Verlag, New York, Berlin, Heidelberg.

Jacobson, M. (1968a), Development of neuronal specificity in retinal ganglion cells of *Xenopus*. *Dev. Biol.*, **17**, 202–218.

Jacobson, M. (1968b), Cessation of DNA synthesis in retinal ganglion cells correlated with the time of specification of their central connections. *Dev. Biol.*, **17**, 219–232.

Jacobson, M. (1970), *Developmental Neurobiology*, Holt, Rinehart and Winston, Inc., New York.

Jacobson, M. (1971), Absence of adaptive modification in developing retinotectal connections in frogs after visual deprivation or disparate stimulation of the eye. *Proc. natn. Acad. Sci. U.S.A.*, **68**, 528–532.

Jacobson, M. and Baker, R.E. (1969), Development of neuronal connections with skin grafts in frogs: behavioural and electrophysiological studies. *J. comp. Neurol.,* **134**, 121–142.

Jacobson, M. and Hirsch, V.B. (1973), Development and maintenance of connectivity in the visual system of the frog I The effects of eye rotation and visual deprivation. *Brain Res.,* **49**, 47–65.

Keating, M.J. (1974), The role of visual function in the patterning of binocular visual connections. *Br. Med. Bull.,* **30** (2), 145–151.

Keating, M.J. (1976), The formation of visual neuronal connections: a appraisal of the present status of the theory of neuronal specificity. In: *Neural and Behaviour Specificity.* pp. 59–109. (Gottlieb, G., ed.), Academic Press, New York, San Francisco, London.

Keating, M.J., Beazley, L., Feldman, J.D. and Gaze, R.M. (1975), Binocular interaction and intertectal neuronal connections: dependence upon developmental stage. *Proc. R. Soc. Lond. Ser. B.,* **191**, 445–466.

Keating, M.J. and Feldman, J.D. (1975), Visual deprivation and intertectal neuronal connections in *Xenopus laevis. Proc. R. Soc. Lond. Ser. B.,* **191**, 467–474.

Keating, M.J. and Kennard, C. (1975), The amphibian visual system as a model for developmental neurobiology. In: *The Amphibian Visual System: A Multi-disciplinary Approach.* pp. 267–316. (Fite, K.V., ed.), Academic Press, New York, San Francisco, London.

Keeton, W.T. (1974), The mystery of pigeon homing. *Sci. Am.,* **231**, (6), 96–107.

Kuffler, S.W. and Nicholls, J.G. (1976), 'From neuron to brain: A cellular approach to the function of the nervous system'. Sinauer Assoc. Inc. Publishers, Sunderland Mass.

Lamb, A.L. (1976), The projection patterns of the ventral horn to the hind limb during development. *Dev. Biol.,* **54**, 82–99.

Landmesser, L. (1976), The development of neural circuits in the limb moving segments of the spinal cord. In: *Neural Control of Locomotion.* pp. 707–733. (Herman, R.M., Grillner, S., Stein, P.S.G. and Stuart, D.G., eds.), Plenum Publishing Corp., New York.

Landmesser, L. and Morris, D.G. (1975), The development of functional innervation in the hind limb of the chick embryo. *J. Physiol.,* **249**, 301–326.

Landmesser, L. and Pilar, G. (1972), The onset and development of transmission in the chick ciliary ganglion. *J. Physiol.,* **222**, 692–713.

Langley, J.N. (1895), Note on regeneration of pre-ganglion fibres of the sympathetic. *J. Physiol.,* **18**, 280–284.

Langley, J.N. (1897), On the regeneration of pre-ganglionic and of post-ganglionic visceral nerve fibres. *J. Physiol.,* **22**, 215–230.

Le Douarin, N.M. and Teillet, M.A.M. (1974), Experimental analysis of the migration and differentiation of neuroblasts of the autonomic nervous system and of neuro-ectodermal mesenchymal derivatives using a biological cell marking technique. *Dev. Biol.,* **41**, 152–184.

Letourneau, P.C. (1975), Cell-to-substratum adhesion and guidance of axonal elongation. *Dev. Biol.,* **44**, 92–101.

Levi-Montalcini, R. (1972), The nerve growth factor. In: *Immunosympathectomy.* (Steiner, G. and Schonbaum, G. eds.), pp. 25–35, Elsevier, New York.

Levi-Montalcini, R. and Chen, J.S. (1971), Selective outgrowth of nerve fibres *in vitro* from embryonic ganglia of *Periplaneta americana. Arch. Ital. Biol.,* **109**, 307–337.

Lopresti, V., Macagno, E.R. and Levinthal, E. (1973), Structure and development of neuronal connections in isogenic organisms; cellular interactions in the development of the optic lamina of *Daphnia. Proc. natn. Acad. Sci. U.S.A.,* **70**, 433–437.

Lund, R.D., Cunningham, T.J. and Lund, J.S. (1973), Modified optic projections after unilateral eye removal in young rats. *Brain Res. Evol.,* **81**, 51–72.

Lynch, G., Deadwyler, S. and Cotman, C. (1973), Postlesion axonal growth produces permanent functional connections. *Science,* **180**, 1364–1366.

McMahon, D. and West, C. (1976), Transduction of positional information during development. In: *The Cell Surface in Animal Embryogenesis and Development.* pp. 449–494. (Poste, G. and Nicolson, G.L. eds.), North Holland Publishing Co., Amsterdam, New York, Oxford.

Marchase, R.B., Pierce, M. and Roth, S. (1977), Complementarity between the ganglioside GM_2 and the enzyme GM_1 synthethase is a possible recognition mechanism in the chick retinotectal projection. Keystone – UCLA membrane meeting (abstract in Press).

Mark, R.F. (1965), Fin movements after regeneration of neuromuscular connections: an investigation of myotypic specificity. *Exp. Neurol.,* **12**, 292–302.

Marotte, L.R. and Mark, R.F. (1970a), The mechanism of selective reinnervation of fish eye muscles I. Evidence from muscle function during recovery. *Brain Res.,* **19**, 41–51.

Marotte, L.R. and Mark, R.F. (1970b), The mechanism of selective reinnervation of fish eye muscle II. Evidence from electron microscopy of nerve endings. *Brain Res.,* **19**, 53–61.

Maturana, H.R., Lettvin, J.Y., McCulloch, W.S. and Pitts, W.H. (1959), Physiological evidence that cut optic nerve fibres in the frog regenerate to their proper places in the tectum. *Science,* **130**, 1709–1710.

Meyer, R.L. (1975), Tests for regulation in the goldfish retinotectal system. *Anat. Rec.,* **181**, 427.

Meyer, R.L. and Sperry, R.W. (1973), Tests for neuroplasticity in the anuran retinotectal system. *Exp. Neurol.,* **40**, 525–539.

Meyer, R.L. and Sperry, R.W. (1974), Explanatory models for neuroplasticity in retinotectal connections. In: *Plasticity and Recovery of Function in the Central Nervous System.* pp. 45–63. (Stein, D.G., Rosen, J.J. and Butters, N. eds.), Academic Press, New York.

Meyer, R.L. and Sperry, R.W. (1976), Retinotectal specificity: chemo-affinity theory. In: *Neural and Behaviour Specificity.* pp. 111–149. (Gottlieb, G. ed.), Academic Press, New York, San Francisco, London.

Miner, N. (1956), Intergumental specification of sensory fibres in the development of cutaneous local sign. *J. comp. Neurol.* **105**, 161–170.

Murray, J.G. and Thompson, J.W. (1957), The occurrence and function of collateral sprouting in the sympathetic nervous system of the cat. *J. Physiol.*, **135**, 133–162.

Nelson, G.A. and Revel, J.P. (1973), Scanning electron microscopy study of cell movements in the corneal endothelium of the avian embryol. *Dev. Biol.*, **42**, 315.

Nornes, H.O. and Das, G.D. (1972), Temporal pattern of neurogenesis in spinal cord: cytoarchitecture and directed growth of axons. *Proc. natn. Acad. Sci. U.S.A.*, **69**, 1962–1966.

Olson, M.I. and Bunge, R.P. (1973), Anatomical observations on the specificity of synapse formation in tissue culture. *Brain Res.*, **59**, 19–33.

Peterson, E.R. and Crain, S.M. (1970), Innervation in culture of fetal rodent skeletal muscle by organotypic explants of spinal cord from different animals. *Z. Zellforsch.* **106**, 1–21.

Prestige, M.C. and Willshaw, D.J. (1975), On a role for competition in the formation of patterned neuronal connections. *Proc. R. Soc. Lond. Ser. B.*, **190**, 77–98.

Purves, D. (1975), Persistent innervation of mammalian sympathetic neurons by native and foreign fibres. *Nature*, **256**, 589–590.

Purves, D. (1976a), Long-term regulation in the vertebrate peripheral nervous system. *International review of Physiology*. Neurophysiology II. pp. 125–177. (Pather, R. ed.), University Park Press, Baltimore.

Purves, D. (1976b), Competitive and non-competitive re-innervation of mammalian sympathetic neurones by native and foreign fibres. *J. Physiol.*, **261**, 433–475.

Rakič, P. (1976), Prenatal genesis of connections subserving ocular dominance in the rhesus monkey. *Nature*, **261**, 467–472.

Rakič, P. and Sidman, R.L. (1973), Weaver mutant mouse cerebellum; defective neuronal migration secondary to specific abnormality of Bergmann glia. *Proc. natn. Acad. Sci. U.S.A.*, **70**, 240–244.

Raisman, G. (1977), Formation of synapses in the adult rat after injury: similarities and differences between a peripheral and a central nervous site. *Phil. Trans. R. Soc. Lond. Ser. B.*, **278**, 349–360.

Raisman, G. and Field, P.M. (1973), A quantitative investigation of the development of collateral reinnervation after partial deafferentation of the septal nuclei. *Brain Res.*, **50**, 241–264.

Ramón, y Cajal (1960), *Studies on Vertebrate Neurogenesis*. Charles C. Thomas, Springfield, Illinois.

Redfern, P.A. (1970), Neuromuscular transmission in new born rats. *J. Physiol.*, **209**, 701–709.

Roth, S. and Marchase, R.B. (1976), An *in vitro* assay for retinotectal specificity. In: *Neuronal Specificity*. pp. 227–248. (Barondes, S.H. ed.), Academic Press, New York and London.

Schlaer, R. (1971), Shift in binocular disparity causes compensatory change in the cortical structure of kittens. *Science*, **173**, 638–641.

Schneider, G.E. (1973), Early lessions of superior colliculus: factors affecting the formation of abnormal retinal projections. *Brain Behav. Evol.*, **8**, 73–109.

Schneider, G.E. and Jhaveri, S.K. (1974), Neuroanotomical correlates of spared or altered function after brain lesions in the new born hamster. In: *Plasticity and Recovery of Function in the Central Nervous System.* pp. 65–109. (Stein, D.G., Rosen, J.J. and Butters, N., eds.), Academic Press, New York.

Scott, S.A. (1975), Persistence of foreign innervation on reinnervated goldfish extra ocular muscles. *Science,* **189**, 644–646.

Sharma, S.C. (1972a), Reformation of retinotectal projections after various tectal ablations in adult goldfish. *Exp. Neurol.,* **34**, 171–182.

Sharma, S.C. (1972b), Redistribution of visual projections in altered optic tecta in adult goldfish. *Proc. natn. Acad. Sci. U.S.A.,* **69**, 2637–2639.

Sperry, R.W. (1943a), Effect of 180 degree rotation of the retinal field on visuomotor coordination. *J. exp. Zool.,* **92**, 263–279.

Sperry, R.W. (1943b), Visuomotor coordination in the newt (*Triturus viridescens*) after regeneration of the optic nerve. *J. comp. Neurol.,* **79**, 35–55.

Sperry, R.W. (1944), Optic nerve regeneration with return of vision in anurans. *J. Neurophysiol.,* **7**, 57–69.

Sperry, R.W. (1945a), Restoration of vision after crossing of optic nerve and after contralateral transplantation of eye. *J. Neurophysiol.,* **8**, 15–28.

Sperry, R.W. (1945b), The problems of central nervous tissue re-organisation after nerve regeneration and muscle transposition. *Q. J. Rev. Biol.,* **70**, 311–369.

Sperry, R.W. (1948), Patterning of central synapses in regeneration of the optic nerve in teleosts. *Physiol. Zool.,* **21**, 351–361.

Sperry, R.W. (1949), Reimplantation of eyes in fishes (*Bathygobius soporator*) with recovery of vision. *Proc. Soc. exp. Biol. Med.,* **71**, 80–81.

Sperry, R.W. (1956), Mechanisms of neural maturation. In: *Handbook of Experimental Psychology* pp. 234–280, (Stevens, S.S., ed.). New York.

Sperry, R.W. (1951), Regulative factors in the orderly growth of neural circuits. *Growth* (Symposium) **10**, 63–87.

Sperry, R.W. (1955), Problems in the biochemical specification of neurons. In: *Biochemistry of the Developing Nervous System.* pp. 74–84. (Waelsch, H. ed.), Academic Press, New York.

Sperry, R.W. (1958) Developmental Basis in Behaviour, In: *Behaviour and Evolution.* pp. 128–138. (Roe, A. and Simpson, G.G. eds), Yale University Press, New Haven.

Sperry, R.W. (1963), Chemoaffinity in the orderly growth of nerve fibre patterns and connections. *Proc. natn. Acad. Sci. U.S.A.,* **50**, 703–710.

Sperry, R.W. (1965), Embryogenesis of behavioural nerve nets. In: *Organogenesis.* pp. 161–186. (De Haan, R.L. and Ursprung, H. eds), Holt, Rinehart and Winston, New York.

Sperry, R.W. and Arora, H.L. (1965), Selectivity in regeneration of the oculomotor nerve in the cichlid fish, *Astronatus ocellatus. J. Embryol. exp. Morph.* **14**, 307–317.

Stanfield, B. and Cowan, M. (1976), Evidence for a change in the retino-hypothalamic projections in the rat following early removal of one eye. *Brain Res.,* **104**, 129–134.

Straznicky, K. (1973), The formation of the optic fibre projection after tectum removal in *Xenopus. J. Embryol. exp. Morph.*, **29**, 397–409.

Straznicky, K., Gaze, R.M. and Keating, M.J. (1971), The retinotectal projections after uncrossing the optic chiasma in *Xenopus* with one compound eye. *J. Embryol. exp. Morph.*, **26**, (3), 523–542.

Székely, G. (1954), Zur Ausbildung der lokalen funktionellen spezifitat der. Retina. *Acta Biol. Acad. sci. hung.*, **5**, 157–167.

Toole, B.P. (1976), Morphogenetic role of glycosaminoglycans (acid mucopolysac-charides) in brain and other tissues. In: *Neuronal Recognition.* pp. 275–330. (Barondes, S.H. ed.), Chapman and Hall, London.

Trinkaus, J.P. (1976), On the mechanism of metazoan cell movements. In: *The Cell Surface in Animal Embryogenesis and Development.* pp. 225–330. (Poste, G. and Nicolson, G.L. eds.), Elsevier, Amsterdam, New York and Oxford.

Van der Loos, H. (1965), The 'improperly' oriented pyramidal cell in the cerebral cortex. *Bull. Johns Hopkins Hosp.* **117**, 228–250.

Wall, P.D. (1977), The presence of ineffective synapses and the circumstances which unmask them. *Phil. Trans. R. Soc. B.* **278**, 361–371.

Wall, P.D. and Werman, K. (1976), The physiology and anatomy of long ranging afferent fibres within the spinal cord. *J. Physiol.*, **255**, 321–334.

Weiss, P. (1926), The relations between central and peripheral coordination. *J. comp. Neurol.*, **40**, 241–251.

Weiss, P. (1934), *In vitro* experiments on the factors determining the course of the outgrowing fibres. *J. exp. Zool.*, **68**, 393–448.

Weiss, P. (1936), Selectivity controlling the central-peripheral relations in the nervous system. *Biol. Rev.*, **11**, 494–531.

Weiss, P. (1939), *Principles of Development.* Henry Holt and Company, New York.

Weiss, P. (1941), Nerve patterns: the mechanics of nerve growth. *Growth* (Third Growth Symposium Suppl.), **5**, 113–203.

Weiss, P. (1945), Experiments on cell and axonal orientation *in vitro*: The role of colloidal exudates in tissue organisation. *J. exp. Zool.*, **100**, 353–386.

Weiss, P. (1956), Special vertebrate organogenesis: nervous system. In: *Analysis of Development.* pp. 346–401. (Willier, B.H., Weiss, P.A. and Hamburger, V. eds.), W.B. Saunders, Philadelphia and London.

Wiesel, T.N. and Hubel, D.H. (1963), Single-cell responses in striate cortex of kittens deprived of cision in one eye. *J. Neurophysiol.*, **26**, 1003–1017.

Wiesel, T.N. and Hubel, D.H. (1965), Comparison of the effects of unilateral and bilateral dye closure on cortical unit responses in kittens. *J. Neurophysiol.*, **28**, 1029–1040.

Willshaw, D.J. and Von der Malsburg, C. (1976), How patterned neural connections can be set up by self-organization. *Proc. R. Soc. Lond. Ser. B.*, **194**, 431–445.

Wolpert, L. (1969), Positional information and the spatial pattern of cellular differentiation. *J. theor. Biol.*, **25**, 1–47.

Wolpert, L. (1971), Positional information and pattern formation. *Current Topics Dev. Biol.,* **6**, 183–224.

Yip, J.W. and Dennis, M.J. (1976), Suppression of transmission of foreign synapses in adult newt muscles involves reduction in quantal content. *Nature,* **260**, 350–352.

Yoon, M. (1971), Reorganization of retinotectal projections following surgical operations on the optic tectum in goldfish. *Exp. Neurol.,* **33**, 395–411.

Yoon, M.G. (1972a), Transposition of the visual projection from the nasal hemiretina onto the foreign rostral zone of the optic tectum in goldfish. *Exp. Neurol.,* **37**, 451–462.

Yoon, M. (1972b), Synaptic plasticities of the retina and of the optic tectum in goldfish. *Am. Zool.,* **12**, 106.

Yoon, M. (1972c) Reversibility of the reorganization of retinotectal projection in goldfish. *Exp. Neurol.,* **35**, 565–577.

Young, J.Z. (1951), Growth and plasticity in the nervous system. *Proc. R. Soc. Lond. Ser. B.,* **139**, 18–37.

9 Formation and Experimental Modification of Chemical Synapses

C. R. SLATER

Acknowledgements

I would like to thank Dr Terje Lømo for many productive discussions on synapse formation during a year's visit to Oslo, and for his willingness to allow the appearance in this chapter of some of the still unpublished results of our work together. My own work is at present financed by the Muscular Dystrophy Association of America Inc. and the Muscular Dystrophy Group of Great Britain.

Intercellular Junctions and Synapses
(*Receptors and Recognition,* Series B, Volume 2)
Edited by J. Feldman, N.B. Gilula and J.D. Pitts
Published in 1978 by Chapman and Hall, 11 New Fetter Lane, London EC4P 4EE
© Chapman and Hall

9.1 INTRODUCTION

Chemical synapses are highly specialized regions of cell contact. Unlike most electrotonic synapses and gap junctions, they are essentially asymmetric in that one of the cells is specialized to secrete, and the other to respond to, a chemical transmitter. Associated with these different functions are characteristic morphological and biochemical features which arise during formation of the synpase (see Matus, Chapter 6). For example, in the pre-synaptic nerve terminal, membrane-bound vesicles are present which contain transmitter and are probably involved in the 'quantal' process of transmitter release in multimolecular packets. On the post-synaptic side, receptors for the transmitter are present in the plasma membrane in the immediate region of synaptic contact. In addition, after a variety of histological procedures, characteristic paramembranous densities are seen to be associated with both the pre- and post-synaptic membranes and the intracellular cleft which separates them.

Some of these specializations are to be found separately in secretory cells and in cells sensitive to circulating hormones. An essential feature of the chemical synapse is that it brings them together in a well-defined organelle where chemical transmission can occur efficiently and rapidly. A major current interest is to learn how such a local differentiation of two separate cells is co-ordinated in development and subsequently maintained.

In this chapter, I want first to consider some aspects of the normal development of synapses in a variety of situations, emphasizing what seem to me to be some of the key events, and the importance of interactions between cells in bringing them about. To investigate the nature of these interactions, the response of cells at synapses to a variety of experimental modifications has been studied. In the second part of the chapter, I will consider some of these experiments, in particular, those dealing with the restoration of neuro-muscular connections in adult animals after experimental intervention.

The range of examples cited in this chapter is intentionally narrow and reflects largely the situations with which I am most familiar. Many of the phenomena I shall discuss occur in other situations in the nervous system and are dealt with in a number of recent reviews (e.g. Bloom, 1972; Jones, 1975; Cotman and Lynch, 1976; Pfenninger and Rees, 1976; Purves, 1976).

9.2 SYNAPSE FORMATION

In this section, I want to consider 3 aspects of synapse formation; the early structural changes in the axon terminal and the post-synaptic cell, the onset of synaptic function, and the local biochemical differentiation of the post-synaptic cell, in particular the muscle fibre at the nerve—muscle junction (n.m.j.). Obviously these are closely related phenomena. They are treated separately because at present, there is not sufficient evidence to show how they are related.

9.2.1 Early structural events in synaptogenesis

In the developing nervous system, synapses generally form between a growing axon and either a cell body or a dendrite, which may itself be growing. The transformation of the axonal growth cone into a secreting pre-synaptic terminal is thus an important feature of synapse formation (see Pfenninger and Rees, 1976).

When viewed with the light microscope, the living growth cone of axons growing in culture appears as an undulating expansion of the tip of the axon where spike-like filopodia are extended and retracted (Harrison, 1910; Pomerat *et al.*, 1967; Bray and Bunge, 1973). In the electron microscope, the growth cones of cultured axons have two particularly noticeable characteristics (Yamada *et al.*, 1971; Bunge, 1973, Rees *et al.*, 1976). The filopodia are seen to be filled almost exclusively with a felt-work of fine filaments, possibly actin-like. More centrally, the expanded region of the axon terminal is filled with a mass of agranular membranous reticulum and vesicles and irregular size and shape, in addition to dense-cored vesicles and mitochondria. In the axon proper, proximal to the growth cone, micotubules and neurofilaments are important components of the cytoplasm.

It has been speculated that the membranous cisternae and vesicles provide a source of new membrane which is inserted at the growth cone as axonal elongation occurs, and that the actin-like filaments in some way provide the motive force for this growth (Wessells *et al.*, 1971; Bray and Bunge, 1973).

In vivo, the identification of growth cones is less certain than in culture. Nonetheless, in situations where growth cones are to be expected, axonal and dendritic terminals are found which have some of the characteristics of those seen in culture (e.g. Bodian, 1966; del Cerro and Snider, 1968; Vaughan *et al.*, 1974; Fox *et al.*, 1976). These include the presence of extensive agranular reticulum and vesicles, varying in diameter from about 40—200 nm, as well as a felt-work of fine filamentous material.

In contrast to the growth cone, the mature pre-synaptic nerve terminal is noted for the presence of a homogenous population of membrane-bound vesicles, 40—50 nm in diameter at many synapses, and for the absence of any obvious filopodia. The synaptic vesicles are often clustered at discrete zones of increased density of the pre-synaptic membrane which is itself opposite a dense region of the post-synaptic membrane.

The transformation of the growth cone into a pre-synaptic terminal has been

studied in detail in cultured sympathetic ganglion cells where the appearance of
individual contacts can be related to the previous history of the cells (Rees *et al.,*
1976). Initial very close contact between the cells is followed by at least a temporary
cessation of membrane movement, suggesting the contact inhibition of movement
seen in cultured fibroblasts (Abercrombie, 1967; Trinkhaus *et al.,* 1971). Some
6–12 h after contact, the post-synaptic membrane in the zone of contact appears
more dense than elsewhere, but synaptic vesicles and a pre-synaptic density cannot
yet be seen. Vesicles similar in appearance to those at mature synapses appear within
the next 12 h or so and are generally clustered together just under the pre-synaptic
membrane opposite the immature post-synaptic density. Later, 24–36 h after the
initial contact, the pre-synaptic densities become apparent. It is not yet clear when
the ability to transmit signals first appears at these synapses.

The sequence of events in synaptogenesis *in vivo* is less clear, particularly as
concerns the interesting question of whether or not post-synaptic densities precede
detectable pre-synaptic specializations (compare, for example, the sequence outlined
by Jones, 1975, p. 38, in which pre-synaptic vesicles are seen in the first stage of
synaptogenesis, with the observations of Gless and Sheppard (1964) and Kelly and
Zacks (1969) who found post-synaptic densities in the absence of pre-synaptic
vesicles). It may well be that these uncertainties arise as much from the technical
difficulties involved in this work as from real variations in the process as it occurs in
different situations.

Studies of a different nature suggest that post-synaptic densities may arise in the
absence of pre-synaptic terminals. In the cerebellum of certain mutant mice, the
granule cells do not develop, but post-synaptic densities appear on the dendritic
spines of the Purkinje cells nonetheless (see Rakič, 1976 for a review). A similar
situation is seen in genetically normal animals in which the development of the
granule cells has been blocked in other ways. Since the chemical composition of the
various 'densities' at the synapse is largely unknown (but see Matus, Chapter 6) it is
not clear that the post-synaptic densities that appear in these experiments are
identical to those which appear normally.

The appearance of synaptic vesicles seems to be a very local phenomenon, which
in some cases occurs while the rest of the nerve terminal still has the appearance of a
growth cone (del Cerro and Snider, 1968). While this may reflect the relative ease of
detecting vesicles when they are clustered, it is notable that in almost all cases, the
clusters appear immediately opposite the post-synaptic densities (but see Fox *et al.,*
1976). This suggests that vesicle clusters, and possibly the vesicles themselves, arise
as a result of a very local surface interaction with a specialized region of the post-
synaptic cell, rather than as a part of a more general transformation of the nerve
terminal as a whole. That such local effects might persist into adult life is suggested
by the existance of so-called 'reciprocal' synapses in the C.N.S. in which one part of a
nerve terminal is pre-synaptic while the adjacent region of the same terminal is
post-synaptic (cf. Reese and Shepherd, 1972).

Although morphologically recognizable synapses can be seen in the fetal and

neonatal brain soon after the initial contact between cells has occurred (Vaughan
et al., 1974), they continue to develop for a period of weeks (e.g. Agajhanian and
Bloom, 1967; Dyson and Jones, 1976). Studies of the paramembranous densities,
for example, show that in the cerebral cortex of the guinea-pig, these increase in
thickness and density for several weeks after birth (Jones *et al.*, 1974).

At the n.m.j. a conspicuous feature of synaptic maturation is the development of
the characteristic folds of the muscle surface. In rodents, physiological signs of
junctional transmission can first be detected in the diaphragm nearly a week before
birth (Bennett and Pettigrew, 1974). At this time, only occasional spot-like contacts
between nerve and muscle are seen, and the nerve terminals contain few synaptic
vesicles (Kelly and Zacks, 1969). At birth the extent of contact is much increased
and the surface of the muscle fibre is slightly indented to accomodate the developing
pre-synaptic boutons. Only 10 days or so after birth are post-junctional folds clearly
seen. The fully mature form of the junction is not present for several weeks after
birth (see Section 9.2.3).

9.2.2 Development of synaptic transmission

The early stages of synaptic function have been best studied at the mammalian
n.m.j.. There, as already suggested, the first signs of transmission in the fetus are seen
when only very primitive synaptic contacts are present. This suggests that by the
time synaptic junctions can be clearly seen in the C.N.S., some degree of function
may have already begun. This is supported by several studies correlating the onset of
spinal reflex activity with synaptic ultrastructure in the spinal cord.

For example, in the rat, reflex movements of the fore limb begin on about the
15th or 16th embryonic day (Windle and Baxter, 1936) and just at this time, a marked
increase in the number of synaptic junctions is seen in the dorsolateral and association
neuropil of the spinal cord (Vaughan and Grieshaber, 1973). Similar correlations
have been found elsewhere in the nervous system (e.g. Bodian, 1966; Bodian *et al.*,
1968; Bloom, 1972) and suggest that the onset of synaptic function occurs within
a day or less of the appearance of recognizable synaptic junctions.

At the developing n.m.j., it has been possible to study the early stages of synaptic
function in more detail. In the rat diaphragm, small end-plate potentials can be
recorded in response to stimulation of the phrenic nerve from about the 15th to
16th embryonic day (Bennett and Pettigrew, 1974). A day or two later, spontaneous
miniature end-plate potentials (min.e.p.p.s.) can be observed which are of normal
size or greater, but are very infrequent (of the order of 0.01 s^{-1} instead of 1 s^{-1}).
While rigorous tests of the quantal nature of transmitter release at such new
synapses have not been made, it seems likely from the small size of the e.p.p.s. that
during the first few days of innervation, only a few packets of transmitter are
released from each nerve terminal by an action potential, instead of the several
hundred at the mature n.m.j. (Hubbard and Wilson, 1973). During the first few
weeks of post-natal life, the frequency of min.e.p.p.s. rises about 100-fold

(Diamond and Miledi, 1962) and a similar increase in quantal content must also occur during this time. Thus, in parallel with the gradual morphological maturation of the n.m.j., there is an increase in the effectiveness of transmission. Many features of this increase in transmission could arise from an increase in synaptic area.

9.2.3 Maturation of the post-synaptic surface of the n.m.j.

Little is known about the molecular organization of the post-synaptic surface of central synapses or of its development. While it has been shown that some of the material in the synaptic cleft is sensitive to proteolytic enzymes (Pfenninger, 1973) and that carbohydrate groups extend from the post-synaptic membrane (Matus *et al.*, 1973; Cotman and Taylor 1974) the functional significance of these groups is not known. Some of the carbohydrate groups may well be associated with receptors for the transmitter. At the n.m.j., the receptor has been extensively studied and is known to bind concanavalin A (Michelson and Raftery, 1974) a substance which binds to a limited range of sugar groups.

Acetylcholine receptor
In recent years, studies of the acetylcholine receptor (AChR), particularly those using snake toxins which bind essentially irreversibly to it, have revealed a good deal about the molecular organization of the post-synaptic surface of the muscle fibre and how that develops.

At the time of innervation, the entire surface of muscle fibres in the rat diaphragm is sensitive to locally applied ACh (Diamond and Miledi, 1962). Recent estimates indicate that at this time (15–16 days of gestation) the density of receptors is of the order of 150 μm^{-2} (Bevan and Steinbach, 1977). In mature muscles, the density of receptors at the n.m.j. is about 30 000 μm^{-2} (Fertuck and Saltpeter, 1976), while that in the extrajunctional region is reduced to less than 5 μm^{-2} (Fambrough, 1974). The junctional receptors are slightly different chemically from those in uninnervated muscle (Brockes *et al.*, 1976) and their estimated half-life in the membrane is much longer, probably one to several weeks (Chang and Huang, 1975; Berg and Hall, 1975; Frank *et al.*, 1975a) as opposed to less than one day in denervated muscle (Chang and Huang, 1975; Berg and Hall, 1975) or cultured myotubes (Devreotes and Fambrough, 1975). Furthermore, while extrajunctional receptors, at least in denervated adult muscles, disappear within a few days if muscles are directly stimulated with chronically implanted electrodes (Lømo and Rosenthal, 1972) a substantial fraction (about 40%) of receptors of denervated end-plates are still present after 6 weeks of stimulation (Frank *et al.*, 1975a).

Studies of n.m.j. formation both in animals and in cultured cells suggest that the zone of high receptor density develops at an early stage in synaptogenesis. Using fluorescent-labelled α-bungarotoxin which binds tightly to the ACh receptors (Anderson and Cohen, 1974), accumulation of receptors in the vicinity of nerve muscle contacts has been observed as synaptic contacts form in culture (Anderson *et al.*, 1976).

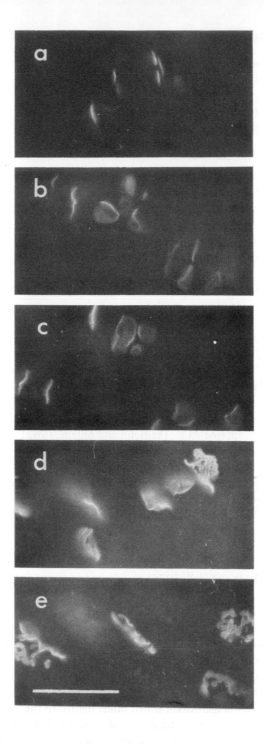

In developing rodent muscle, n.m.j.s can be clearly stained with ^{125}I-labelled toxin as early as 16 days gestation (Bevan and Steinbach, 1977). This is probably not more than 1–2 days after e.p.p.s. can first be recorded in response to nerve stimulation (Bennett and Pettigrew, 1974). I have recently obtained similar results with fluorescent-labelled toxin (Anderson and Cohen, 1974) (Fig. 9.1). As the junctions develop, the pattern of staining changes markedly. At birth, each end-plate appears as a roughly elliptical spot typically about 8 x 14 μm which is uniformly stained. During the following month or so, the receptors become grouped into a cluster of smaller spots or bands, each 2–4 μm wide, covering a region roughly 15–25 μm in the adult. Since the methods used are not quantitative ones, the absolute density of receptors in these structures is not yet known.

To see whether the accumulations of receptors at new n.m.j.s are stable in the absence of the nerve, the phrenic nerve was cut within 24 h of birth. As much as 5 weeks later, it was still possible to stain the end-plates with toxin, although the staining was much more diffuse and apparently weaker than that seen in normally innervated muscle either at birth or 5 weeks later (Fig. 9.2). Thus, although the persistance of a local high density of AChR does not require the continued presence of the nerve during the first weeks after birth, at least in rodents, the normal pattern of staining apparently does. This is in contrast to the adult n.m.j. where denervation leads to a reduction in toxin-binding sites but not to any marked change in their spatial extent (Frank *et al.*, 1975a; Slater, unpublished observations).

Important questions remain about how the ACh receptor becomes localized and stabilized at developing junctions. One possibility is that receptors which are present all over the membranes of uninnervated muscle fibres are 'trapped' at the site of nerve-muscle contact (Anderson *et al.*, 1976; Edwards and Frisch, 1976). It has been suggested that at central synapses the post-synaptic density might play a role in stabilizing membrane components (see Matus, Chapter 6). At the mature n.m.j., filamentous structures in the sub-synaptic cytoplasm have recently been described (Ellisman *et al.*, 1976) which might play a similar role. However, the appearance of these structures during development of the n.m.j. has not yet been reported.

Acetylcholinesterase

Like the ACh receptor, the enzyme acetylcholinesterase (AChE) is present in high density in the vicinity of the motor nerve terminal. At least 3 forms of the enzyme

Fig. 9.1 Changing distribution of ACh receptors at n.m.j.s in the mouse diaphragm during development. Muscles from animals of different ages were incubated with α-bungarotoxin which had been labelled with a fluorochrome (tetramethyl-rhodamine isothiocyanate) according to the methods of Anderson and Cohen (1974). The pattern of fluorescence was recorded using incident illumination. The ages of the animals were; (a) 16/17 days gestation, (b) 2 days, (c) 9 days, (d) 1 month, (e) 4 months. Calibration bar in (e) represents 100 μm and applies to all frames.

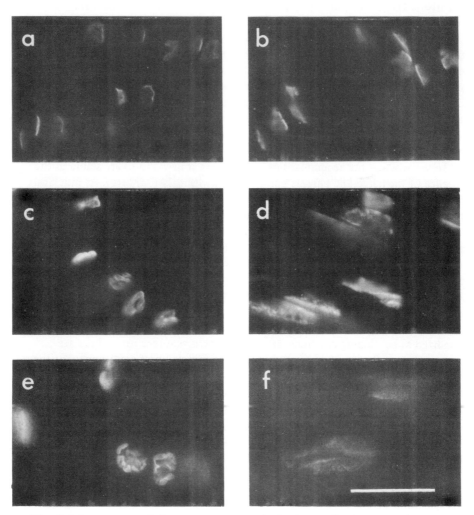

Fig. 9.2 Response to ACh receptors at n.m.j.s in the rat diaphragm to denervation on the first day after birth. Staining method as in Fig. 9.1. Innervated
control muscles are on the left and denervated muscles are on the right. The
ages of the animals were; (a,b), 5 days, (c,d) 2 weeks, (e,f) 5 weeks, The
calibration bar in (f) represents 100 μm and applies to all frames.

are present in skeletal muscle, one of them being found only in regions containing
end-plates (Hall, 1973; Rieger and Vigny, 1976). Using histochemical methods,
which probably do not distinguish between these 3 forms, AChE can first be
detected at developing rodent n.m.j.s within a day or so of the onset of rudimentary

junctional transmission (Bennett and Pettigrew, 1974; Chiapinelli *et al.,* 1976).
Biochemical studies show that the end-plate-specific form of the enzyme appears at
about the same time (Vigny *et al.,* 1976). As the n.m.j. matures, the spatial pattern
of AChE distribution increases in complexity in a manner closely paralleling that of
AChR (see above) (Zelena, 1962; Filogamo and Gabella, 1967).

The development of AChE at the end-plate depends upon the nerve, since
denervation a few days before birth results in the absence of stainable plaques of
enzyme activity a few days later (Zelená, 1962). If, however, denervation is delayed
for 3 weeks after birth, histochemically demonstrable AChE persists for weeks. This
persistent AChE activity apparently does not include the end-plate-specific form,
however, which virtually disappears within 2 weeks of denervation (Vigny *et al.,*
1976).

While it is still difficult to correlate the results of histochemical and biochemical
studies of AChE, it seems clear that the induction of junctional AChE is induced by
a local interaction with the nerve. Within the first few weeks after birth, at least some
of components of the AChE at the n.m.j. lose their immediate dependence upon
that interaction. The mechanism of the localization and fixation of AChE, like that
of AChR, is unknown. Unlike the receptor, which is an integral protein of the muscle
fibre plasma membrane, AChE is solubilized by treatment with colleagenase (Betz
and Sakmann, 1971; Hall and Kelly, 1971) and seems to be fixed to the basement
membrane which surrounds the muscle fibre (Betz and Sackmann, 1971). The
possibility that the basement membrane in the junctional region may be further
specialized is a topic of considerable current interest.

9.2.4 Conclusions

The essential outcome of synaptogenesis is the elabotation in adjacent cells of the
specialization for the release of, and response to, a chemical transmitter. In many
ways, our knowledge of how this co-ordinated differentiation comes about is poorly
understood. Even at a descriptive level, much needs to be done to define the
sequence of events in the formation of synapses. Still less is known about the causal
relations between those events. In spite of these uncertainties, some general
conclusions about synaptogenesis do emerge.

One of these is that from the earliest recognizable stages in synaptogenesis, the
process appears to be an extremely local one. In the brain, primitive synaptic
contacts are rarely more than a micron or so in extent, and may represent only a
fraction of the zone of 'contact' between the cells. Nonetheless, pre- and post-
synaptic specializations are generally found together. In the earliest stages of
synapse formation, this apparent coincidence may be one of definition, since only
when specializations of both cells are seen together is it clear that one is looking at
a synapse. But it seems likely that this coincidence also reflects the existance of
very local interactions between the cells which are involved in building a synapse.
These interactions, whatever their molecular basis, operate in both directions at the

developing synapse; differentiation of the nerve terminal occurs only opposite local specializations of the post-synaptic cell, and vice versa.

It is possible that the main feature of the initial interaction between cells at the synapse is to bring about the localization and fixation of cellular components, be they transmitter-containing vesicles or membrane receptors, which are synthesised elsewhere. This seems particularly likely in the case of post-synaptic receptors at the n.m.j., since these are clearly present throughout the cell membrane in the absence of the nerve, and become grouped in high concentration only at sites of interaction with the nerve. The accumulations of readily staining paramembranous material, so characteristic of the chemical synapse, may represent a framework which serves to fix synaptic components in place, and by interactions across the cleft, to ensure the alignment of pre- and post-synaptic differentiation.

A second general feature of synapse formation is that it seems to operate on two time scales. During the first days, and possibly hours, after the process is initiated, a marked change in both pre- and post-synaptic cells occurs which allows information transmission, even if only rather inefficiently, across the synaptic cleft. Then, over a period as long as several weeks, this primitive contact develops into a fully mature synapse. This raises the possibility that the factors which control the initial formation of a synaptic contact differ from those which bring about its subsequent maturation and possibly even its survival.

9.3 EXPERIMENTAL MODIFICATION OF SYNAPSES AND SYNAPTOGENESIS

The ordered appearance of the mature synapse gives the impression of a stable structure in which various components are held more or less rigidly in place. This view is supported by the mechanical strength of the junction which allows its physical isolation as synaptosomes and intact junctional complexes from brain homogeneates (see Jones, 1975). However, in a number of experimental situations, the normal relations and behaviour of the cells at the synapse can be greatly altered, leading in some cases to disruption of the synapse, and in others to marked change in the properties and behaviour of its constituent cells.

The most obvious of these is the destruction of the synaptic terminal which follows its isolation from the cell body after afferent nerve section (Gray and Guillery, 1966). A second instance is the disruption of the synaptic junction following retrograde changes in the soma and dendrites of a post-synaptic cell after its own efferent axon has been cut (cf. Watson, 1976). For example, after section of the hypoglossal nerve, about half of the pre-synaptic boutons terminating on the hypoglossal motorneurons withdraw from their contacts (Sumner and Sutherland, 1973; Sumner, 1975a,b), and only return if the hypoglossal axons restore their peripheral connections (Sumner, 1976). In this case, no clear degenerative process occurs, though there is a major change in the metabolic state of the post-synaptic cells. Regression of apparently well-formed synaptic contacts also occurs as a normal event in the development of some parts of the nervous system (see for example Ronnevi and Conradi, 1974; Brown *et al.,* 1976).

In addition to these degenerative alterations of synapses, there are also circumstances in which the behaviour of the cells is modified so as to favor the formation of new synaptic contacts. This modification includes the initiation of growth of pre-synaptic axons by sprouting, and in some cases the development of the ability of post-synaptic cells to enter into synaptic relations with pre-synaptic terminals. The occurrence of these events in adults, both in the C.N.S. (Cotman and Lynch, 1976) and in the periphery (Edds, 1953), provides an opportunity to study the factors which control synapse formation in situations often much more easily manipulated than those in immature animals. In the rest of this section, I shall consider a number of experiments, made for the most part on the nerve-muscle junction of adult mammals, in which those factors have been investigated.

9.3.1 Control of sprouting from motor axon terminals

Partial deafferentation of an isolated structure often causes sprouting of the intact pre-synaptic axons, and thus provides an example of an important change in the behaviour of one number of a synapse in the absence of direct insult to either.

The consequences of motor nerve section, whether partial or complete, are many and complex. They involve not only degeneration of the distal parts of the cut axons, and the phagocytosis of their remnants by Schwann cells, but also the complex response of the muscle fibre to inactivity and denervation (Gutmann, 1962; see Purves, 1976, for a useful recent review). Which of these various events triggers axonal sprouting?

In an effort to answer this question, the normal relationship of nerve and muscle cells has been altered in different ways by a variety of chemical agents. These experiments provide some insight into the situation but their interpretation is complicated by incomplete knowledge of the sites and mechanisms of the actions of the chemicals used.

Local injection of botulinum toxin into mammalian limbs at a sub-lethal dose causes paralysis within less than one day (Guyton and MacDonald, 1947; Tonge, 1974a). The principal action of this toxin seems to be to reduce the amount of transmitter (Burgen *et al.,* 1949; Brooks, 1956) and possibly other substances (Bray and Harris, 1975) released from the motor axon terminal by neural activity. Within 4 days of toxin injection into mouse legs, local sprouting from many motor nerve terminals can be seen in the soleus muscle, which contains predominantly slow-twitch muscle fibres (Duchen and Strich, 1968; Duchen, 1970). In primarily fast-twitch muscles, such as gastrocnemius, sprouting begins only 3–4 weeks after toxin injection (Duchen, 1970).

Tetanus toxin, in addition to its well-known central effects which lead to the simultaneous contraction of antagonistic muscles, also causes block of transmitter release at n.m.j.s in the soleus muscle of mice, but not in the predominantly fast extensor digitorum longus (EDL) (Duchen and Tonge, 1973). This action is paralleled by axonal sprouting which begins about a week after toxin injection in the soleus, but not in the EDL.

These toxins might induce sprouting by a direct action on the nerve terminal, or more indirectly, as a result of blocking transmission. To examine the latter possibility, action potentials in muscle nerves were blocked by local application of tetrodotoxin at some distance from the soleus muscles of mice (Brown and Ironton, 1977). When this was done, sprouting occurred in the soleus within a few days of the onset of paralysis, even though most nerve terminals in these preparations were intact.

In the conditions used, there was no sign that these various toxins caused degeneration of nerve terminals. It seems, therefore, that the degenerative process which occurs as a result of partial denervation is not required to induce sprouting, though it may of course play some role when it does occur. What these toxin treatments do have in common with partial denervation is that they lead to paralysis of muscle fibres, thus suggesting that muscle activity might be an important factor in the control of local axonal sprouting.

The sprouting induced by botulinum toxin can be prevented in two ways. The first is to implant an additional nerve into the muscle prior to toxin injection. After a single injection of toxin, such a transplanted nerve forms new functional n.m.j.s with the intoxicated muscle (Fex *et al.*, 1966). This new innervation effectively prevents sprouting of the original axons (Duchen *et al.*, 1975).

To see whether the muscle activity generated by a transplanted nerve might suppress sprouting on its own, the effect on botulinum-induced sprouting of direct stimulation of muscles, by means of chronically implanted electrodes, has recently been tested (Brown *et al.*, 1977). When mouse soleus muscles were adequately stimulated (as determined by their lack of hypersensitivity to acetylcholine after the paralysis induced by the toxin) fewer than 10% of nerve terminals showed signs of sprouting, as opposed to more than 40% in unstimulated contralateral muscles.

These experiments suggest that in mature mammalian muscles, sprouting from axon terminals can indeed be held in check by some effect of muscle activity. However, in some circumstances, this suppressing effect of activity can be overcome. For example, it has been shown that sprouting may occur in regions of muscle in which an inflammatory response has been induced, although muscle activity is probably still quite normal (Jones and Tuffery, 1973). Furthermore, a number of experiments on the peripheral nerves of lower vertebrates show that brief exposure of spinal roots to colchicine, a drug whose best-known actions are to interfere with the integrity of microtubules and with axonal transport, can induce peripheral sprouting without preventing neural activation of muscle (Diamond *et al.*, 1976).

What these procedures have in common with denervation and muscle paralysis is their ability, at least in some circumstances, to induce a number of 'denervation-like' changes in the surface of mammalian muscle fibres. These changes include increased sensitivity to acetylcholine (Jones and Vrbová, 1974; reviewed in Lømo, 1974) and the presence of tetrodotoxin-resistant action potentials (Cangiano and Fried, 1977). It seems likely, therefore, that sprouting of mammalian motor nerve terminals can be induced by some property of the muscle fibre whose control closely resembles that of, for example, extrajunctional sensitivity to acetylcholine. The potent effect of induced muscle activity in preventing sprouting in botulinum-poisoned muscles may well result from its ability to suppress such denervation-like changes (Lømo and Westgaard, 1976).

In the context of the argument just put forward, it may be relevant that the soleus muscle, where sprouting is relatively easily induced, responds more quickly to denervation than do fast muscles (Albuquerque and McIsaac, 1970). In addition, however, the selective action of botulinum and tetanus toxins on neuromuscular transmission in the soleus suggests that the nerve terminals in slow and fast mammalian muscles may differ inherently in their sensitivity to the toxins.

While the initiation of sprouting from intact pre-synaptic terminals can in some cases be inhibited by muscle activity, the growth of axons exploring the surface of a muscle apparently is not. Thus, if a muscle nerve is transplanted onto the surface of a normally innervated muscle, it will grow extensively in spite of the continuing activity of the immediately adjacent muscle (Aitken, 1950). This suggests that the exploratory growth of axons prior to synapse formation differs in important ways from the sprouting of nerve terminals which are already part of an established synapse.

9.3.2 Control of ectopic innervation

Axons exploring the surface of muscle fibres are not always able to make synaptic junctions with them. The second group of experiments I want to describe is aimed at learning what factors determine the outcome of encounters between nerves and muscles.

It has been known for some time that when a muscle nerve is cut away from its normal target and placed over the surface of a normally innervated muscle, the transplanted axons grow out from their cut ends and onto the surface of the host muscle. But unless the host muscle is denervated, synapses with such foreign nerves rarely form (Elsberg, 1917; Aitken, 1950; reviewed in Bennett and Pettigrew, 1976). Fex and Thesleff made the important discovery that if a period of several weeks is allowed after transplantation for growth to take place, new synapse formation occurs within a few days of denervating the host muscle (Fex and Thesleff, 1967).

Further studies of the development of this form of ectopic innervation have recently been made using the rat soleus and the transplanted fibular nerve. Regenerating fibular nerve axons appear on the surface of the soleus about a week after the transplant (Lømo and Slater, unpublished observations). Among these growing axons, no profiles have been found which resemble pre-synaptic terminals in the electron microscope (Korneliussen and Sommerschild, 1976). Furthermore, the growing nerve has no obvious effect on the surface of the underlying muscle fibres. Unlike the situation during an inflammatory response, for example, there is no obvious increase in sensitivity to ACh of the muscle fibres associated with the dense cellular growth accompanying the axons (Lømo and Slater, unpublished observations).

If the soleus nerve is cut 2 weeks or more after implanting the fibular nerve, extensive synapse formation occurs with the transplanted nerve. Within 2–3 days after denervation, end-plate potentials, which in some cases are large enough to evoke muscle fibre action potentials and contraction, can be seen in response to stimulation of the fibular nerve. The extent of innervation increases over a period of a week or two until most (70–100%) of the fibres in the vicinity of the foreign nerve sprouts are well innervated.

When transmission is first detectable, the new synapses cannot be recognized in the light microscope in methylene blue preparations. In muscles studied with the electron microscope, 2 days after the first signs of transmission are detected, structures which are apparently rudimentary synaptic junctions have been found with characteristic synaptic vesicles and increased density of the post-synaptic membrane (Korneliussen and Sommerschild, 1976). The gradual maturation of the functional properties of these extopic junctions is paralleled by increasing structural complexity as the post-synaptic folds develop and the area of synaptic contact is increased. Fully mature n.m.j.s are not seen for several weeks after the initiation of new synapse formation (cf. Koenig, 1973).

This experimental model presents very clearly the question of how the normal nerve prevents innervation by a foreign nerve. One possibility is that the muscle activity which results from normal synaptic activity plays some role. To test this, the sciatic nerve was anaesthetised several weeks after the fibular nerve transplant was made. New functional n.m.j.s with the foreign nerve were promptly made even though the soleus nerve terminals were still intact and capable of transmitting (Jansen *et al.*, 1973).

To test further the possible effect of muscle activity, electrodes were implanted in the legand used to stimulate the muscles directly. When the host nerve was then cut, stimulation almost completely prevented the formation of new n.m.j.s with the foreign nerve (Jansen *et al.*, 1973). These important results show that activity of the muscle can control some property which is necessary to allow the formation of new n.m.j.s with overlying nerve sprouts.

To learn more about when such a factor might operate in the sequence of events leading to synapse formation, we have recently looked to see when the new n.m.j.s become resistant to the effects of renewed muscle activity, such as they will generate by their own action. If stimulation of a denervated rat soleus muscle is delayed as little as 2 days after cutting the soleus nerve, then even though the new junctions were not yet functional at the time stimulation started, a significant number of previously transplanted axons make functional n.m.j.s which persist for at least the week or so of the intense stimulation we used (Lømo and Slater, in preparation). In these experiments, about 25% of the surface muscle fibres under-lying the foreign nerve became innervated, as opposed to about 75% in the unstimulated controls.

Thus, at an early stage of their development, some at least of these new ectopic junctions are able to withstand the suppressing effects of imposed muscle activity. In trying to interpret this result, it is important to consider that the full effect of imposed activity may only be expressed a day or two after it begins, as is the case with ACh sensitivity (Lømo and Westgaard, 1976). Thus, in these experiments, though the new n.m.j.s are not yet functional when stimulation begins, they may be by the time it becomes fully effective.

In summary, these experiments indicate that the state of activity of a muscle plays an important role in determining whether or not it will make ectopic synapses with a transplanted nerve. Soon after synapse formation begins, however, the new junction is resistant to the effects of activity. This suggests that the ability to make ectopic synapses is controlled in a manner similar to that of extrajunctional ACh sensitivity (see Section 9.2.3). Some further support for this is given by the observation that local injury to frog muscle induces both increased ACh sensitivity (Katz and Miledi, 1964) and allows the formation of new innervation, even though the normal nerve remains intact (Mildedi, 1963).

9.3.3 Reinnervation of previously formed end-plates

In the previous section, I described the ability of direct stimulation to prevent the innervation of the extrajunctional region of denervated soleus muscle fibres. But at the site of the original n.m.j. quite a different situation exists. For there, muscle activity is not so effective in preventing reinnervation. This is true whether the stimulus is electrical (Jansen *et al.,* 1973) or neural, by means of a previously implanted foreign nerve (Gutmann and Hanzliková, 1967). That this is not exclusively a property of end-plates formed during normal development is shown by the ability of a crushed foreign nerve to reinnervate previously formed ectopic n.m.j.s on a muscle fibre which has been reinnervated by the normal nerve (Frank *et al.,* 1975b).

Special features of established end-plates are further suggested by the very rapid morphological maturation of the nerve terminal when they are being reinnervated. Whereas in the formation of new ectopic n.m.j.s the mature appearance of the nerve terminal may not develop for some weeks after transmission begins (see Section 9.3.3), this can occur in a few days during reinnervation of old end-plates (Koenig and Pecot-Dechavesine, 1971; Jansen and van Essen, 1975). Furthermore, Tonge (1974b) has shown that the properties of denervated mouse soleus muscles are restored to normal more rapidly when the soleus nerve reinnervates its original end-plates than when new ectopic ones have to be formed.

In some experiments, particularly on lower vertebrates, stable reinnervation of a denervated muscle by a regenerating nerve occurs predominantly at the original end-plates, even if the regenerating axons grow over the surface of denervated muscle fibres on the way (Miledi, 1960; Bennett and Pettigrew, 1976). Mammalian muscles, and the soleus in particular, may thus be unusually susceptible to ectopic innervation after denervation.

All these observations suggest that once a n.m.j. becomes established, the surface of the muscle fibre becomes locally specialized so as to favour reinnervation, and that this property is relatively stable to the effects of muscle activity and innervation which repress it elsewhere (but see Frank *et al.*, 1975b and Brown *et al.*, 1976 for some possible exceptions).

9.3.4 ACh sensitivity and n.m.j. formation

In every case where innervation of a muscle fibre has been observed the complex molecules which bear the receptor sites for ACh are present at much higher concentrations than in the extrajunctional region of normally innervated mature muscle fibres. As has been described above, this is true of muscle fibres at the time of original innervation, denervated adult muscle fibres and denervated mature endplates, as well as at sites of local injury.

These parallels between ACh sensitivity and the susceptibility to innervation naturally suggest that the ACh receptors themselves might play a role in the early stages of synapse formation (Katz and Miledi, 1964). At one level, this is clearly true, for a functioning n.m.j. must have an adequate number of receptors. But do the receptors play some other part, such as inducing changes in the behaviour of the regenerating nerve terminal ? Although this question has not been conclusively answered, there are two lines of evidence which suggest that sensitivity to ACh is neither necessary nor sufficient to induce synapse formation.

The first comes from experiments in which synapse formation in the presence of a blocker of ACh receptors was studied. Both during new n.m.j. formation *in vitro* (Cohen, 1972) and reinnervation of old end-plates *in vivo* (Jansen and van Essen, 1975) agents which fully blocked the pharmacological sensitivity of the muscle to ACh failed to prevent the development of the transmitter release system of the nerve terminal. While these experiments are subject to the difficulty that reversal of the effects of these blockers may take several hours, during which time changes in the nerve terminal might occur, they nonetheless suggest that critical steps in the differentiation of the nerve terminal can take place in the absence of detectable ACh sensistivity.

The second line of evidence is drawn from situations in which regions of muscle fibres which have appreciable ACh sensitivity do not form n.m.j.s with exploring nerves. One of these is in neonatal mammalian muscle which will not form ectopic n.m.j.s with a transplanted foreign nerve (Brown *et al.*, 1976) in spite of its general sensitivity to ACh (Diamond and Miledi, 1972). Another is in muscles which have been experimentally innervated by a foreign nerve and the original nerve allowed to regenerate only after a delay of several months. In such cases, reinnervation of the old end-plates is greatly impaired though localized ACh sensitivity persists (Frank *et al.,* 1975b; see also Gutmann and Young, 1944).

None of these experiments is without difficulties of interpretation. At present, however, the weight of the available evidence favours the view that while the sensitivity to ACh seems to vary in concentration roughly in parallel with the ability of a site to accept innervation, it plays no direct role in initiating the events of nerve terminal differentiation and n.m.j. formation. Since the receptors themselves are part of complex glycoproteins which may have numerous ligand binding sites in addition to the ACh binding sites that are blocked in the experiments sited above, the possibility remains that some other part of the molecule plays a key role in synapse formation.

9.3.5 Discussion

These experimental studies confirm that both of the principal cellular components of the mature n.m.j. are capable of considerable plasticity in their behavior. In a variety of circumstances in which synaptic function is interfered with, or peripheral injury inflicted, the properties of both nerve and muscle may be dramatically modified so as to favour the formation of new nerve-muscle contacts. It seems likely that this co-ordinated response to insult normally helps to restore adequate muscle innervation after a partial loss of motor neurons or their axons after injury, disease or senescence.

The manner in which this regenerative response is controlled and co-ordinated may be multifactorial. However, at least one set of conditions seems to promote both axonal sprouting and the increased susceptibility of muscles to accept new innervation at sites other than at the original end-plates. These conditions are most commonly encountered as the response to partial denervation, and include changes in many properties of the muscle. Recently, however, it has become clear that denervation *per se* is not a necessary stimulus for these changes, since they can be caused by anaesthesia of the intact nerve on the one hand, or the induction of an inflammatory response of a normally innervated muscle on the other. While in experimental circumstances, it may be possible to separate these various factors, in more natural circumstances, they may often be combined to provide a potent stimulus to regeneration, possibly by acting on some common process in the muscle fibre which triggers the various aspects of cell behaviour leading to synaptic regeneration.

In contrast to the plasticity of cell properties which underlies the ability to reform synaptic connections, the mature motor end-plate stands out as a relatively stable structure whose properties are little influenced by the factors considered above. The ability to enter into a synaptic relationship with an exploring motor axon, like the sensitivity to ACh and the presence of AChE, is a property of the end-plate which persists after denervation and is relatively resistant to the effects of muscle activity which suppress it elsewhere. The persistance of these properties after denervation ensures that functional transmission can be quickly restored if a regenerating axon finds its way to a denervated end-plate. Failing this, the increased ability of the extrajunctional region to accept new innervation may ultimately allow new n.m.j.s to form away from the original end-plate (see, for example, Gutmann and Young, 1944).

The molecular basis of this 'innervatability' is unknown. Though ACh sensitivity seems to vary in rough proportion to the ease of innervation, the two properties seem to have different chemical bases. At present, however, it is not even clear what the role of any putative 'innervatability factor' of the muscle fibre would be. Would it cause adhesion of the nerve terminal, induce the apparatus for transmitter release, allow accumulation of ACh receptors, or play some other role? Whatever its cellular effect might be the early stability of ectopic n.m.j.s suggests that this pro- perty need only be present generally in the muscle fibre during the first stages of synaptogenesis. It may be that it triggers a response in the nerve terminal which is self-perpetuating. Alternatively, like the ACh receptor, it may be that a surface molecule conferring 'innervatability' becomes stabilized by virtue of its interaction with the nerve terminal, and at the same time stabilizes the developing n.m.j. This raises the question of whether the process by which synaptic components become localized is the same as that which confers long-term stability upon them.

The observations described in Section 9.2.3. suggest that the stability of ACh receptors at the end-plate, and possibly of post-synaptic components more generally, may be of two forms. The first is a chemical stability which would allow junctional receptors as molecules or groups of molecules to persist for weeks after denervation. This form of stability appears to be built into the receptors at an early stage of synapse formation, at least in the rodent muscles studied. The second is a morphological stability which determines the detailed spatial distribution of these molecules. This appears to be built in more gradually, as the mature form of the n.m.j. itself develops. It will be interesting to see, as this field develops, whether such a distinction holds true and if so, what molecular events underly it.

A further implication of these experiments is that the process of muscle innerva- tion, at least as it occurs in adult mammals, is a self-limiting one, in that activity of the muscle generated by newly forming n.m.j.s renders the muscle incapable of accepting further innervation. It is natural to ask whether this self-limitation plays any role during normal development in establishing patterns of innervation in muscle.

At one level, the pattern of innervation concerns the distribution of sites of synaptic contact. While mammalian skeletal muscle fibres are innervated at a single site, in lower vertebrates and invertebrates it is common for innervation to be distributed along the fibre at intervals of several contacts per millimetre. It is generally true that fibres with such distributed innervation do not generate action potentials, relying instead on local depolarization of the muscle fibre in the vicinity of the n.m.j.s to activate contraction. It has been suggested that as muscles develop, innervation is suppressed by the post-synaptic effects of neural activity and that where this is only local, multiple innervation develops (see Gordon *et al.*, 1976). Some evidence in favour of this view comes from experiments in which partial block of neuromuscular transmission during the development of chick embryos apparently leads to the formation of multiple sites of innervation in a normally focally innervated muscle (Gordon and Vrbova, 1975). On the other hand, it has been shown that multiple sites of innervation of frog sartorius muscle fibres develop after the first contact is able to elicit muscle action potentials (Bennett and Pettigrew, 1975).

A second level of the pattern of muscle innervation concerns the morphology of individual nerve-muscle contacts. Very little is known about how the spatial features of the n.m.j. are specified, though it seems that these are largely determined by the neuron rather than the muscle (e.g. Bennett *et al.,* 1973). As noted in Section 9.2.3, maturation of mammalian n.m.j.s involves a considerable increase in synaptic area. Furthermore, in mature animals, ageing is accompanied by an increase in terminal axonal branching (Tuffery, 1971) which seems to imply a continuing, if slow, process of nerve terminal degeneration and sprouting (Barker and Ip, 1966). These changes in the extent and pattern of individual synaptic contacts are of considerable interest since they occur in active muscle fibres which are not able to make completely new synapses with implanted axons exploring the extrajunctional region.

Both these examples suggest that to explain the development of patterns of muscle innervation, we must look beyond a simple mechanism in which post-synaptic activity shuts off continuing synaptogenesis.

The relevance of experiments on the formation of new synapses in adult muscle to events at neuronal synapses in the peripheral or central regions of the nervous system is of course difficult to assess. Many features of synaptic regeneration in muscle also occur at neuronal synapses (cf. Cotman and Lynch, 1976) where additional complications of the specificity of induction of axonal sprouting and post-synaptic receptivity are present. One feature which regeneration at neuronal synapses seems to have in common with that in muscle is that a quantitatively similar pattern of innervation is re-established (cf. Raisman and Field, 1973). Associated with this is the possibility that, as in muscle, post-synaptic sites, once formed, survive denervation to remain as favoured sites of reinnervation (Raisman, 1969).

Whether the activity of neurons in any way determines their ability to make synapses remains unknown. Clearly, individual pre-synaptic inputs are in most cases too weak to have a dominant effect on the activity of a post-synaptic cell. But the possibility that during development, groups of pre-synaptic inputs which tend to be active at the same time, and thus successfully activate the post-synaptic cell, might exclude the formation of dissimilar inputs cannot be ruled out.

9.4 SUMMARY

I have considered what seem to me to be the primary events in the formation of chemical synapses; the transformation of the axonal growth cone into a secreting nerve terminal, and the development of local sensitivity to the transmitter in the post-synaptic cell. These events occur in immediate proximity across the intercellular cleft, and it seems possible that they are co-ordinated by direct interaction of surface molecules in the two cells. While the initial stages of synaptogenesis seem to occur in a day or so, leading to a structurally recognizable synaptic junction capable of detectable transmission and possessing relatively stable post-synaptic receptors, the final form of the synapse may take as long as several weeks to develop.

From experiments on the regeneration of nerve-muscle synapses in adult muscle, it seems clear that changes in the muscle fibre are capable of initiating events which favour new synapse formation, including axonal sprouting and the appearance of some unidentified property of the muscle which allows synapse formation. While this co-ordinated response can in some cases be suppressed by artificially maintained muscle activity, muscle paralysis is not the only way it can be elicited. As yet, it is not clear how this apparent self-limitation of synapse formation relates to the control of patterned innervation during the normal development of muscle or of neuronal synapses.

REFERENCES

Abercrombie, M. (1967), *Nat. Cancer Inst. Monograph,* **26**, 249–277.

Agajhanian, G.K. and Bloom, F.E. (1967), *Brain Res.,* **6**, 716–727.

Aitken, J.T. (1950), *J. Anat.,* **84**, 38–48.

Alburquerque, E.X. and McIsaac, R.J. (1970), *Exp. Neurol.,* **26**, 183–202.

Anderson, M.J. and Cohen, M.W. (1974), *J. Physiol.,* **237**, 385–400.

Anderson, M.J., Cohen, M.W. and Zorychta, E. (1976), *Neurosci. Abst.,* **2**, 707.

Barker, D. and Ip, M.C. (1966), *Proc. R. Soc. (Lond.). Ser. B.,* **163**, 538–554.

Bennett, M.R. and Pettigrew, A.G. (1974), *J. Physiol.,* **241**, 515–545.

Bennett, M.R. and Pettigrew, A.G. (1975), *J. Physiol.,* **252**, 203–239.

Bennett, M.R. and Pettigrew, A.G. (1976), *Cold Spring Harbor Symp.,* **40**, 409–424.

Bennett, M.R., Pettigrew, A.G. and Taylor, R.S. (1973), *J. Physiol.,* **230**, 331–357.

Berg, D. and Hall, Z.W. (1975), *J. Physiol.,* **252**, 771–789.

Betz, W. and Sakmann, B. (1971), *Nature New Biol.,* **232**, 94–95.

Bevan, S. and Steinbach, J.H. (1977), *J. Physiol.,* **267**, 195–213.

Bloom, F.E. (1972), In: *Structure and Function of Synapses* (Pappas, G.D. and Purpura, D.P., eds), Raven Press, New York.

Bodian, D. (1966), *Bull. Johns Hopkins Hosp.,* **119**, 129–149.

Bodian, D., Melby, E.C. and Taylor, N. (1968), *J. comp. Neurol.,* **133**, 113–166.

Bray, D. and Bunge, M.B. (1973), *Ciba Found. Symp.,* **14**, 195–209.

Bray, J.J. and Harris, A.J. (1975), *J. Physiol.,* **253**, 53–77.

Brockes, J.B., Berg, D.K. and Hall, Z.W. (1976), *Cold Spring Harbor Symp.,* **40**, 253–262.

Brooks, V.B. (1956), *J. Physiol.,* **134**, 264–277.

Brown, M.C., Goodwin, G.M. and Ironton, R. (1977), *J. Physiol.,* **267**, 42P.

Brown, M.C. and Ironton, R. (1977), *Nature,* **265**, 459–461.

Brown, M.C., Jansen, J.K.S. and Van Essen, D.C. (1976), *J. Physiol.,* **261**, 387–422.

Bunge, M.B. (1973), *J. Cell Biol.*, **56**, 713–735.

Burgen, A.S.V., Dickens, F. and Zatman, L.J. (1949), *J. Physiol.*, **109**, 10–24.

Cangiano, A. and Fried, J.A. (1977), *J. Physiol.*, **265**, 63–84.

Chang, C.C. and Huang, M.C. (1975), *Nature*, **253**, 643–644.

Chiapinelli, V., Giacobini, E., Pilar, G. and Uchimura, H. (1976), *J. Physiol.*, **257**, 749–766.

Cohen, M.W. (1972), *Brain Res.*, **41**, 457–463.

Cotman, C.W. and Lynch, G.S. (1976), In: *Neuronal Recognition*, (Barondes, S.H., ed.), Chapman and Hall, London.

Cotman, C.W. and Taylor, D. (1974), *J. Cell Biol.*, **62**, 236–242.

del Cerro, M.P. and Snider, R.S. (1968), *J. comp. Neurol.*, **133**, 341–362.

Devreotes, P. and Fambrough, D.M. (1975), *J. Cell Biol.*, **65**, 335–358.

Diamond, J., Cooper, E., Turner, C. and MacIntyre, L. (1976), *Science*, **193**, 371–377.

Diamond, J. and Miledi, R. (1962), *J. Physiol.*, **162**, 393–408.

Duchen, L.W. (1970), *J. Neurol. Neurosurg. Psychiat.*, **33**, 40–54.

Duchen, L.W., Rogers, M., Stolkin, C. and Tonge, D.A. (1975), *J. Physiol.*, **248**, 1–2P.

Duchen, L. and Strich, S.J. (1968), *Quart. Rev. J. exp. Physiol.*, **53**, 84–89.

Duchen, L.W. and Tonge, D.A. (1973), *J. Physiol.*, **228**, 151–172.

Dyson, S.E. and Jones, D.G. (1976), *Cell Tissue Res.*, **167**, 363–371.

Edds, M.V. (1953), *Quart. Rev. Biol.*, **28**, 260–276.

Edwards, C. and Frisch, H.L. (1976), *J. Neurobiol.*, **7**, 377–381.

Ellisman, M.H., Rash, J.E., Staehelin, A. and Porter, K.R. (1976), *J. Cell Biol.*, **68**, 752–774.

Elsberg, C.A. (1917), *Science*, **45**, 318–320.

Fambrough, D.M. (1974), *J. gen. Physiol.*, **64**, 468–472.

Fertuck, H.C. and Saltpeter, M.M. (1976), *J. Cell Biol.*, **69**, 144–158.

Fex, S., Sonesson, S., Thesleff, S. and Zelená, J. (1966), *J. Physiol.*, **184**, 872–882.

Fex, S. and Thesleff, S. (1967), *Life Sci.*, **6**, 635–639.

Filogamo, G. and Gabella, G. (1967), *Archs Biol. (Liege)*, **78**, 6–90.

Fox, G.Q., Pappas, G.D. and Purpura, D.P. (1976), *Brain Res.*, **101**, 411–425.

Frank, E., Gautvik, K. and Sommerschild, H. (1975a), *Acta Physiol. Scand.*, **95**, 66–76.

Frank, E., Jansen, J.K.S., Lømo, T. and Westgaard, R. (1975b), *J. Physiol.*, **247**, 725–743.

Glees, P. and Sheppard, B.L. (1964), *Z. Zellforsch.*, **62**, 356–362.

Gordon, T., Jones, R. and Vrbová, G. (1976), *Prog. Neurobiol.*, **6**, 103–136.

Gordon, T. and Vrbová, G. (1975), *Pflügers Arch.*, **360**, 349–364.

Gray, E.G. and Guillery, R.W. (1966), *Int. Rev. Cytol.*, **19**, 111–182.

Gutman, E. (ed.), (1962), *The Denervated Muscle*, Czechoslovak Acad. Sci., Prague.

Gutman, E. and Hanzlikova, V. (1967), *Physiol. Bohemoslov.*, **16**, 244–250.

Gutman, E. and Young, J.Z. (1944), *J. Anat.*, **78**, 15–43.

Guyton, A.C. and MacDonald, M.A. (1947), *Arch. Neurol. Psychiat., (Chicago)*, **57**, 578–592.

Hall, Z.W. (1973), *J. Neurobiol.*, **4**, 343–361.

Hall, Z.W. and Kelly, R. (1971), *Nature New Biol.*, **232**, 62–63.

Harrison, R.G. (1910), *J. exp. Zool.*, **9**, 787–846.

Hubbard, J.I. and Wilson, D.F. (1973), *J. Physiol.*, **228**, 307–325.

Jansen, J.K.S., Lømo, T., Nicolaysen, K. and Westgaard, R.H. (1973), *Science*, **181**, 559–561.

Jansen, J.K.S. and Van Essen, D.C. (1975), *J. Physiol.*, **250**, 651–667.

Jones, D.G. (1975), *Synapses and Synaptosomes,* Chapman and Hall, London.

Jones, D.G., Dittmer, M.M. and Reading, L.C. (1974), *Brain Res.*, **70**, 245–259.

Jones, R. and Tuffery, A.R. (1973), *J. Physiol.*, **232**, 13–15P.

Jones, R. and Vrbová, G. (1974), *J. Physiol.*, **236**, 517–538.

Katz, B. and Miledi, R. (1964), *J. Physiol.*, **170**, 389–396.

Kelly, A.M. and Zacks, S. (1969), *J. Cell Biol.*, **42**, 154–169.

Koenig, J. (1973), *Brain Res.* **62**, 361–365.

Koenig, J. and Pecot-Dechavassine, M. (1971), *Brain Res.*, **27**, 43–57.

Korneliussen, H. and Sommerschild, H. (1976), *Cell Tissue Res.*, **167**, 439–452.

Lømo, T. (1974), *Nature*, **249**, 473–474.

Lømo, T. and Rosenthal, J. (1972), *J. Physiol.*, **221**, 493–513.

Lømo, T. and Westgaard, R.H. (1976), *Cold Spring Harbor Symp.*, **40**, 263–274.

Matus, A., de Petris, S. and Raff, M. (1973), *Nature New Biol.*, **244**, 278–280.

Michaelson, D.M. and Raftery, M.A. (1974), *Proc. natn. Acad. Sci., U.S.A.*, **71**, 4768–4772.

Miledi, R. (1960), *J. Physiol.*, **151**, 1–23.

Miledi, R. (1963), *Nature*, **199**, 1191–1192.

Pfenninger, K.H. (1973), *Prog. Histochem. Cytochem.*, **5**, 1–86.

Pfenninger, K.H. and Rees, R.P. (1976), In: *Neuronal Recognition* (Barondes, S.H. ed.), Chapman and Hall, London.

Pomerat, C.M., Hendelman, W.J., Raiborn, C.W. and Massey, J.F. (1967), In: *The Neuron,* (Hyden, H. ed.), American Elsevier Publishing Co. Inc., New York.

Purves, D. (1976), *Int. Rev. Physiol., Neurophysiol. II*, **10**, 125–177.

Raisman, G. (1969), *Brain Res.*, **14**, 25–48.

Raisman, G. and Field, P.M. (1973), *Brain Res.*, **50**, 241–264.

Rakič, P. (1976), *Cold Spring Harbor Symp.* **40**, 333–346.

Rees, R.P., Bunge, M.B. and Bunge, R.P. (1976), *J. Cell Biol.*, **68**, 240–263.

Reese, T.S. and Shepherd, G.M. (1972), In: *Structure and Function of Synapses,* (Pappas, G.D. and Purpura, D.P. eds.), Raven Press, New York.

Rieger, F. and Vigny, M. (1976), *J. Neurochem.*, **27**, 121–129.

Ronnevi, L.O. and Conradi, S. (1974), *Brain Res.*, **80**, 335–339.

Sumner, B.E.H. (1975a), *Exp. Neurol.*, **46**, 605–615.

Sumner, B.E.H. (1975b), *Exp. Neurol.*, **49**, 406–417.

Sumner, B.E.H. (1976), *Exp. Brain Res.*, **26**, 141–150.

Sumner, B.E.H. and Sutherland, F.I. (1973), *J. Neurocytol.*, **2**, 315–328.

Tonge, D.A. (1974a), *J. Physiol.*, **241**, 127–139.

Tonge, D.A. (1974b), *J. Physiol.*, **241**, 141–153.

Trinkhaus, J.P., Betchaku, T. and Krulikowski, L.S. (1971), *Exp. Cell Res.*, **64**, 291–300.

Tuffery, A.R. (1971), *J. Anat.*, **110**, 221–247.

Vaughan, J.E. and Grieshaber, J.A. (1973), *J. comp. Neurol.*, **148**, 177–210.

Vaughan, J.E., Henrikson, C.K. and Grieshaber, J.A. (1974), *J. Cell Biol.,* **60**, 664–672.

Vigny, M., Koenig, J. and Rieger, F. (1976), *J. Neurochem.,* **27**, 1347–1353.

Watson, W.E. (1976), *Cell Biology of Brain,* Chapman and Hall, London.

Wessells, N.K., Spooner, B.S., Ash, J.F., Bradley, M.O., Luduena, M.A., Taylor, E.L., Wrenn, J.T. and Yamada, K.M. (1971), *Science,* **171**, 135–143.

Windle, W.F. and Baxter, R.E. (1936), *J. comp. Neurol.,* **63**, 189–209.

Yamada, K.M., Spooner, B.S. and Wessells, N.K. (1971), *J. Cell Biol.,* **49**, 614–635.

Zelena, J. (1962), In: *The Denervated Muscle,* (Gutmann, E., ed.), Czechoslovak Acad. Sci., Prague.

Index